W9-CWS-847

AIDS: The Impact On
The Criminal Justice System

ATLANTIC COMM. COLLEGE

Mark Blumberg
Central Missouri State University

MERRILL PUBLISHING COMPANY
Columbus   Toronto   London   Melbourne

To Peggy

Published by Merrill Publishing Company
Columbus, Ohio 43216

This book was set in Palatino.

Administrative Editor: Steven Helba

Production Editor: Jan Hall

Cover Designer: Russ Maselli

Text Designer: Debra Fargo

Copyeditor: Jan Brittan

Library of Congress Catalog Card Number: 89-64404

International Standard Book Number: 0-675-21183-2

Printed in the United States of America

1 2 3 4 5 6 7 8 9—94 93 92 91 90

Preface

This text examines how AIDS affects the criminal justice system. It is designed to provide students and practitioners with information on a wide range of topics about AIDS.

All too often discussions about AIDS are based on misinformation and prejudice. In selecting the articles in *AIDS: The Impact on the Criminal Justice System*, I have attempted to present the most accurate information as is currently available.

This text has been divided into sections that examine topics relevant to persons working in or studying the criminal justice system. Material has been selected that students will find interesting and easy to comprehend.

Finally, because this is an area where the body of knowledge has expanded rapidly in the last few years, only readings that contain the most recent information have been included.

Many persons provided assistance in bringing this project to fruition. Unfortunately, space limitations do not permit me to acknowledge the contribution of each one of these individuals. However, I do wish to express my gratitude to those who were especially helpful in making this text a reality.

I wish to say "thanks" to all my colleagues at Central Missouri State University who encouraged me to pursue this project. Richard Holden deserves special recognition for creating an academic environment that encourages scholarship and research. Allen Sapp took the time to review many of the original contributions in this reader and provided valuable feedback. And to Donald Wallace, thank you for contributing, on short notice, an article about AIDS as it affects the courts.

I also appreciate the comments and thoughtful guidance of those who reviewed the manuscript. The reviewers were: Raymond Ellis, Coppin State College; James Farris, California State University—Fullerton; Aric Frazier, Vincennes University; Ron Kazorski, Pensacola Junior College; Peter Kratcoski, Kent State University; Kenneth Peak, University of Nevada—Reno; Laurin Wollan Jr., Florida State University.

A number of people at Merrill Publishing Company have been very helpful and deserve a word of gratitude. I want to say "Thank you," to Steve Helba for encouraging me to consider a book of readings on this topic; to Joyce Rosinger, who skillfully answered my questions about the mechanics of securing permission to reprint copyrighted articles; and to Jan Hall and Jan Brittan, who made numerous suggestions that greatly enhanced the quality of this reader.

This list would not be complete if I did not also thank the following individuals: Douglas Heckathorn for providing helpful advice in the preparation of this text; Scott Christianson for his willingness to spend several hours familiarizing me with the New York State corrections system's experience with AIDS; and the librarians at the Kansas University Medical Center, who were always eager to help me locate material (and patient in answering my questions). Finally, I want to express special appreciation to my wife, Peggy, who not only provided valuable proofreading assistance, but also was willing to surrender me to the library and the word processor for much of the past year.

Contents

CONTENTS

INTRODUCTION

An Overview of AIDS in the U.S. and Its Significance for Criminal Justice Agencies

1

AIDS and the Criminal Justice System: An Overview

Mark Blumberg

THE NATURE OF THE AIDS EPIDEMIC

AIDS was first identified in the United States among gay men in 1981 (Moran and Curran, 1986:459). During the eight-year period subsequent to this date, over 100,000 cases were reported to the U.S. Public Health Service (Centers for Disease Control, 1989:9). In addition, it is estimated that as many as 1.4 million Americans have become infected with the human immunodeficiency virus (HIV) (Centers for Disease Control, 1987:15). By the year 1991, it is projected that approximately 270,000 Americans will develop full-blown AIDS and that 179,000 people will have died from this disease (Morgan and Curran, 1986:461).

In 1984 scientists identified the human immunodeficiency virus as the cause of AIDS. This virus attacks the body's immune system and leaves the person vulnerable to a wide array of opportunistic infections that are not usually found in persons with a properly functioning immune system. There is no vaccine to prevent HIV infection. To date, most persons who have contracted full-blown AIDS have eventually died. However, the drug aziodothymidine (AZT) has shown some promise as a means of prolonging the lives of persons with AIDS as well as in preventing the onset of illness in certain asymptomatic individuals who are infected with HIV (Fackelmann, 1989:135).

There are only three ways that the AIDS virus can be transmitted (Friedland and Klein, 1987): by sexual contact, through contact with infected blood, and perinatally (i.e., from an infected mother to a newborn infant). Studies of persons who have lived in the same household as seropositive[1] individuals for a prolonged period of time have concluded that HIV cannot be transmitted through casual

3

contact (Friedland, Saltzman, Rogers, et al., 1986). In addition, there is no evidence that the virus can be spread by insects or in the preparation of food (Lifson, 1988:1355).

In the United States, approximately 90 percent of AIDS cases have been found among two risk groups: homosexual/bisexual males and intravenous drug users (Centers for Disease Control, 1989:8). Despite exaggerated claims to the contrary (Masters and Johnson with Kolodny, 1988), there is little evidence that the virus is breaking out of these high-risk groups into the general population (Fumento, 1987). To date, only 5 percent of adult/adolescent cases have been linked to heterosexual transmission (Centers for Disease Control, 1989:8), and the great majority of these have been among the sex partners of IVDUs (Haverkos and Edelman, 1988:1925).

Two facts have greatly influenced the nature of public response to this epidemic: that a lethal, sexually transmitted disease (STD) appeared in an era when it was widely believed that medical science had brought such ailments under control; and the fact that most AIDS cases have been found among members of already stigmatized groups—gay males and IVDUs. Persons with AIDS have had to confront not only the debilitating physical effects of the virus, but also ostracism and rejection on the part of family members and friends, in some cases. Despite repeated assurances from scientists and government officials that AIDS is not transmitted through casual contact, infected children have been barred from the classroom in some communities, some employers have terminated infected employees, and certain landlords have evicted tenants suffering from this ailment (Altman, 1987:61). A recent survey indicates that fewer than a third of the nation's 140,000 dentists are willing to treat patients with AIDS (Hinds, 1989:A14). In addition, it has been reported that the number of assaults directed at gay individuals has increased (National Gay and Lesbian Task Force, 1988) due to a belief on the part of some that homosexuals are somehow responsible for the AIDS epidemic (Altman, 1987:65–70).

With the passage of time, the level of public hysteria over AIDS has gradually subsided. However, complaints regarding various forms of discrimination continue to be received by government agencies that monitor this problem (Watkins, 1988:120). Persons with AIDS and seropositive individuals still experience difficulties in the areas of housing, employment, insurance coverage, and in obtaining social service benefits. In addition, a substantial number of citizens continue to hold serious misconceptions regarding how the AIDS virus is transmitted. Many still believe that HIV can be contracted as a result of being sneezed on, from a drinking fountain, or through various other forms of casual contact that present no danger whatsoever (Blendon and Donelan, 1988:1024). Most disturbing of all, a substantial proportion of the population voices approval for measures that almost all public health authorities agree are inappropriate for dealing with AIDS (e.g., tattooing or isolating seropositive individuals—Blendon and Donelan, 1988:1023).

THE IMPACT ON SOCIETY

The AIDS crisis has raised many important issues that our society must address. Receiving considerable attention are questions such as whether HIV testing should be mandatory or voluntary, how to pay the enormous medical costs associated with this epidemic, whether physicians may refuse to treat seropositive patients, the appropriate content of educational programs designed to reduce high-risk behavior on the part of adolescents, and whether schools may deny admission to infected children. In the pages that follow, these controversies are examined in order to give the reader a basis for appreciating the issues that the AIDS crisis poses for the criminal justice system. From this discussion, it will become clear that many of the questions facing the justice system are concerns that society is already grappling with.

The Medical Profession

The AIDS crisis has forced the medical profession to confront a number of difficult issues: including whether physicians and surgeons who fear for their safety may refuse to treat seropositive patients. Until the appearance of this disease in the early 1980s, modern clinicians were able to practice medicine without any serious concern for their physical well-being. Although there is general agreement that providing routine medical care presents little risk of HIV transmission,[2] there have been a small number of documented cases in which health care workers became infected on the job either as a result of needle-stick wounds or through contact with contaminated blood (Centers for Disease Control, 1988:232). For this reason, the question of physicians' and surgeons' ethical obligation to provide medical care for patients infected with the AIDS virus has been raised.

This debate has been fueled by several prominent surgeons who publicly announced that they would not treat seropositive individuals (Gruson, 1987). In addition, a survey of 258 doctors in New York City reported that 25 percent believe it is ethical for a physician to refuse treatment to a patient who has AIDS (Link, Feingold, Freeman, and Shelov, 1988). These views run counter to the position of the American Medical Association that a physician "may not ethically refuse to treat a patient whose condition is within the physician's current realm of competence" merely because the patient has AIDS or is seropositive (AMA, 1987:4).

The medical profession also has had to reconsider the issue of confidentiality as it relates to the doctor-patient relationship. Traditionally, physicians have been expected not to divulge information that patients may reveal in the course of receiving medical care. However, the AIDS virus is sexually transmitted and physicians may be concerned that the activities of certain patients are putting other individuals (i.e., spouses or lovers) at risk. What is the ethical obligation of the doctor under these circumstances? Does concern for the well-being of the third party outweigh the requirements of confidentiality?

The AMA has adopted guidelines that are designed to assist physicians in resolving this difficult ethical dilemma. In those jurisdictions that have no statute either mandating or prohibiting physicians from reporting seropositive individuals to public health authorities, when the physician knows that an infected patient is endangering the health of a third party, the following course of action has been recommended:

1. An attempt should be made to persuade the infected individual to cease endangering the third party.
2. If such persuasion is ineffective, the physician may notify public health officials.
3. If no action is taken, the physician may personally notify the endangered third party (AMA, 1987).

Educational Institutions

Educational institutions have also had to confront a number of important questions as a result of the AIDS crisis. Probably no issue has received as much attention as whether seropositive children should be allowed to attend school. Despite repeated assurances from public health officials that the virus cannot be transmitted by normal classroom activities, infected children have sometimes been denied admission to school or met with boycotts and protests by parents concerned for the safety of their children. Perhaps the most tragic incident of all occurred in Arcadia, Florida, where the home of three seropositive hemophiliac brothers was burned after they tried to attend school (*New York Times*, 1987:1).

The debate over admitting infected children to school has gradually subsided. However, another issue that has not gone away is the question of what educational materials are appropriate for teaching schoolchildren how to avoid exposure to HIV. Because there is no vaccine currently available to prevent infection with the AIDS virus, it is generally agreed that education is the only tool for fighting the epidemic. However, there is a great deal of disagreement over the form that these educational campaigns should take. Dr. C. Everett Koop, former Surgeon General of the United States, has suggested that students be taught the proper use of condoms as a means of preventing viral transmission. However, many conservatives are critical of this approach, arguing that condom education promotes immorality, and that school children should be encouraged to abstain from sex as a means of avoiding AIDS and other sexually transmitted diseases (Barol, Hager, and Wingert, 1987:64).

Financing Medical Care

AIDS can be a debilitating ailment from a financial as well as a medical perspective. One study concluded that the average lifetime cost of treating a single patient with AIDS is approximately $61,000 (Hellinger, 1988:309). In addition, many persons with AIDS, as well as many asymptomatic individuals, must continually take the drug AZT, which currently costs between seven and eight thousand dollars per year (Fackelmann, 1989:135).[3] According to one estimate, the cost of finding and treating the hundreds of thousands of persons infected with HIV who could benefit from this medication could reach five billion dollars or more per year (Hilts, 1989:11). Who is going to pay the bill for these expensive treatments?

In the United States, medical care is financed through a combination of private and public insurance programs. Most, but not all, persons in the work force receive health insurance coverage through their employers. In addition, there are federal and state programs such as Medicare and Medicaid that assist individuals who are elderly, disabled, or indigent with their medical bills. Despite these programs, persons with AIDS often have a difficult time paying the bills that accrue as a result of this costly illness.

There are several factors that account for the serious financial hardship that these individuals encounter. For one thing, a considerable number of patients with full-blown AIDS are no longer able to work. Because many of these individuals cannot afford the premiums that would be required to continue coverage after leaving their employer, they lose their health insurance coverage. Second, it is estimated that as many as 35 million Americans may be without any form of health insurance whatsoever (Watkins, 1988:145). As the proportion of AIDS cases attributable to intravenous drug use has increased, so has the proportion of AIDS patients who have lacked private health insurance. Third, many private insurance carriers are taking steps to limit their liability for costs resulting from HIV infection (Institute of Medicine, 1988:112–113). Some companies are screening applicants for the virus, others are adding questions about AIDS to their enrollment application or refusing to sell coverage to persons who have a history of sexually transmitted diseases (STDs). In addition, insurers sometimes classify new drugs that are developed for AIDS patients as "experimental." Such treatments do not qualify for reimbursement. Fourth, the waiting period to receive social security disability may be quite lengthy in some cases. Because of the enormous expense associated with catastrophic illness, the patient's financial obligation under these circumstances can increase very rapidly. Finally, the requirements to qualify for Medicaid (a combined federal and state program designed to provide insurance coverage for the poor) are not uniform in all states (Institute of Medicine, 1988:111). Thus, many AIDS patients may be denied coverage or forced to "spend down" to near-poverty level in order to be eligible for benefits.

As a consequence, society faces a number of critical questions as it attempts to come to terms with the economic costs that result from the AIDS epidemic. Policy makers will be forced to decide such issues as

- How much of the burden should be placed on public hospitals to provide care for uninsured patients?

- What are the responsibilities of private insurance carriers?
- Should these companies be forbidden to screen prospective applicants for HIV infection?
- What role should the federal government play?
- Should it pay more of the costs for AIDS patients than it does at present?

However, the biggest issue is who is going to pay the enormous cost of providing AZT to the hundreds of thousands of asymptomatic individuals who could benefit from taking it. Because AZT is able to delay the onset of illness for many, does society have a moral obligation to ensure that this drug is available to all who need it, regardless of their financial situation?

Mandatory HIV Screening

In 1985, scientists developed a blood test that could detect antibodies to HIV. Persons who have been exposed to the virus will usually develop these antibodies and therefore test positive within six to twelve weeks (Petricciani and Epstein, 1988:237).[4] These individuals are presumed to be capable of transmitting the virus for the rest of their lives. Although the vast majority of seropositives manifest no symptoms of illness, researchers are uncertain what proportion eventually will develop full-blown AIDS. One study reported that 40 percent of the members of an infected cohort developed AIDS within 8.5 years (Institute of Medicine, 1988:2). Others estimate that this number may eventually reach 99 percent (Lui, Darrow, and Rutherford, 1988:1334).

The most controversial issue that has faced public health officials since the development of this blood test is who should be screened for HIV, and whether screening should be done on a mandatory or voluntary basis. Although a number of states have enacted statutes that authorize mandatory testing for certain individuals,[5] these measures have generally been opposed by public health officials (Gostin, 1989), who argue that a more effective strategy is to encourage members of high-risk groups to seek voluntary testing and counseling to reduce high-risk behaviors (i.e., unsafe sex and needlesharing). Mandatory testing is seen as counterproductive because of the fear that it will discourage persons at risk from cooperating with public health officials, and therefore serve to drive the epidemic underground. Gay-rights advocates and civil libertarians are also opposed to compulsory HIV screening on the grounds that persons who test positive may be subjected to discrimination.

The nature of the debate over HIV testing is likely to change dramatically. In 1989, medical researchers announced that the drug AZT could delay the onset of symptoms in certain asymptomatic individuals who are infected with the AIDS virus (Fackelmann, 1989:135). For the first time, science has something to offer individuals who test positive. Persons and organizations that have opposed all testing in the past may modify this stance as a result of this finding. Concern that a positive test result will lead to discrimination is now likely to be outweighed by the medical benefits of learning one's HIV status.

Opposition to the concept of *mandatory* testing is likely to continue from civil libertarians. The rationale for compulsory screening is weak now that persons at risk have a strong incentive to come forward for voluntary testing and treatment.

THE IMPACT OF AIDS ON THE CRIMINAL JUSTICE SYSTEM

Against the background of the controversies that AIDS poses for society, attention can now be directed toward the questions that the epidemic raises for persons studying or working in the criminal justice system. The articles in this reader are divided into seven sections designed to give the reader some familiarity with the range of issues that the criminal justice system must confront. Articles of a general nature will be of interest to all persons, regardless of whether their specialty is law enforcement, the courts, or corrections. Other articles address more specific topics, such as the risk of HIV infection faced by rape survivors, the legal issues for correctional administrators designing policies for working with infected inmates, and programs that may slow the transmission of the virus among IVDUs. We have attempted to select readings that address important issues and that provide the most recent and comprehensive information on a given topic.

AIDS and Criminal Justice Agencies

Persons working in the criminal justice system have had to confront many of the issues discussed in this introduction. Because agency personnel come in contact with IVDUs and others who may be infected with HIV, they have often expressed anxiety about becoming infected as a result of their employment. Consequently, police departments, courts, correctional institutions, and probation/parole agencies have all had to develop educational programs for their staff and guidelines to be followed in situations that involve contact with seropositive individuals. The readings in Section One examine some of the issues that criminal justice agencies have had to confront as a result of the AIDS crisis. The discussion focuses on the risk of occupational transmission that agency personnel realistically face and the appropriate precautionary measures that should be followed by all persons whose work brings them in contact with seropositive individuals.

AIDS and the Courts

The articles in Section Two examine some of the issues that the courts have been forced to confront as a result of the AIDS crisis. The first article discusses some of the controversies that the courts have been asked to settle: disputes regarding mandatory HIV testing, the question of whether infected children may be denied admission to public school, and allegations of discrimination raised by persons with AIDS and seropositive individuals. These are just a few of the issues that have been dropped in the lap of the courts. The second article explores concerns that have been raised by courtroom officials in some jurisdictions with respect to the dangers posed by seropositive defendants. The author examines the risk of infection to judges, lawyers, bailiffs, and other court personnel. In addition, there is a discussion of the constitutionality of various protective measures that have been used by some courts in the belief that they could prevent viral transmission. Both articles make the point that there are well-established legal precedents available to guide the courts as they seek answers to the issues raised by the AIDS epidemic.

AIDS and Rape Survivors

Because AIDS is transmitted through sexual contact, many rape survivors are concerned about the possibility of HIV infection. The first article in this section presents the recommendations of the Presidential Commission on the Human Immunodeficiency Virus Epidemic regarding sex offenses and offenders. The second article in Section Three examines the risk of viral transmission faced by sexually assaulted persons. This discussion is followed by the implications of these findings for counseling programs and for proposals for mandatory testing of offenders.

AIDS and Female Prostitution

Section Four examines whether prostitution is a source of viral transmission. The readings focus on the risks posed by this activity and discuss issues surrounding control of prostitution.

Currently AIDS is primarily a sexually transmitted disease. Concern has therefore been expressed that prostitutes (who are often IVDUs and generally have numerous sex partners) may become a major source of HIV infection for the general population. In the states in which prostitution is illegal (all states except Nevada), some people would like to have tougher laws to better curtail the business of prostitutes and their customers. The readings in this section examine whether tougher legal measures are warranted.

AIDS and the Law

A common response to crisis in the United States is to pass a law. Not surprisingly, state legislatures have enacted a substantial number of measures designed to control HIV transmission by proscribing certain types of conduct on the part of seropositive individuals (Gostin, 1989). For example, some of these statutes make it a criminal offense to knowingly expose another person to HIV. Others authorize forced isolation (i.e., quarantine) of infected individuals who continue to engage in high-risk behavior.

Both articles in Section Five examine the utility of these measures. The first article considers the legal and evidentiary hurdles that must be overcome if the criminal law were to be successfully employed against HIV-infected persons who continue to engage in unsafe sex. The author presents several reasons that criminal measures should not be involved. The second reading discusses the various forms of quarantine that could be implemented to slow the spread of the virus. The practical and ethical difficulties that would be part of quarantine are examined.

AIDS and Intravenous Drug Users

Section Six examines the link between HIV infection and IVDU. Twenty-seven percent of the adult/adolescent AIDS cases in the United States have IVDU as a risk factor (Centers for Disease Control, 1989:8). Because the criminal justice system has been given a mandate by Congress and the various legislatures to control illicit drug use, a number of states have banned over-the-counter sales of hypodermic needles except by doctor's prescription. This prohibition has resulted in considerable needlesharing on the part of IVDUs and extensive HIV infection among members of this group. As a consequence, there has been considerable attention devoted to efforts to modify the behavior of IVDUs. Many jurisdictions have developed outreach programs designed to reach these individuals; others have attempted to teach IVDUs how to clean their needles and syringes as a means of avoiding infection. A few, despite intense opposition, have taken the extraordinary step of providing IVDUs with sterile needles. The readings in this section look at some of the programs that have been developed to change the behavior of IVDUs.

AIDS and Corrections

The readings in the final section focus on the impact of AIDS on corrections. Jails and prisons have been viewed by some as likely contributors to the spread of the virus, because they house a substantial number of persons at risk for AIDS (e.g., IVDUs) and often provide inmates with opportunities for illicit homosexual activity. As a consequence, correctional administrators have been forced to deal with the issues of mandatory testing, whether infected inmates should be segregated, prevention information and condom distribution, and adequacy of medical care.

The impact of this epidemic on corrections is not limited to staff and administrators working in correctional facilities. Community corrections (probation and parole) agencies have also had to confront a number of difficult questions. For example, who should have access to the medical records of infected clients? Should seropositive probationers and parolees be required to refrain from high-risk sexual behavior as a condition of their release? Should agencies warn third parties who may be placed at risk as a result of unsafe conduct on the part of probationers and parolees? These and related issues are examined in the final section of the reader.

REFERENCES

Altman, Dennis. (1987). *AIDS in the Mind of America: The Social, Political, and Psychological Impact of a New Epidemic.* Garden City, N.Y.: Anchor Books.

American Medical Association. (1987). *Report of the Council on Ethical and Judicial Affairs: Ethical issues involved in the growing AIDS crisis.* Chicago, American Medical Association.

Barol, Bill, Mary Hager, and Pat Wingert. (1987). Koop and Bennett agree to disagree. *Newsweek.* Feb. 16, p. 64.

Blendon, Robert J. and Karen Donelan. (1988). Discrimination against people with AIDS: The public's perspective. *The New England Journal of Medicine.* Vol. 319, No. 15, 1022–1026.

Centers for Disease Control. (1989). *HIV/AIDS Surveillance.* U.S. Department of Health and Human Services, August.

Centers for Disease Control. (1988). Update: Acquired immunodeficiency syndrome and human immunodeficiency virus infection among health-care workers. *Morbidity and Mortality Weekly Report.* Vol. 37, No. 15 (April 22).

Centers for Disease Control. (1987). Human immunodeficiency virus infection in the United States: A review of current knowledge. *Morbidity and Mortality Weekly Report.* Vol. 36, No. S-6 (December 18).

Fackelmann, K. A. (1989). Early AZT use slows progression to AIDS. *Science News.* Vol. 136, No. 9, 135.

"Firm cutting its price for AIDS drug." *Kansas City Times.* September 19, 1989, p. A1.

Friedland, Gerald H., Brian R. Saltzman, Martha F. Rogers, et al. (1986). Lack of transmission of HTLV-III/LAV infection to household contacts of patients with AIDS or AIDS-related complex with oral candidiasis. *The New England Journal of Medicine.* Vol. 314, No. 6, 344–349.

Friedland, Gerald H. and Robert S. Klein. (1987). Transmission of the human immunodeficiency virus. *The New England Journal of Medicine.* Vol. 317, No. 18, 1125–1135.

Fumento, Michael A. (1987). AIDS: Are heterosexuals at risk? *Commentary.* November, 21–27.

Gostin, Larry O. (1989). Public health strategies for confronting AIDS: Legislative and regulatory policy in the United States. *Journal of the American Medical Association.* Vol. 261, No. 11, 1621–1630.

Gruson, L. (1987). AIDS fear spawns ethics debate as some doctors withhold care. *New York Times.* July 11, p. A1.

Hammett, Theodore M. (1988). *AIDS in correctional facilities: Issues and options, third edition.* Washington, D.C.: National Institute of Justice, April.

Hammett, Theodore M. (1989). *1988 Update: AIDS in correctional facilities.* Washington, D.C.: National Institute of Justice, June.

Haverkos, Harry W. and Robert Edelman. (1988). The epidemiology of acquired immunodeficiency syndrome among heterosexuals. *Journal of the American Medical Association.* Vol. 260, No. 13, 1922–1929.

Hellinger, Fred J. (1988). Forecasting the personal medical care costs of AIDS from 1988 through 1991. *Public Health Reports.* Vol. 103, No. 3, 309–319.

Hilts, Philip J. (1989). Cost of early AIDS treatment estimated at $5 billion a year. *New York Times.* Sept. 15, 11.

Hinds, Michael deCouray. (1989). Amid fears over AIDS, one dentist offers care. *New York Times*. Sept. 13, Section A, p. 14.

Institute of Medicine. (1988). *Confronting AIDS: Update 1988*. Washington, D.C.: National Academy Press.

Lifson, Alan R. (1988). Do alternate modes for transmission of human immunodeficiency virus exist? A review. *Journal of the American Medical Association*. Vol. 259, No. 9, 1353–1356.

Link, R. N., A. R. Feingold, M. H. Charap, et al. (1988). Concerns of medical and pediatric house officers about acquiring AIDS from their patients. *American Journal of Public Health*. Vol. 78, 455–459.

Lui, Kung-Jong, William W. Darrow, and George W. Rutherford, III. (1988). A model-based estimate of the mean incubation period for AIDS in homosexual men. *Science*. Vol. 240, 1333–1335.

Masters, William and Virginia Johnson with Robert Kolodny. (1988). *Crisis: Heterosexual behavior in the age of AIDS*. New York: Grove Press.

Morgan, W. Meade and James W. Curran. (1986). Acquired immunodeficiency syndrome: Current and future trends. *Public Health Reports*. Vol. 101, No. 5, 459–465.

National Gay and Lesbian Task Force. (1988). *Anti-gay violence, victimization and defamation in 1987*. Washington, D.C.: NGLTF.

New York Times. (1987). Family in AIDS case quits Florida town after house burns. Aug. 30, p. 1.

Petricciani, John C. and Jay S. Epstein. (1988). The effects of the AIDS epidemic on the safety of the nation's blood supply. *Public Health Reports*. Vol. 103, No. 3 (May–June), 236–241.

Watkins, James. (1988). *Report of the presidential commission on the human immunodeficiency virus*. Submitted to the President of the United States, June 24.

NOTES

[1] The term "seropositive" is used to refer to persons infected with the human immunodeficiency virus (HIV), regardless of whether they exhibit symptoms of illness.

[2] Certain types of medical care may place the provider at some risk of infection. For example, surgeons often experience some contact with blood from patients even in those situations where they have taken appropriate precautionary measures (e.g., wearing surgical gloves and masks).

[3] The manufacturer of AZT (Burroughs Wellcome) has announced that the wholesale price of this drug will be cut by 20 percent. This step, along with the recent finding that AZT is effective at lower dosages, may significantly reduce the cost of this drug for patients (Associated Press, 1989: A1).

[4] In some individuals, the length of time required to produce antibodies is much greater. There have been reports of cases in which this did not occur until 6 to 30 months after exposure (Petricciani and Epstein, 1988: 237).

[5] Mandatory testing has been authorized by certain state legislatures for a wide assortment of groups. These include marriage applicants, prison inmates, prostitutes, intravenous drug users, sex offenders, hospital patients, mentally ill and mentally retarded patients, pregnant women, and newborns. The federal government requires that military personnel, applicants for the Peace Corps and new immigrants to the United States be tested for HIV (Gostin, 1989: 1625).

2

The Causes of AIDS
and Its Transmission

Dana Eser Hunt with assistance from Saira Moini and Susan McWhan

AIDS, or Acquired Immunodeficiency Syndrome, is a condition in which the immune system becomes so compromised that the individual is unable to fight off a host of infections. It was first identified in 1981 among previously healthy homosexual or bisexual men in New York and San Francisco, although it has been found in banked blood of IV drug users in New York donated as early as 1978.[1] The first cases involved a rare form of bacterial pneumonia (*Pneumocystis carinii* pneumonia), or a type of skin cancer (Kaposi's sarcoma), which had previously been seen only in a far less virulent form among elderly men of eastern European or Mediterranean origins. In the absence of other causes, the appearance of these rare diseases pointed to an underlying problem with the immune system. Those affected were simply unable to fight off infection naturally and, often after a series of illness episodes, died. In addition to these two diseases, identified early in the epidemic, persons with AIDS may also suffer from a wide range of "opportunistic infections." These infections, often from common viral or bacterial sources, are not life-threatening in a healthy individual but become deadly in persons with seriously compromised immune systems.

The diagnosis of AIDS involves the appearance of one of the known AIDS-related diseases and clinical evaluation of severe immune suppression unrelated to other factors (such as chemotherapy). . . . Since AIDS was first recognized, New York City reports an unusually high incidence of fatalities from diseases such as

Reprinted from *AIDS in Probation and Parole* (Chapter 1), Washington, D.C.: National Institute of Justice, June, 1989.

bacterial endocarditis, non-pneumocystic pneumonia and tuberculosis among intravenous drug users,[2] leading to speculation about the specific role of the AIDS virus in other diseases as well. As information develops, these or other diseases may be added to the CDC definition.

There are a number of "indicator diseases" associated with AIDS. The anomalous presence of one or more of them helps to identify AIDS. For example, some diseases are often not seen in a given age group, such as Kaposi's sarcoma or severe candidiasis ("thrush"). Others are not typically found in the organ affected, such as cytomegalovirus or tuberculosis in areas other than the lung. Some are even diseases not usually manifested in humans. The AIDS virus may also produce encephalopathy or "AIDS dementia," which involves increasing neurological problems, or a condition known as HIV "wasting syndrome," involving uncontrolled weight loss and deterioration.

The name "AIDS" is really an umbrella term, referring to a syndrome, or a group of diseases caused by a virus. Moreover, it actually refers to the end state of the illness. Some persons infected with the virus may remain asymptomatic for many years, perhaps indefinitely. Others progress from infection to a condition known as AIDS-Related Complex (ARC), a milder condition characterized by weight loss, swollen lymph glands, continuous or intermittent diarrhea and fever, severe fatigue and tests indicating immune suppression. It is only recently, in fact, that scientists have argued that ARC should be considered an early form of AIDS, rather than a separate complex or condition. From ARC, patients usually progress to full-blown manifestation of the disease. In the end state, the individual has marked laboratory indications of immune suppression and has developed one or more of the indicator diseases associated with the syndrome.

However, AIDS does not always mean an orderly progression to an end state, as the definition might imply. Persons may become infected and quickly develop the end stage of the illness. Others may never progress beyond ARC symptoms. What determines the rate or sequence of progression is the subject of current investigation. It is believed, though, that AIDS is nearly always fatal. Of the 80,000 cases of AIDS diagnosed since June of 1981, 56 percent have died. In the early stages of the epidemic, life expectancy for a person diagnosed with AIDS was approximately two years. Due to the development of life-extending treatments, patients may live as long as five or more years after diagnosis.[3] Expectancy nationwide also varies with a number of co-factors, which are discussed in the next section.

WHAT CAUSES AIDS?

AIDS is caused by a virus generally known as the Human Immunodeficiency Virus (HIV), a human retrovirus which was discovered by scientists at the Institute Pasteur in Paris and further defined by Dr. Robert Gallo and his associates at the National Institutes of Health in 1983 and 1984. The virus infects certain white blood cells known as T-4 cells, rendering them incapable of combating infections. Once the virus has entered a host cell, it may remain dormant for long periods of time. When stimulated into action, though, the virus reproduces rapidly, causing the depletion of T-4 cells that is the hallmark of AIDS diagnoses, and thus leaving the individual vulnerable to a number of opportunistic infections which would not normally harm a healthy person.

It is not known definitely what stimulates the dormant virus into activity. However, it is believed that a number of "co-factors" influence one's susceptibility to the development of AIDS once exposed: continued high-risk behaviors such as intravenous drug use, poor nutrition, alcohol and drug consumption, and continued unprotected sexual contact with infected persons; additional infections such as hepatitis B or cytomegalovirus; and genetic predisposition.[4] Research continues on the co-factors involved with AIDS, but the exact role they play is as yet unknown. A factor such as heavy alcohol use, for example, may act as a catalyst for HIV action or may simply further suppress the immune system.

Exposure, Seroconversion and Manifestation of AIDS Symptoms

It is important to distinguish among the various stages of HIV-related illness and to understand their relationships to one another. Exposure to the virus, for example, does not guarantee infection, and infection does not necessarily cause symptoms to appear.

Exposure means that the person has had high-risk contact with someone infected with the AIDS virus, which may have resulted in his or her own infection. The ratio of exposure to actual infection is not known. However, research with homosexuals and intravenous drug users indicates that those who engage in high-risk activities frequently and with multiple partners are the most likely to become infected.

Tests are usually done in series, consisting of an "ELISA test," which is repeated if positive, and a confirmatory "Western Blot test." Table 1 explains the relationships among exposure, infection, HIV seropositivity, ARC, and AIDS.

The term "seropositivity" refers to a positive result, indicating a person's infection with the virus. All of the standard tests, it is crucial to note, detect *antibodies* to the virus in the blood of those infected, not the virus itself. Thus an infected individual is accurately referred to as "HIV antibody-positive" or alternately, seropositive. Moreover, since seropositivity refers to infection, the progression from exposure to infection is known as "seroconversion." As was discussed, seropositivity does not imply current or active illness. But it is generally agreed that seropositivity *does* indicate the ability to transmit the virus to others.

One factor which may complicate the identification of a particular stage is the "window," or period of time between exposure and development of antibodies or subsequent detectable infection. This window, or time to conversion, may not occur for as long as weeks or even months after exposure.[5] Thus, an infected person may

TABLE 1

Relationships Among Exposure, Infection, HIV Seropositivity, ARC, and AIDS

Stage	Meaning	Relationship to Previous Stage(s)
Exposure	Individual has contact with HIV in a way that makes transmission possible (e.g., sexual contact or needle-sharing activity).	———
Infection	Individual is infected with HIV. Infection is assumed to be permanent.	Unknown, although multiple exposures probably increase the risk of infection.
Seropositivity	Individual has antibodies to HIV, meaning that infection has occurred at some time in the past. Antibody tests cannot pinpoint date of infection. It usually takes 3–12 weeks from the time of infection for the antibodies to appear, although lag-times significantly longer have been reported.	CDC considers double ELISA test confirmed with a Western Blot to be an accurate indicator of infection status; however, there continues to be concern about false positives, particularly in populations with a low prevalence of infection
ARC	Presence of a combination of conditions together giving evidence of symptomatic infection with HIV. (Note: New CDC definition of AIDS incorporates many individuals previously classified as ARC patients).	National Academy of Sciences estimates that 90% of seropositive individuals show some immunodeficiency within 5 years.
AIDS	Illness characterized by one or more "indicator diseases" listed by CDC.	It is generally believed that at least one-half of seropositive individuals and individuals with ARC will develop AIDS. However, all estimates are uncertain due to the lengthy incubation period.

Source: T. M. Hammett, *Aids in Correctional Facilities: Issues and Options, Third Edition* (Washington, D.C.: National Institute of Justice, U.S. Department of Justice, 1986).

test negative because antibodies to the virus have not yet developed, but in this critical period, the individual would still be able to transmit the virus. For this reason, tests should be repeated up to six months after exposure to ensure the validity of the results.

There is limited evidence as to the amount of the virus and/or the number of exposures required for infection to occur. There is also limited evidence as to the amount of the virus or the number of exposures required to transmit infection. It does appear that a large dose of tainted blood given intravenously, as occurs during a blood transfusion, poses an extremely high risk; small doses, as with an

accidental needle-stick, pose a fairly small one. On the other hand, repeated exposure even to small amounts of blood or other body fluid, as with intravenous drug
use involving shared needles, ultimately will present a serious risk.[6]

There also appears to be a relationship between continued exposure and
development of the disease. In studies of HIV-infected intravenous drug users in
New York, the best predictor of manifestation of the disease is continued intravenous use of drugs.[7] This may be related to continued assaults on the immune system, lessening its ability to combat the virus, or to the accumulation of active virus
in the system.

The number of seropositive persons who will eventually manifest the disease
is unknown. It is believed, however, based on data gathered by tracking infected
persons, that the majority of those infected will eventually develop AIDS.
The National Academy of Science estimates that 25–50 percent of HIV seropositives will develop AIDS within five to 10 years of infection and that 90 percent of
seropositives will show some immune system deficiency within five years of
seroconversion.[8]

One of the difficult aspects of AIDS for epidemiological study is the long
incubation period of the disease, or the long time between infection and the appearance of symptoms. In most cases the incubation period ranges from two and a half
to five years, although there are reported cases of incubation as long as eight or 10
years.[9] This long period of uncertainty presents some of the most difficult problems
for managing infected persons and for estimating seroprevalence, or prevalence of
seropositivity in a given population. Persons who are infected may not know they
are HIV-infected until symptoms of illness appear. Persons who are aware of their
HIV antibody-positive status, but are otherwise healthy, may spend many anxious
years anticipating and fearing the appearance of symptoms.

While AIDS is believed to be universally fatal, survival time varies in length
according to the particular illness manifested, and to genetic factors, the availability of treatment, and the general health of the patient. Table 2 indicates the rates
of survival by year of diagnosis. As this figure shows, fatality for cases diagnosed
in 1981 is over 90 percent. Survival after the first year of diagnosis also varies considerably with the specific illness contracted. Persons who develop Kaposi's
sarcoma seem to survive almost twice as long as those with *Pneumocystis carinii*
pneumonia, though short-term survival with this disease is improving.[10]
Factors such as concurrent intravenous drug use also influence the length of
survival. Intravenous drug users, for example, are more likely to contract
Pneumocystis and/or opportunistic infections, are more likely to continue high-risk
activity, and are more likely to have both poor nutrition and health care.

HOW IS THE AIDS VIRUS TRANSMITTED?

While a great deal of media attention has been paid to AIDS, the question para-
mount in the public's mind, "Can someone give it to me?" is still not adequately

TABLE 2
Breakdown of AIDS Survival Rates in the U.S. by Year of Diagnosis

		Number of Cases	Number of Known Deaths[1]	Case-Fatality Rate
1981	Jan–June	89	82	92%
	July–Dec	181	168	93%
1982	Jan–June	368	326	89%
	July–Dec	655	577	88%
1983	Jan–June	1238	1112	90%
	July–Dec	1608	1429	89%
1984	Jan–June	2501	2064	83%
	July–Dec	3258	2670	82%
1985	Jan–June	4536	3586	79%
	July–Dec	5846	4379	75%
1986	Jan–June	7361	4963	67%
	July–Dec	8675	4723	54%
1987	Jan–June	10306	4394	43%
	July–Dec	10534	3008	29%
1988	Jan–May 02	3620	542	15%
	Total[2]	60852	34088	56%

[1]Reporting of deaths is incomplete.
[2]Table totals include 76 cases diagnosed prior to 1981. Of these 76 cases, 65 are known to have died.
Source: CDC, AIDS Weekly Surveillance Report–United States, May 2, 1988.

understood by a great number of people. A survey conducted by the United States Public Health Service's Weekly National Health Interview revealed that a number of people still think AIDS can be transmitted through sharing kitchen utensils, from public toilets or by donating blood.[11]

There are three known methods of transmission of the virus: sexual contact, inoculation with blood, and perinatal events. The latter term refers to pregnancy and childbirth, and may include breast-feeding. Empirical evidence from the CDC and other sources speaks strongly against the probability of transmission through body fluids other than blood, semen, vaginal secretions, and breast milk. In the 10 years of the AIDS epidemic, there have been no documented cases of transmission through any other sources.

Moreover, studies of over 14,000 persons with AIDS have found no cases of transmission to family members through non-sexual casual contact. These findings hold true even in the case of children or infants with AIDS where daily contact with urine, tears and saliva is part of the care of the child.[12]

Since the epidemic began, epidemiologists have carefully tracked all cases, and the three known routes outlined have remained the only means of transmission identified. With almost 75,000 cases of AIDS and many more ARC and seropositivity data, the consistency of these findings is extremely compelling. Except for a small number of cases lost to follow-up, all known cases of AIDS can be attributed to one of the three methods of transmission. Table 3 summarizes the risk of infection through the various transmission modes.

As the data indicate, transmission of HIV is difficult and does not occur through casual contact. Though it is a blood-borne disease like hepatitis B, HIV is far more difficult to transmit than hepatitis B,[13] and precautions or clean-up procedures developed for hepatitis B are more than adequate for dealing with the AIDS virus.

The following sections briefly describe the three known transmission modes:

- transmission through inoculation with blood
- transmission through sexual contact
- perinatal transmission

Transmission through Inoculation with Blood or Blood Products

There are four instances in which contaminated or HIV-infected blood is inoculated into a non-infected person, making transmission of HIV possible:

1. injection of the blood of someone else during sharing of intravenous drug use equipment;
2. transmission during transfusion with contaminated blood or blood products;
3. transmission through accidental needle-sticks with contaminated needles; and
4. transmission through an open wound or mucous membrane exposure.

1. Transmission through intravenous drug use.   Transmission which occurs during sharing of intravenous drug use equipment is the most common method of transmission by inoculation. Eighteen percent of all AIDS cases in this country come from this source. In areas of high incidence of intravenous drug use, the numbers are even higher. For example, in New York and northern New Jersey, almost 50 percent of all AIDS cases are found among intravenous drug users.

TABLE 3
Breakdown of Total AIDS Cases in the U.S. by Transmission Frequency

Transmission Categories[1]	Year Ending May 2, 1987		Year Ending May 2, 1988		Cumulative Cases and Deaths Since June 1981			
	Number	(%)	Number	(%)	Number	(%)	Deaths	(% Cases)
Adults/Adolescents								
Homosexual/Bisexual Male	9949	(66.1)	14990	(60.0)	37999	(63.4)	21010	(62.7)
Intravenous (IV) Drug Abuser	2446	(16.3)	5113	(20.5)	11045	(18.4)	6203	(18.5)
Homosexual Male and IV Drug Abuser	1081	(7.2)	1752	(7.0)	4438	(7.4)	2637	(7.9)
Hemophilia/Coagulation Disorder	166	(1.1)	256	(1.0)	591	(1.0)	349	(1.0)
Heterosexual Cases[2]	615	(4.1)	1072	(4.3)	2463	(4.1)	1320	(3.9)
Transfusion, Blood/Components	386	(2.6)	752	(3.0)	1467	(2.4)	988	(2.9)
Undetermined[3]	402	(2.7)	1038	(4.2)	1894	(3.2)	1027	(3.1)
Subtotal	15045	(100.0)	24973	(100.0)	59897	(100.0)	33534	(100.0)
Children[4]	Number	(%)	Number	(%)	Number	(%)	Deaths	(% Cases)
Hemophilia/Coagulation Disorder	14	(6.3)	26	(5.9)	53	(5.5)	32	(5.8)
Parent with/at risk of AIDS[5]	181	(80.8)	329	(74.9)	735	(77.0)	422	(76.2)
Transfusion, Blood/Components	22	(9.8)	63	(14.4)	131	(13.7)	79	(14.3)
Undetermined[3]	7	(3.1)	21	(4.8)	36	(3.8)	21	(3.8)
Subtotal	224	(100.0)	439	(100.0)	955	(100.0)	554	(100.0)
Total	15269		25412		60852		34088	

[1] Cases with more than one risk factor other than the combinations listed in the tables or footnotes are tabulated only in the category listed first.

[2] Includes 1460 persons (321 men, 1139 women) who have had heterosexual contact with a person with AIDS or at risk for AIDS and 1003 persons (780 men, 223 women) without other identified risks who were born in countries in which heterosexual transmission is believed to play a major role, although precise means of transmission have not yet been fully defined.

[3] Includes patients on whom risk information is incomplete (due to death, refusal to be interviewed, or loss to follow-up), patients still under investigation, men reported only to have had heterosexual contact with a prostitute, and interviewed patients for whom no specific risk was identified; also includes one health-care worker who seroconverted to HIV and developed AIDS after documented needle-stick to blood.

[4] Includes all patients under 13 years of age at time of diagnosis.

[5] Epidemiologic data suggest transmission from an infected mother to her fetus or infant during the perinatal period.

Source: CDC, AIDS Weekly Surveillance Report–United States, May 2, 1988.

The cases in this region constitute almost 75 percent of the nation's total IV drug-related AIDS cases.[14]

The AIDS virus is spread among intravenous users through sharing the needles, syringes and heating elements ("cookers") used in injection. Users traditionally will draw their own blood up into the syringe to mix with the dissolved drug and re-inject it into their veins, in order to use all traces of the drug mixture. The next user will continue in the same way, but will inject any traces of blood remaining from the previous user, as well as his own blood with his drug injection. Since needles are only cleaned in the most perfunctory way—traditionally this means only blowing into the needle or manually clearing a clogged tip of the hypodermic with a wire—traces of the prior user's blood remain in the equipment. When a needle is shared among many users, as is often the case, the possibility of HIV infection is multiplied again and again.

Sharing equipment is common. A study in San Francisco indicates that 90 percent of addicts reported that they had shared needles with an average of 37 different people in the prior year,[15] and a New York/New Jersey study found that one-third of users reported sharing daily.[16] Data from the Drug Use Forecasting System (DUF) indicates that almost half of all drug injectors arrested in Los Angeles report that they currently share needles with one or more people;[17] other cities report lower incidence of sharing, 20 to 25 percent. DUF, a program sponsored by the National Institute of Justice, conducts voluntary and anonymous urine screening of male and female arrestees nationally every three months. Differences found across the country may be attributable to changes in the behavior of addicts in response to AIDS or to basic regional differences in the drug culture.

Why do users share equipment? There are several reasons. First, initiation into drug use is often the occasion for sharing "works." New IV users are unlikely to have their own injection equipment, as initiation is not generally a planned event. Consequently, they are most often "turned on" with friends who share their equipment with them.

Second, sharing "works" with a "running partner," a friend or a spouse, is a common feature of the drug-use world. Sharing is seen in this context as a social activity, a sign of trust and friendship as well as a convenience. Only one party need carry the equipment when both go to buy and use drugs. And both parties may share the drugs purchased by pooling them into the same "cooker" and into the same syringe. Researchers have found that failure to share can be seen as a serious sign of mistrust or disloyalty among IV users and a serious breach of drug world etiquette.[18]

Sharing needles may also be a convenience if equipment is scarce. While only 12 states make possession of a hypodermic needle a punishable offense, they are in many cases the states in which IV drug use is very common. Addicts may share or rent "works" because they have no access to their own or because they do not wish to be caught with the equipment in their possession. This is the underlying motivation for the use of shooting galleries. Shooting galleries can vary from highly commercial operations, such as those found in New York City, to the more prevalent informal renting of works done by other users in their apartments or in areas where drugs are bought. In a shooting gallery or similar place, a set or several sets of works are rented out to users so that they can use their drugs quickly and leave the area.

For the obvious reasons, the spread of HIV has been linked to the use of shooting galleries or similar operations. It is clear that the more one injects drugs, and consequently the more one is likely to rent, borrow, or share contaminated works, the more likely one is to become infected.

2. Transmission during transfusion. HIV infection can also occur when contaminated blood or blood products such as plasma are administered to a patient. Since the blood supply has been screened for the presence of HIV since 1985, the number of cases from this source has been dramatically reduced. Only 3 percent of the total AIDS cases reported since 1981 have come from this source, and the majority of these cases stem from infection prior to 1985. The CDC estimates that only about 100 transfusion-associated infections will occur annually out of a total of 16 million units of blood transfused, and the National Academy of Sciences estimates that the risk of transfusion infection is less than 1 in 34,000 for those receiving packed red blood cells.[19]

3. Transmission through accidental needle-sticks. The fear of accidental puncture with a contaminated needle causes great concern among both health care workers and correctional personnel who worry that they may inadvertently come into contact with a needle used by an HIV antibody-positive individual through routine delivery of care, or during law enforcement procedures such as pat-downs or searches. While at first glance the risk of infection through accidental puncture seems similar to that of needlesharing among IV users, there are important differences. First, in the case of IV drug use, blood is thoroughly mixed with drugs and possibly with contaminated blood before the injection. In the case of a needle-stick, the infected traces of blood are not thoroughly blended with the second person's blood and in most cases enter only under the skin rather than intravenously, reducing the likelihood of transmission. Second, IV drug users share contaminated needles repeatedly, multiplying the risk of transmission, while the accidental needle-stick is a solitary risk event.

For these reasons, the number of transmissions from accidental needle-sticks has been very small. In studies of 887 health care workers who have received needle-sticks or puncture wounds from HIV-contaminated needles, only four have been infected as a result.[20] These data strongly suggest that, while not an impossible event, infection from these sources is not common.

4. Transmission through an open wound or mucous membrane exposure. Exposure through contact with certain contaminated mucosa (eyes, nose, mouth) is also of concern to those working closely with or caring for HIV-infected persons. Fortunately, transmission from this source is even less likely than transmission from accidental needle-sticks. In CDC studies of health care workers who have had open wounds or mucous membrane exposure to infected patients, no cases of transmission have appeared. There are four instances reported in the literature, however, which have involved open wound or mucous membrane exposure to contaminated blood.

In these cases, all four of whom were health care workers, the individuals became infected after direct contact between HIV-infected blood of a patient and their own broken skin or mucosa.[21] In the first instance, a health care worker with seriously chapped hands came into direct contact with the blood of an HIV-infected patient for 20 minutes. In the second case, an individual using a high-speed centrifuge spilled HIV-contaminated blood over ungloved hands and forearms. In the third case, a health care worker was splashed with infected blood in the face and mouth. In the last case, a laboratory researcher became infected after regular and extended contact with concentrated preparations of the virus. It is believed that in the course of the work, an incident of unprotected contact occurred between the preparations and the researcher's broken skin or mucosa.

It should be emphasized that these instances might all have been prevented had precautions been taken—gloves, masks, covering broken skin. In the many laboratory situations across the country where staff are working daily with HIV, often in highly concentrated forms, and in the many hospital settings in which infected patients are treated, there have not been additional cases of transmission. This evidence strongly suggests that this fourth form of inoculation transmission is uncommon and preventable with adequate precautions.

Perinatal Transmission

Perinatal transmission, apparently occurring during pregnancy or childbirth, is the most common cause of AIDS infection in infants and small children. These cases result from the mother's HIV infection, often stemming from her intravenous drug use. Seventy-seven percent of the pediatric AIDS cases reported to the CDC are from perinatal events. In these cases, the virus is passed to the unborn child in utero, during childbirth, or through breast milk. The mechanism of perinatal transmission has not completely been identified, and the timing has not been pinpointed. But there appears to be a 40–50 percent chance that an HIV-infected mother will give birth to a child who will be HIV antibody-positive at birth.[22] There has only been one known case of confirmed transmission of the virus through breast milk.[23] In this case, the mother was infected by a blood transfusion after delivery, and the child became infected through nursing. About a third of children who test HIV antibody-positive at birth will also test negative months later; this happens because infants shed their mothers' antibodies and form their own.

Thus an infant may have tested positive because it retained some of its mother's *antibodies*, but was not itself harboring the virus. When its own immune system begins to mature, and the mother's antibodies naturally degrade and disappear, the infant will no longer test positive. Infants may change from positive to negative status as long as 15 months after birth; it is crucial, therefore, that they be re-tested until then, according to some clinicians.[24]

The majority of pediatric cases have come from New York City, New Jersey, and Florida—areas with high concentrations of IV drug users. Perinatal transmission cases also come disproportionately from minority populations, as these populations are over-represented among IV drug users. Eighty-five percent of the total cases of perinatal transmission occurred among blacks or Hispanics, a figure which represents 65 percent of all pediatric AIDS cases.[25]

Transmission through Sexual Contact

The AIDS virus can be transmitted through either homosexual or heterosexual contact. Activities that may produce small breaks in mucosa, such as anal intercourse, appear to be the most risky. However, vaginal intercourse is also a mode of male-to-female or female-to-male transmission.

Unprotected homosexual activity remains the single largest risk behavior for transmission of the AIDS virus. Homosexual or bisexual males constitute 64 percent of the total number of AIDS cases reported. Having receptive anal intercourse as well as having many partners are both linked to increased chances of contracting infection.[26] Both factors increase the likelihood of contact with another infected male and the likelihood of producing small fissures in the anal mucosa.

The extent of heterosexual transmission has been widely discussed. While the proportion of total cases stemming from heterosexual transmission has remained constant at 4 percent, the *number* of heterosexual cases has increased more rapidly than the numbers in other categories. For example, in September 1984, only 25 cases of heterosexual transmission to women were reported to the New York City Health Department; just two years later that figure had multiplied more than five times. The number of AIDS cases among female IV drug users also increased dramatically during this time, to three and a half times the 1984 figure.[27] These data do not necessarily predict an explosion of AIDS into the non-IV drug-using population, but they do suggest increasing numbers of cases among those in regular sexual contact with IV users and/or bisexual men.

The question of the efficiency of heterosexual transmission is an important one. Most of the data on heterosexual transmission comes from studies of the sexual partners of intravenous drug users, prostitutes, or other persons with AIDS and from American military samples.

Small studies of the sexual partners of persons with AIDS indicate that regular unprotected sexual activity results in a high rate of infection in the partners.

In a U.S. study of 24 seronegative partners of persons with AIDS, of the 10 pairs who used condoms over the 12–36 month study period, only one partner became infected. By comparison, of the 14 pairs who engaged in unprotected sexual activity, 12 partners (88%) became infected.[28] Padian reports that the risk of heterosexual transmission from vaginal intercourse increases with frequency of contact, but seems to remain stable after a threshold of 10–20 exposures.[29] This is not true for anal intercourse in her sample. In this small sample, 88 percent of partners of persons with AIDS became infected, and 30 percent of persons who were seropositive but asymptomatic got the disease. Similar findings have been reported among sexual partners of IV drug users in New York. Since 60 to 75 percent of IV users are male, and approximately 95 percent are heterosexual, the number of non-IV drug-using sexual partners for this population is significant.[30] One study in particular found that nearly half the female partners of male IV users did not themselves use IV drugs.[31]

Studies of American military recruits report that nationally, the ratio of male-to-female seropositivity is 2.7 to 1, but almost one-to-one in areas of highest population prevalence of seropositivity.[32] Among this group were numerous married couples in which both parties were HIV antibody-positive. The areas where male-to-female ratios are almost equal are areas in which substantial portions of the cases involve IV drug use—highlighting again the strong link between heterosexual transmission and intravenous drug use. The largest subgroup of heterosexual transmission cases involves partners of IV users from the New York metropolitan area and South Florida. To date there is little evidence of major transmission in the "second wave"; for example, infection from IV user to non-drug-using partner to another non-drug-using sexual partner.

For criminal justice agencies, the case of heterosexual transmission from prostitutes is a particularly important issue. In both European and U.S. studies of prostitutes, the percentage of seropositivity is high, due primarily to the large number of IV drug users in this group. In a New York study, for example, 42 percent of street prostitutes were IV drug users,[33] and in a New Jersey study, half of the IV drug-using prostitutes were seropositive.[34] There is some speculation that prostitutes may also be more susceptible to HIV infection, due to high rates of other sexually transmitted diseases.[35] Prostitutes also come into contact with both IV drug users and persons who have multiple sexual partners. In the CDC multi-city study of prostitutes, 11 percent of the prostitutes who engaged in unprotected sex with customers tested positive for HIV, compared to *none* of the 22 who always used condoms for vaginal intercourse.[36]

Transmission from infected prostitutes appears to be surprisingly low, however. First, many prostitutes both here and abroad practice safer sex techniques in response to both AIDS and other sexually transmitted diseases.[37] In addition, the frequency of contact with an infected prostitute may be too low to produce effective transmission to any one customer. As a result, only a handful of reported cases involve transmission through heterosexual contact with a prostitute.

It is important to note that single-contact heterosexual transmission does occur, but it appears less likely than was first thought. Padian's results, the prostitution data, and the overall case distribution material all suggest that regular or repeated sexual contact with an infected individual is required for heterosexual transmission. It should be emphasized, however, that the possibility exists of single-contact transmission between heterosexuals.

Common Misconceptions about Transmission

It is critical for education and training programs to address some of the common misconceptions about AIDS transmission. Here, we will briefly review some of the most common areas of confusion.

- *Can I get infected from kissing, hugging, or sharing dishes, silverware, toothbrushes, razors, with a person with AIDS or who is seropositive?*

    There is strong evidence that HIV infection does not occur from sharing household items, even those intimate household items such as a toothbrush or razor. Seven separate studies totaling almost 500 family members of persons with AIDS in daily intimate contact show *no* cases of infection which did not come from one of the known risk factors.[38] In some cases, toothbrushes, razors, toilets, and such intimate household items were routinely shared with the infected party. In addition, family members and health care workers often kiss or hug AIDS patients, and no cases of infection through this route have been reported. CDC does recommend avoidance of deep kissing, however, due to the possibility of small breaks in skin or sores which may contact mucosa and, although highly unlikely, result in transmission. Similarly, though no cases exist, sharing razors and toothbrushes should be avoided as the possibility exists that small amounts of blood could be transferred.

- *Can I contract HIV on the job? What if I have to administer emergency first aid to a co-worker?*

    There is absolutely no evidence to support fears of transmission in the normal course of job performance. Again, in a study of persons with several years of close personal contact in a residential school setting with hemophiliac children who were seropositive, no non-hemophiliac children became infected.[39] There have been no cases of infection among law enforcement personnel, paramedics, or firemen as a result of giving mouth-to-mouth resuscitation to an infected person. Hammett also finds no cases of infection reported in correctional personnel through occupational contact in the three years of examination of AIDS in correctional settings.[40] As a general precaution, however, masks or resuscitation cups should be used in *all* cases of resuscitation to protect both parties from this and numerous other contagious infections.

■ *I have heard that the AIDS virus is in saliva. Can I get infected if an infected person bites me?*

HIV can be isolated in a number of body fluids—saliva, tears, urine—though the concentrations in these fluids is low and, in recent culture studies, very rarely viable.[41] It has been estimated, therefore, that it would take one quart of saliva or urine entering the bloodstream to produce infection.[42]

Biting or spitting generally involves small amounts of saliva which, as has been discussed, poses no real threat. Biting which breaks the skin may bring saliva of an infected person in contact with the blood of the person bitten. But only if the person biting has an open sore or wound in his or her mouth can blood mix with the blood of the person bitten. Thus, given both the low frequency of the usually one-time event, and the unlikelihood of enough infected blood being involved, it is not surprising that there have been no reported infections among persons who have been bitten by someone with AIDS.

■ *Is there risk of transmission to staff who conduct urine testing?*

Again, the concentration of the virus in HIV-infected urine is so small that transmission would require exposure to a much larger quantity of urine than is handled in routine testing. Moreover, good hygiene would indicate that staff should be wearing gloves to handle urine samples, to avoid any contact with the many other, far more readily transmitted infectious agents found in human urine.

■ *Should I allow an HIV-positive probationer or parolee to work in a food-handling job?*

Much of the same evidence holds here. HIV antibody-positive individuals have undoubtedly been employed in food handling, and no cases of transmission have appeared as a result. Persons with AIDS have also prepared food as members of a family with no cases of infection resulting. Hypothetically, an individual could bleed or spit into food preparations, which could be eaten by someone with a cut or sore in the mouth. Even in this unlikely scenario, any virus would almost certainly be killed by the stomach acids. Therefore, CDC specifically recommends against screening food service workers for HIV.

■ *Since the AIDS virus is a blood-borne virus, can I get it from an insect that has bitten someone who is infected?*

Important evidence about insect transmission comes from areas where the virus is well-established, and prevalence of HIV infection is high. In studies of areas of Africa where large portions of the adult population are infected, and in Belle Glade, Florida, where there is an unusually high concentration of HIV infection, there is no evidence of infection outside the known risk groups—IV drug users, homosexuals and their partners.[43] If insects transmitted the infection, one would expect children, the elderly, and all segments of the population to be affected. In addition, the insect must be able to replicate the virus in its own system before it could transmit it to humans; it has been found that mosquitoes are unable to do this with the AIDS virus.

CURRENT TREATMENTS AND VACCINE RESEARCH

A great deal of scientific attention has been focused on the AIDS virus. To date, no cure for the underlying immune suppression caused by the virus has been found. There are, however, a few treatments currently available which appear to prolong life and make the AIDS patient more comfortable. There are also more than 100 studies of 40 or more substances under study by the Food and Drug Administration for use in the treatment of AIDS.[44]

Treatments center around two types of drugs. Anti-viral agents attack or inhibit the growth of the virus; immunomodulating agents work to boost or restore the immune system. As of this writing, only azidothymidine (AZT) is approved by the Food and Drug Administration specifically for treatment of AIDS or advanced ARC, although many more agents are under study. Other drugs, which are already approved for other uses, may be included in AIDS treatment; an example is pentamidine, used to treat *Pneumocystis carinii* pneumonia (PCP). AZT is an anti-viral drug that attacks the replication cycle of the virus and has had considerable success in extending the life of persons with AIDS. While still an expensive therapy, the price of AZT has been reduced from about $10,000 to $7,500 per patient per year. It is also a drug approved for use only in seriously immune-compromised persons, those with T-4 cell counts below 200. In a healthy individual, the T-4 cell count ranges from 700 to 1,400; in a person with ARC or AIDS, the count can range from 50 to 200.[45] AZT, therefore, could not be used to retard the virus among asymptomatic seropositive persons or those in the very early stages of illness.*

Other drugs, like pentamine isethionate or Ampligen, are designed to stimulate the immune system (increase the number of T-4 cells), and inhibit the spread of the virus. Some treatments under study involve the combination of types of drugs. For example, researchers report encouraging results in the treatment of PCP using pentamidine, an anti-cancer drug which interferes with the metabolism of the organism causing PCP, and a vitamin-like substance, called Trimextrate, which protects normal cells from destruction.[46]

In all of these therapies, the illness is retarded or thwarted somewhat, rather than cured. To date, no therapy has provided a cure or complete remission. Therefore, a great deal of effort is being made in the search for a vaccine.

Scientists report that the AIDS virus presents a particularly difficult vaccine problem in that "it hides in cells, it mutates rapidly, and it survives despite many immune responses that would normally rid the body of an invading virus."[47]

---

*The drug AZT has recently been shown to delay the onset of illness in certain asymptomatic seropositives.—*Ed.*

It appears, for example, that people infected with the live AIDS virus develop antibodies which, in the laboratory, inactivate the virus. These people, however, may still become sick and die, indicating that the kind of immune response which will protect a person from AIDS infection is unknown, and that vaccines, like those used in the development of the polio or measles immunizations, may not work. There are also no animal models appropriate for vaccine research. Chimps who can be infected successfully with the virus never develop the disease.

The goal of the vaccine research is to find a vaccine that will produce a strong group-specific antibody that could protect against the diverse AIDS virus strains. Estimates as to the timetable for vaccine availability reflect these problems, and range from several years to decades. There are currently several AIDS vaccines in clinical trials in humans. However, a recent article in *Science* concluded: "Scientists have known since they began to work on an AIDS vaccine that it would not be easy, but perhaps no one realized it would be so difficult."[48]

NOTES

[1] D. C. Des Jarlais and S. R. Friedman, "HIV Infection Among Intravenous Drug Users: Epidemiology and Risk Reduction,"*AIDS* 1987: 1:67–76.

[2] *Ibid.*

[3] A. Ranki et al., "Long Latency Precedes Overt Seroconverstion in Sexually-Transmitted HIV Infection," *Lancet*, September 12, 1987: 2:589–93.

[4] H. W. Haverkos, "Factors Associated with the Pathogenesis of AIDS," *Journal of Infectious Diseases*, July 1987: 156:251–7.

[5] J. S. Schwartz, P. E. Dans, and B. P. Kinosian, "Human Immunodeficiency Virus Test Evaluation, Performance and Use," *Journal of the American Medical Association* 259 (May 6, 1988): 17:2574–79.

[6] G. H. Friedland and R. S. Klein, "Transmission of the Human Immunodeficiency Virus," *New England Journal of Medicine*, October 29, 1987: 317:1125–35.

[7] D. C. Des Jarlais and D. Hunt, "AIDS Bulletin: AIDS and Intravenous Drug Use" (Washington, D.C.: National Institute of Justice, U.S. Department of Justice, 1988).

[8] Institute of Medicine, National Academy of Sciences, *Confronting AIDS: Directions for Public Health, Health Care, and Research* (Washington, D.C., 1986).

[9] J. J. Goedert, presentation, "Heterosexual Spread of HIV Infection and AIDS in the U.S.," National Institute on Drug Abuse Technical Review, January 1988.

[10] Rothenburg et al., "Survival with AIDS," *New England Journal of Medicine*, November 19, 1987: 317:1297–1302.

[11] "AIDS Fears Persist," *Medical World News*, November 23, 1987: 39.

[12] Friedland and Klein, *op. cit.*

[13] *Ibid.*

[14] Centers for Disease Control, "AIDS Weekly Surveillance Report–United States," May 2, 1988.

[15] J. Watters, D. Iura and K. Iura. "AIDS Prevention Services to Intravenous Drug Users through the Mid-City Consortium to Combat AIDS: Administrative Report," December 1986.

[16] H. Ginsberg, J. French, J. Jackson, et al., "Health Education and Knowledge Assessment of HTLV-III Disease Among Intravenous Drug Users," *Health Education Quarterly* 13 (Winter 1986): 4:373–82.

[17] E. Wish, J. O'Neil, and V. Baldau, "Lost Opportunity to Combat AIDS: Drug Abusers in the Criminal Justice System," presented at National Institute of Justice Drug Abuse Technical Review on AIDS and IV Drug Use, July 1988.

[18] D. C. Des Jarlais, S. Friedman, and D. Strug, "AIDS Among Intravenous Drug Users: A Sociocultural Perspective," in *The Social Dimensions of AIDS*, ed. D. Feldman and T. Johnson (New York: Praeger Press, 1985).

[19] Institute of Medicine, National Academy of Sciences, *op. cit.*

[20] Friedland and Klein, *op. cit.*
[21] Update: "HIV Infections in Health-care Workers Exposed to Blood or Infected Patients," *Morbidity and Mortality Weekly Report,* May 22, 1987: 36:285–88.
[22] G. B. Scott, M. A. Fischl, N. Klimas, M. A. Fletcher, G. M. Dickinson, R. S. Levine, and W. P. Parks, "Mothers of Infants With the Acquired Immunodeficiency Syndrome," *JAMA* 1985a: 253:363.
[23] J. B. Ziegler, et al., "Post-natal Transmission of AIDS-Associated Retrovirus from Mother to Infant," *Lancet,* 1985: 1:896–98.
[24] K. Speger, R. N., M.P.H., epidemiologist, Boston City Hospital, personal communication, September, 1988.
[25] Centers for Disease Control, *op. cit.*
[26] Haverkos, *op. cit.*
[27] Friedland and Klein, *op. cit.*
[28] M. A. Fischl, G. M. Dickinson, G. B. Scott, N. Klimas, M. A. Fletcher, and W. Parks, "Evaluation of Heterosexual Partners, Children, and Household Contacts of Adults With AIDS," *JAMA* 257:640–44.
[29] N. Padian, "Male to Female Transmission in San Francisco Heterosexual Spread of HIV Infection and AIDS in the U.S.," *NIDA Technical Review,* January 1988.
[30] Des Jarlais and Hunt, *op. cit.*
[31] D. C. Des Jarlais, E. Wish, S. R. Friedman, R. Stoneburner, et al., "Intravenous Drug Use and Heterosexual Transmission of Human Immunodeficiency Virus: Current Trends in N.Y.C.," *New York State Journal of Medicine* 87 (1987): 283–85.
[32] "HTLV-III/LAV Antibody Prevalence in U.S. Military Recruit Applicants," *MMWR,* July 4, 1986: 35:421–24.
    D. S. Burke et al., "HIV Infections among Civilian Applicants for U.S. Military Service, October 1985 to March 1986," *New England Journal of Medicine,* July 16, 1987: 317:131–6.
[33] E. Wish and B. Johnson, "The Impact of Substance Abuse on Criminal Careers," in *Criminal Careers and Career Criminals,* ed. A. Blumstein, J. Cohan, and C. Visher (Washington, D.C.: National Academy Press, 1986), 2:52–58.
[34] H. Ginsberg, J. French, J. Jackson, et al., "Health Education and Knowledge Assessment of HTLV-III Disease Among Intravenous Drug Users," *Health Education Quarterly* 13 (Winter 1986) 4:373–82.
[35] Des Jarlais and Friedman, *op. cit.*
[36] *MMWR,* July 4, 1986, *op. cit.*
[37] Des Jarlais, Wish, Friedman, et al., *op. cit.*
[38] Friedland and Klein, *op. cit.*
[39] A. Bertheir et al., "Transmissibility of HIV in Hemophiliac and Non-Hemophiliac Children Living in a Private School in France," *Lancet,* September 13, 1986: 598–601.
[40] T. M. Hammett, *AIDS in Correctional Facilities: Issues and Options, Third Edition* (Washington, D.C.: National Institute of Justice, U.S. Department of Justice, 1988).
[41] D. D. Ho et al., "Letter: Infrequency of Isolation of HTLV-III Virus from Saliva in AIDS," *New England Journal of Medicine,* December 19, 1985: 1606.
[42] Alvin Novick, M.D., Yale University, presentation at National Institute on Sentencing Alternatives/National Institute of Corrections Workshop on AIDS—Policy and Treatment Dilemmas for Residential Community Corrections Programs, Newton, Mass., September 21, 1987.
[43] "AIDS in Western Palm Beach County, Florida," *MMWR,* 1986: 35:609–12.
[44] G. McBride, "Impact of AIDS Drugs on Hospitals Unclear," *Modern Health Care,* January, 1988: 40–41.
[45] M. Chase, "Researchers to Report Results of Study on Drug Intended to Delay Onset of AIDS," *The Wall Street Journal,* December 4, 1987: 42.
[46] "Extending AIDS Patients' Lives," *Newsweek,* November 2, 1987: 85.
[47] D. Barnes, "Obstacles to an AIDS Vaccine," *Science,* May 1988, 719–21.
[48] *Ibid,* p. 721.

SECTION ONE

AIDS and Criminal Justice Agency Personnel

$\mathbf{A}$IDS raises important questions for institutions in our society. Some businesses, schools, hospitals, and other employers already have been forced to confront such issues as

- Should seropositive employees (who are otherwise qualified to perform their duties) be terminated?
- Would termination be a violation of current antidiscrimination statutes?
- Should employers test employees for HIV infection?
- What responsibilities do employers have for providing AIDS education and training for their personnel?
- May employees refuse to perform work that brings them in contact with seropositives or persons diagnosed with full-blown AIDS?

These are just a few of the questions that administrators in both the public and the private sectors have been forced to confront as the number of HIV-infected individuals rises.

Criminal justice agencies are like other employers. In fact, in this field the issue of education and training takes on added importance because persons working in the criminal justice system routinely come in contact with intravenous drug users and others who may be infected with the virus. Indeed, there have been police officers, court personnel, and correctional officers who, because they fear infection, have either refused to perform work assignments or have insisted upon taking precautionary measures that almost all medical authorities agree are not necessary. This anxiety persists despite the fact that not a single case of occupational HIV transmission has been reported among employees of criminal justice agencies in the United States.

These general issues are examined in the first article, "The Impact of the HIV Epidemic on Criminal Justice Agencies," by Ann Eichelberger and Mark Blumberg. The authors discuss why criminal justice agencies must stress employee education and training. The second article, by Theodore M. Hammett, summarizes specific recommendations from the National Institute of Justice. These focus on such areas as staff training, how to minimize the likelihood of employee exposure to the virus, and legal and labor relations issues that could arise. Although these recommendations are directed toward law enforcement personnel, they apply to persons working in other components of the criminal justice system as well.

3

The Impact of HIV on Criminal Justice Agencies

Ann Eichelberger and Mark Blumberg

INTRODUCTION

This article examines the impact of the human immunodeficiency virus (HIV) epidemic on criminal justice agencies. Several issues are explored that are germane to persons who work in the field, whether their specialization is law enforcement, the courts, or corrections. The chapter is divided into five sections. The discussion begins with an examination of the occupational risks that criminal justice personnel actually face. Next, the responsibilities of criminal justice agencies with respect to HIV education and training are explored. The third section examines whether agencies may terminate seropositive staff persons or those who have been diagnosed with full-blown AIDS. The legal ramifications of this course of action are explored in a review of the anti-discrimination statutes relating to HIV and AIDS that have been enacted. The final section discusses whether criminal justice agencies should test employees for HIV.

THE RISK OF OCCUPATIONAL HIV TRANSMISSION

Many defendants who pass through the criminal justice system have a history of intravenous drug use (IVDU) or have engaged in other behavior that puts them at increased risk of AIDS. As a consequence, police officers, prison guards and others who work in the system often express anxiety that they will become infected

Pat Stark is owed a debt of gratitude for her helpful editorial assistance.

with HIV as a result of their employment. Although the AIDS virus cannot be transmitted through casual contact (Friedman, Saltzman, Rogers et al., 1986), agency personnel remain concerned about bites, spitting incidents, needle-sticks, and other acts that they believe could put them in danger.

Most of the fears that agency personnel have are unrealistic. The best evidence in support of this view is the fact that at least a decade after appearance of the AIDS virus in the U.S., not a single case has been reported in which a police officer, prison guard, or any other worker in the field of criminal justice has become infected with HIV as a result of duties performed as part of their job (Hammett, 1988:22). Furthermore, there are no documented cases in which viral transmission has occurred due to a bite[1] or spitting incident (Gostin, 1989a:1023; Lifson, 1988:1353–1354). In fact, the Centers for Disease Control no longer recommend that health care workers be required to follow universal precautions when contact with saliva is anticipated (Centers for Disease Control, 1988).

The only serious danger to persons working in the criminal justice system comes from needles that may be contaminated with the blood of HIV-infected individuals. Agency personnel may be placed at risk through either an accidental needle-stick that occurs in the course of conducting a search, or as a result of an assault perpetrated by a seropositive assailant who seeks to harm the officer with a dirty needle. Fortunately, even under these circumstances, the risk of infection is minimal. Studies of health care workers who have accidentally pricked themselves with contaminated needles indicate that the likelihood of viral transmission in these cases is less than 1 percent (Friedland and Klein, 1987:1127). Nonetheless, police officers and others who have contact with seropositive offenders must take steps to avoid this kind of injury. Agencies should train their personnel to exercise extreme caution when conducting searches that may uncover contaminated needles and in dealing with violent individuals, particularly IVDUs.

EDUCATION AND TRAINING

Rationale

AIDS education and training can serve a number of important functions for criminal justice agencies.[2] Training can teach staff how and when to take precautionary measures to avoid infection with the virus. Second, a comprehensive educational effort will reduce anxiety on the part of agency personnel. By highlighting the fact that many routine activities pose no danger of viral transmission, the likelihood that employees will overreact or respond inappropriately to situations involving infected clients should be reduced. Third, HIV education can be useful for clearing up misinformation. Studies have shown that a substantial proportion of the population, including persons who work in the field of criminal justice (Hammett, 1987:21), hold erroneous beliefs regarding the AIDS virus and the ways in which it can be transmitted (Blendon and Donelan, 1988). Fourth, education and training can teach agency personnel to avoid the types of high-risk activities that can lead to infection (i.e., unsafe sex and needlesharing) in their personal lives. Finally, education and training are necessary to minimize the risk of civil liability. Employees who file suit alleging that they became infected with HIV on the job are less likely to prevail if they have been provided with education and training that is designed to familiarize them with infection control procedures.

Content

Educational programs should teach persons who work in criminal justice agencies how the AIDS virus is and is not transmitted, the relative risks that various work assignments may entail, and the procedures to be followed for minimizing these risks. It is important that information be presented in a clear and understandable manner. In addition, the material should be updated periodically to ensure that personnel are kept abreast of the latest developments.

The Centers for Disease Control have published detailed guidelines for avoiding HIV infection in health care settings and other workplaces (Centers for Disease Control, 1987a). They recommend that agency personnel take "universal precautions" in order to avoid exposure to blood and certain other body fluids that may be infected with HIV. Universal precautions means that all blood and semen, regardless of source, should be treated as if they were infectious. The rationale behind such an approach is that most seropositive individuals do not display any symptoms of illness. As a consequence, any policy that encourages staff to follow precautionary measures only in situations where the individual is believed to be seropositive would not be effective.[3]

Occasionally, criminal justice agencies have been confronted with personnel who refuse to carry out work assignments that involve contact with persons who have AIDS or are seropositive (Hammett, 1988:39). This raises the question of whether law enforcement officers and other justice system personnel have a right to refuse duties that bring them in contact with infected co-workers or clients. May a deputy sheriff, for example, refuse to transport a prisoner known to have AIDS?

There is a strong consensus of opinion that agency personnel may *not* refuse these assignments. This is true for two reasons: 1) law enforcement personnel and correctional officers have consented when they were hired to assume a certain degree of risk, and 2) the danger of occupational HIV transmission is minimal. In fact, police officers and prison guards face far greater hazards on a daily basis as a result of other routine aspects of their job (e.g., confronting armed suspects). It has not been suggested that they may walk away from these duties.

A more difficult question is how agency heads should respond when their personnel insist on employing protective measures that are unnecessary and send the wrong message to the public. For example, police officers in Washington, D.C. have worn yellow gloves during demonstrations by gay rights and AIDS activists (Blumberg, 1989:210). Although this practice may seem harmless and does not infringe on the rights of the protestors, it can be interpreted as a signal that the police believe AIDS is transmitted through casual contact. Such a message will not be conducive to the development of a good working relationship between the police department and gay rights activists. Administrators must take steps to ensure that agency personnel refrain from using measures that are not really necessary.

HIV TESTING IN THE WORKPLACE

Ever since the development in 1985 of a blood test that could determine whether an individual had been exposed to the AIDS virus, there has been extensive debate over the issue of HIV screening. Policymakers have been forced to address such questions as:

1. Who should be tested for HIV?
2. Should testing be done on a mandatory or voluntary basis?
3. Under what circumstances is testing appropriate?

However, there has been little debate over the propriety of HIV screening in the workplace.

Criminal justice agencies and other civilian employers do not presently test applicants or current employees for the AIDS virus. HIV screening by employers would be inappropriate for several reasons. For one thing, infected staff persons present no danger to others because this virus is not transmitted by the types of activities that normally occur in the workplace. Second, testing would not provide agencies with useful information. Because the mean incubation period for developing full-blown AIDS is between seven and eight years from the date of infection (Lui, Darrow, and Rutherford, 1988:1334), a positive blood test would not indicate to the employer whether the individual would be likely to fall ill anytime soon. Third, agency screening would not be cost-effective. Because the prevalence of HIV infection is extremely low among exclusively heterosexual individuals who do not inject drugs (Centers for Disease Control, 1987b:18), very few seropositive individuals would be identified through this procedure. Fourth, employees who tested positive might be subjected to discrimination. Indeed, there have been cases in which HIV-infected persons have been evicted from their apartments, denied insurance coverage, or fired from their jobs (Altman, 1987:58–65). Finally, employer testing may be illegal. California, Massachusetts, New York, Wisconsin, and a number of other jurisdictions prohibit screening unless informed consent is specifically obtained from the individual being tested (Hammett, 1988:67).

In 1989, medical researchers reported that the drug AZT could delay the onset of illness for some asymptomatic seropositive individuals (Fackelmann, 1989:135). Therefore, as part of their educational message, criminal justice agencies should encourage employees who believe that they may be at risk to seek voluntary testing and treatment. Although treatment with AZT is expensive, it could forestall the need for more costly medical intervention at a later date. In addition, such therapy might enable the employee to remain on the job for a longer period of time.

SEROPOSITIVE EMPLOYEES

Criminal justice agencies are no different from other employers who must address the issue of how to respond when it becomes known that an employee is either infected with HIV or has actually developed full-blown AIDS. Despite considerable sentiment that such individuals be terminated (Blendon and Donelan, 1988:1024), this course of action is clearly inadvisable in cases where the employee is still able to perform his or her duties.

Termination would be inappropriate for several reasons. For one thing, HIV-infected employees do not pose any danger either to co-workers or the public. For example, it is difficult to imagine that a seropositive police officer could present a danger to those with whom he or she comes in contact. Health care workers have much greater contact with blood from patients, yet no cases have been reported in which a patient became infected as a result of treatment provided by a seropositive caregiver (Institute of Medicine, 1988:100). Second, it would be unfair to deny qualified seropositive employees the opportunity to work merely because of their HIV status. Firing persons under these circumstances would result in the loss not only of needed employment, but also of important health and life insurance benefits in many cases. Third, the agency would be denied the services of a valuable employee for no legitimate reason. Fourth, this policy would set a bad example for the community and undermine the basic educational message that public health officials have been trying to convey: that HIV is not transmitted except through certain types of high-risk behavior. Clearly, criminal justice agencies should be in the forefront of efforts to develop rational policies for dealing with the AIDS crisis. Finally, terminating an HIV-infected employee without cause is likely to be illegal and may therefore subject the agency to costly litigation.

ANTIDISCRIMINATION STATUTES AND HIV

Employees who believe that they were discharged on account of their HIV status are likely to file suit. If successful, these claims could force municipalities to pay large damage awards. For this reason, agencies have a strong interest in avoiding personnel decisions that result in civil liability. Administrators should therefore be familiar with the various antidiscrimination statutes that have been enacted.

To date, the most important piece of antidiscrimination legislation for handicapped individuals is Section 504 of the Rehabilitation Act of 1974. This statute was designed to outlaw discrimination against handicapped persons in any program or activity that receives federal assistance. Because many criminal justice agencies receive federal funds, they are required to meet the requirements of Section 504.

However, there has been some controversy over whether this provision applies to persons with AIDS and asymptomatic seropositive individuals. Some have argued that discrimination that is based on an irrational fear of contagion is not prohibited by the statute (Cooper, 1987).

In recent years, the federal courts have resolved this question. The major ruling in this area was a decision by the U.S. Supreme Court in *School Board of Nassau County v. Arline*, 107 S. Ct. 1123, 1987. Although this case did not involve AIDS or HIV infection, the ruling had enormous implications for persons with AIDS and asymptomatic seropositives. Arline was a teacher who had been fired after testing positive for tuberculosis. There was no evidence presented which suggested that this woman could not perform her job. Instead, the school board defended its action on the grounds that she might transmit the disease to her pupils. The Supreme Court, in deciding for Arline, noted that she posed no danger to others, that she was otherwise qualified for her position, and that an irrational fear of contagion is the type of prejudice that the legislation was designed to counteract.

Although this case did not address the issue of HIV infection, the court's rationale strongly suggested that otherwise qualified persons who have AIDS would receive protection under Section 504. Despite this ruling, it was not immediately clear whether asymptomatic seropositives would also be defined as "handicapped," since they were not actually physically impaired. However, this uncertainty was short-lived. In several recent decisions, the federal courts have extended the scope of Section 504 to include both persons with full-blown AIDS and seropositive individuals who manifest no symptoms of illness (Hevesi, 1988).[4]

In addition to the federal Rehabilitation Act, all fifty states have antidiscrimination statutes that are similar in nature. Forty-five states go further than federal legislation by protecting private as well as public employees from discrimination. In 34 states, there have been rulings that these statutes apply to persons diagnosed with AIDS or infected with HIV (Gostin, 1989b:1628).

Antidiscrimination legislation that protects handicapped persons is not always the sole remedy available for injured parties. Several states and municipalities have also enacted AIDS-specific statutes or ordinances that protect HIV-infected individuals (Gostin, 1989b:1628). This legislation, generally found in those communities that have a substantial number of AIDS cases (e.g., San Francisco), prohibits a wide range of injustices.

Despite these measures, the Presidential Commission on AIDS stated that there is a pressing need for national legislation that would ban all forms of discrimination directed against HIV-infected individuals (Watkins, 1988:chapter 9). The commission charged that the lack of a comprehensive federal antidiscrimination statute not only denies justice to those who suffer with this illness, it also makes the task of combating the epidemic more difficult. In the view of commission members, persons who are unprotected against discrimination are less likely to cooperate with public health officials and come forward for voluntary testing and counseling.

The Presidential Commission recommended that AIDS not be treated differently from other handicapping illnesses. Instead, it suggested that federal legislation be enacted that would unequivocally bar discrimination against any handicapped person, including those suffering from HIV infection (Watkins, 1988:121). The Disabled Americans Act that is pending before the 101st Congress contains provisions that closely parallel these recommendations. This proposal, which would protect both seropositives and persons with AIDS, bars discrimination in employment, accommodations, restaurants, and stores (Gostin, 1989b:1628). Because it has the backing of the Bush administration, its chances for passage are favorable (Nash, 1989).

CONCLUSION

This chapter reviewed a number of important concerns that administrators in criminal justice agencies are likely to face as the number of AIDS cases grows over the next few years. We examined such issues as the importance of developing an appropriate HIV education and training policy, the danger posed to police officers and others who work in the system by seropositive offenders, whether criminal justice agencies should test employees for the AIDS virus, how infected personnel should be handled with respect to continued employment, and the current status of antidiscrimination legislation as it has been applied to AIDS.

There are several important points that administrators must recognize:

1. Education is the key to avoiding unnecessary difficulties and possible civil liability.
2. There have been no reported cases in which criminal justice personnel became infected with HIV as a result of their employment.
3. There is no justification for terminating seropositive employees who are otherwise qualified to perform their work assignments.
4. This course of action is likely to be illegal in most cases.
5. Criminal justice agencies have no legitimate reason to test employees for HIV.

REFERENCES

Altman, Dennis. 1987. *AIDS in the Mind of America: The social, political, and psychological impact of a new epidemic.* Garden City, N.Y.: Anchor Books.

Blendon, Robert J. and Karen Donelan. (1988). Discrimination against people with AIDS: The public's perspective. *The New England Journal of Medicine.* Vol. 319, No. 15, 1022–1026.

Blumberg, Mark. 1989. The AIDS epidemic and the police. In Roger G. Dunham and Geoffrey Alpert (eds.), *Critical issues in policing: Contemporary readings*, pp. 205–215. Prospect Heights, Ill.: Waveland Press, Inc.

Centers for Disease Control. (1988). Update: Universal precautions for prevention of transmission of human immunodeficiency virus, hepatitis B virus, and other bloodborne pathogens in health-care settings. *Morbidity and Mortality Weekly Report.* Vol. 37, No. 24 (June 24).

Centers for Disease Control. (1987a). Recommendations for prevention of HIV transmission in health-care settings. *Morbidity and Mortality Weekly Report.* Vol. 36, No. 2S (August 21).

Centers for Disease Control. (1987b). Human immunodeficiency virus infection in the United States: A review of current knowledge. *Morbidity and Mortality Weekly Report.* Vol. 36, No. S–6 (December 18).

Cooper, Charles J. (1987). Discrimination against the handicapped. In William H. L. Dornette (ed.), *AIDS and the Law*, pp. 141–147. New York: John Wiley and Sons.

Fackelmann, K. A. (1989). Early AZT use slows progression to AIDS. *Science News.* Vol. 136, No. 9, p. 135.

Friedland, Gerald H. and Robert S. Klein. (1987). Transmission of the human immunodeficiency virus. *The New England Journal of Medicine.* Vol. 317, No. 18, pp. 1125–1135.

Friedland, Gerald H., Brian R. Saltzman, Martha F. Rogers, et al. (1986). Lack of transmission of HTLV-III/LAV infection to household contacts of patients with AIDS or AIDS-related complex with oral candidiasis. *The New England Journal of Medicine.* Vol. 314, No. 6, pp. 344–349.

Gostin, Larry. (1989a). The politics of AIDS: Compulsory state powers, public health, and civil liberties. *Ohio State Law Journal.* Vol. 49, No. 4, pp. 1017–1058.

Gostin, Larry O. (1989b). Public health strategies for confronting AIDS: Legislative and regulatory policy in the United States. *Journal of the American Medical Association.* Vol. 261, No. 11, pp. 1621–1630.

Hammett, Theodore M. (1988). *AIDS in correctional facilities: Issues and options, third edition.* Washington, D.C.: National Institute of Justice, April.

Hammett, Theodore M. (1987). *AIDS in correctional facilities: Issues and options, second edition.* Washington, D.C.: National Institute of Justice, May.

Hevesi, Dennis. (1988). AIDS carriers win a court ruling. *New York Times.* July 9, 1988, p. 6.

Institute of Medicine. (1988). *Confronting AIDS: Update 1988.* Washington, D.C.: National Academy Press.

Lifson, Alan R. (1988). Do alternate modes for transmission of human immunodeficiency virus exist? A review. *Journal of the American Medical Association.* Vol. 259, No. 9, pp. 1353–1356.

Lui, Kung-Jong, William W. Darrow, and George W. Rutherford, III. (1988). A model-based estimate of the mean incubation period for AIDS in homosexual men. *Science.* Vol. 240, pp. 1333–1335.

Nash, Nathaniel C. (1989). Bush and Senate leaders support sweeping protection for disabled. *New York Times.* August 3, p. 1.

Watkins, James. (1988). *Report of the presidential commission on the human immunodeficiency virus.* Submitted to the President of the United States, June 24.

CASES

Chalk v. Orange County Dept. of Education (1987) 832 F2d 1158 (9th Cir).
Doe v. Centinela Hospital (1988) 57 USLW 2034 (USDC DC Cal).
Ray v. School District of DeSoto County (1987) 666 F Supp 1524 (MD Fla).
School Board of Nassau County v. Arline (1987) 107 S. Ct. 1123.

NOTES

[1] When a person is bitten, it is generally the assailant, not the victim, who comes in contact with blood. The only way for the victim to be exposed to the blood of the assailant would be if the latter were bleeding from the mouth.

[2] Hammett (1988) presents an excellent discussion of the many issues that must be confronted when an agency implements an AIDS education program.

[3] At one point, police and fire personnel in Albany, New York received intense criticism for maintaining a list of persons with AIDS. This practice, now abandoned, was justified on the grounds that precautionary measures are necessary when dealing with infected individuals. Not only does this procedure raise a number of civil liberty concerns, it is also likely to engender a false sense of security because most persons who can transmit the virus do not manifest any symptoms of illness (Blumberg, 1989: 210).

[4] *Chalk v. Orange County Dept. of Education* 832 F2d 1158 (9th Cir 1987); *Doe v. Centinela Hospital*, 57 USLW 2034 (USDC DC Cal 1988); and *Ray v. School District of DeSoto County*, 666 F Supp 1524 (MD Fla 1987).

4

Summary of Recommendations, AIDS and the Law Enforcement Officer: Concerns and Policy Responses

Theodore M. Hammett

T he major recommendations to law enforcement agencies for addressing AIDS-related issues are summarized below.

OPERATIONAL ISSUES

Most AIDS-related concerns among law enforcement staff relate to contact with individuals known or suspected to be infected with HIV and with potentially contaminated objects. The following recommendations address these concerns:

- **Provide education and training on AIDS for law enforcement officers and other department staff.**
- **Issue specific AIDS policies and procedures, or revise existing communicable disease policies to address AIDS issues.** Such policies may help to avoid incidents caused by overreaction and fear. On the other hand, promulgating specific AIDS policies may heighten concern by calling attention to the issue. The alternative is simply to apply existing communicable disease policies, based on experience with Hepatitis-B and other infections—i.e., emphasizing basic hygiene and cleanup of body fluid spills.
- **Educate officers on the low risk of HIV infection associated with assaults, human bites, and other disruptive behavior by subjects but recommend reasonable precautions.** To establish low risks, emphasize saliva and

Reprinted from the *Issues and Practices in Criminal Justice* series, by Theodore M. Hammett. Washington, D.C.: National Institute of Justice, June, 1987.

needlestick studies. Reasonable precautions include polishing "defensive skills" to minimize physical contact and practicing good hygiene if contact occurs.

- **Ensure careful supervision of lockup areas to prevent incidents in which HIV infection may be transmitted among prisoners.**

- **Counsel caution and use of gloves in searches and evidence handling, but educate on low risk of infection.** Needlestick studies establish the extremely low risk of infection, but officers should wear gloves and use mirrors when possible to examine places hidden from direct view. Puncture-proof containers should be provided for evidence and potentially infectious materials should be labelled.

- **Use masks or airways for CPR, but educate on low risk of infection.** Saliva studies establish the low risk of infection, but protective devices make sense from the point of view of general hygiene.

- **Follow infection control procedures for first aid.** When there is likely to be contact with blood, all cuts or open wounds should be covered with clean bandages and gloves worn. There should be careful handwashing after contact and spills should be cleaned up promptly with a household bleach solution.

- **Ensure that no staff touch bodies of deceased individuals unless authorized or necessary.** If contact is necessary, infection control procedures should be followed.

- **Provide clear education on the fact that HIV infection is not transmitted by any form of casual contact.** Departments should keep continuously abreast of research developments in this area and pass all new information on to staff.

- **Coordinate educational efforts with public health departments, hospitals, emergency medical services, fire departments, community-based AIDS action groups and gay/lesbian organizations.** Cooperative ties with the last two organizational categories are currently rare in law enforcement agencies and probably should be expanded.

KEY ELEMENTS OF AIDS TRAINING FOR STAFF

Effective staff training must be the cornerstone of law enforcement agencies' response to AIDS. Key elements of AIDS training are presented in the following recommendations:

- **Involve staff in the development of training programs and training materials.** This lends credibility to the program and allows it to respond to specific issues raised by the staff.

- **Training should be timely.** Ideally, it should begin before staff begin to raise serious concerns about AIDS.

- **Training should be presented frequently.** One-time segments during recruit training are insufficient. Regular in-service training is necessary to present new information promptly and to prevent misinformation from taking hold. Printed materials should be continuously available.
- **Live training (lectures, seminars, discussions) is the most effective format if trainers are highly knowledgeable.** It is critical that staff have ample opportunity to ask questions and receive answers from experts in the field. Videotapes can be effective but they should be followed by live question-and-answer periods.
- **Training should be keyed to specific law enforcement issues and situations.** It is not enough to distribute generic informational materials. Training topics should include arrest procedures, searches, CPR, first aid, evidence handling, transportation of prisoners, crime scene processing, disposal of contaminated materials, lockup supervision, and body removal procedures.
- **Training should avoid the extremes of alarmism and complacency.** An alarmist tone might foster misinformation and undue fear, while a complacent tone might not provide sufficiently strong recommendations regarding the care and caution appropriate for all staff to practice in all situations.
- **Recognize the role of law enforcement officers as AIDS educators in the community.** Because officers frequently deal with intravenous drug users, prostitutes, and others at high risk of being infected with HIV, they may have a unique opportunity to provide frank, practical educational messages on the disease.

LEGAL AND LABOR RELATIONS ISSUES

Law enforcement agencies have expressed concern about a number of AIDS-related legal and labor relations issues. Most of these issues are still hypothetical because few actual cases have arisen as yet. However, the following recommendations address key concerns that have been raised by agencies:

- **Establish formal procedures for the timely reporting of incidents in which transmission of HIV infection may have occurred.** Such reporting facilitates prompt an appropriate medical intervention.
- **Develop policies on HIV antibody testing.** Departments may wish to require, recommend or make available testing for officers and other individuals involved in incidents in which infection may have been transmitted. Department policies should reflect careful consideration of all of the complex, countervailing issues surrounding HIV antibody testing. Policy statements should specify the rationale for the policy position and the procedures to be used in any testing program.

- Consider potential liability claims against the department (as distinct from worker's compensation claims) arising from job-related HIV infection. The probability of such liability being found appears low because of the officer's "assumption of risk" in accepting the job and would be minimized by providing regular training which recommends specific precautions against infection.
- Emphasize officers' obligation to perform duties involving HIV-infected individuals.
- Consider the department's potential responsibility for preventing HIV transmission by its treatment of potential carriers of the virus. This might apply to prostitutes and intravenous drug users, but it would seem that departmental liability would be very hard to establish if the conduct resulting in infection was consensual—e.g., shooting drugs or patronizing a prostitute. Nevertheless, departments should develop policies for dealing with prostitutes and others in police custody who may be infected with HIV.
- Consider the department's responsibility to prevent HIV transmission among prisoners in the lockup. This represents a potentially very serious legal problem, particularly if HIV transmission occurs as a result of coerced conduct in the lockup. Although none of these cases relate specifically to HIV transmission, correctional departments have been held liable for damages arising from homosexual rapes and other inmate-on-inmate assaults where it was established that supervision had been inadequate.

AIDS poses a range of complicated and potentially serious problems for law enforcement agencies. However, timely and rational policy choices, regular staff training keyed to specific law enforcement concerns, and careful consideration of possible legal liabilities can go far toward minimizing the effects of these problems on the delivery of police services to the public.

SECTION TWO

AIDS
and the Courts

The AIDS crisis presents the courts with important challenges. The first is to the traditional role of the courts in resolving important legal questions. The judiciary has been asked to decide such issues as:

- May persons ever be forced to undergo HIV testing? Under what circumstances?
- What are the limits of the state's power to restrict the liberty of individuals whose behavior may place others at risk?
- What policies may correctional administrators pursue to control the spread of the AIDS virus in prisons and jails?

Courts bear responsibility for balancing the rights of the individual against those of the community. Persons with AIDS have sought protection from discrimination, while institutions have sought to clarify allowable measures to safeguard the community. The courts have been guided by traditional constitutional standards as they seek to evaluate whether public policy meets or exceeds legitimate public health needs.

Persons working in the judicial branch of government may hold fears and misconceptions about AIDS. The courts have therefore been forced to examine the question of what protective measures, if any, may be constitutionally employed with defendants who have AIDS (or who are merely seropositive). Despite overwhelming scientific evidence that HIV cannot be transmitted through casual contact, some courts have employed protective measures that are not only inappropriate, but also jeopardize the defendant's right to a fair trial.

The first article in this section, "AIDS: A Judicial Perspective," by Peter J. Messitte, emphasizes the responsibility that the courts have in resolving legal issues raised by the AIDS crisis within statutory definitions. "AIDS in the Courtroom," by Donald Wallace, examines the constitutional issues that have arisen when courts have altered their normal working environment by requiring protective measures for defendants infected with HIV. Both authors note that ample precedents exist to guide the judiciary in interpreting questions raised by AIDS.

5

AIDS:
A Judicial Perspective

Peter J. Messitte

A IDS presents a full-blown crisis, but this perspective exists: The period of the Middle Ages had its bubonic plague; the nineteenth century its typhoid fever; and the mid-twentieth century its polio epidemic. Mankind eventually surmounted the problems of those diseases and there is no doubt that in time, we will prevail over AIDS. Although talk of a cure is still scant, intensive global research is under way, and experiments with promising drugs continue to be reported.

A distinguishing feature of this epidemic of the 1980s is that our medical research is far more organized and sophisticated than ever before. Another distinguishing feature is the sensitivity of our social institutions to the human dimensions of the disease. We are concerned that fundamental rights of individuals do not get trampled in the process of coming to terms with this disturbing phenomenon. Our challenge as judges is to define those concerns more particularly. I would like to summarize my perspective:

First, the AIDS crisis, for the most part, does not present new legal issues. Second, the issues it presents can be grouped into fairly straightforward categories. Third, while there are some unique aspects to AIDS in the courtroom setting, even those issues are not entirely unfamiliar. And fourth, judges are up to the task of confronting whatever legal challenges AIDS presents.

Reprinted from *Judicature*, Vol. 72, no. 4 (December-January 1989), pp. 205–209.

NO NEW ISSUES

Issues involving marriage, the family, education, employment, discriminatory treatment of individuals, torts and crimes are at the heart of a court's concern. We deal every day in constitutions, statutes and cases, abstracting general principles and deducing specific applications. We may be called upon to decide:

- who can or cannot marry;
- which parent should have custody of or visitation with a child;
- who can be kept out of school or must be allowed back in;
- who can or cannot be fired from a job;
- what constitutes "just cause" for the termination of employment;
- who is eligible for workers', unemployment or disability compensation;
- what the reaches are of such torts as battery, negligence, intentional infliction of emotional distress and fraud; and
- what the reaches are of malicious acts that tend to injure the public in a criminal manner.

AIDS, in a sense, is another spin on the curve balls that judges see all the time. Consider this reformulation of those issues:

- when should disease be a factor in a custody or visitation decision?
- what limitations on custody or visitation are appropriate in the presence of disease?
- when can disease be the basis of a decision to exclude a child from public school?
- is disease ever a proper basis for terminating someone's employment?
- does a particular disease make one eligible for workers' compensation or disability benefits?
- can someone who knowingly transmits a disease be liable in tort?
- can such a person be found criminally liable?

In the special setting of a prison:

- in general, is medical screening of inmates ever appropriate?
- once the medical test results of inmates are known, who is entitled to know about them?
- what is to be done about those inmates who test positive for a disease, *e.g.*, do you segregate them? Are they entitled to special medical treatment?
- On the other hand, what are the rights of the inmates who are compelled to live in such quarters with those individuals?

Lord Bacon observed that law develops following the example of time itself "which, indeed, innovateth greatly, but quietly, and by degrees, scarce to be perceived."[1] Without exhausting the list, there are obviously "quietly" developed precedents discussing disease as a factor in custody or visitation decisions.[2] Virtually every state regulates admission to school of students and employees with communicable diseases.[3] There is ample precedent suggesting that illness, when it is contagious and affects competency, may have consequences for one's right to hold a job.[4]

Maryland, for example, has for some time had a statute which makes transmission of a communicable disease a crime under certain circumstances.[5] Recently, the Maryland Court of Appeals held that knowing transmission of herpes can give rise to liability in tort for fraud, intentional infliction of emotional distress or negligence.[6] For procedural reasons, battery was not part of that case, but in 1917, a Delaware court held a husband criminally liable in battery for infecting his wife with a venereal disease.[7] In the prison setting, courts have held for a number of years that new inmates may be screened for communicable disease.[8] And Maryland has had among its statutes for some time a statute making medical records confidential,[9] as well as another that provides for special treatment of sick offenders who are in prison.[10]

This list could go on, but the point is that judges do not face something so very new and different in the AIDS phenomenon. It comes as no great surprise, then, that an Indiana trial judge overturned a conviction on three counts of attempted murder, where an HIV (human immunodeficiency virus)-infected defendant smeared his blood on, bit, scratched and spit at law enforcement officials. Given the state of knowledge about AIDS and mortality, the judge reasoned that death could not result in the year and a day which the common law requires before homicide will be recognized.[11] Nor is it unexpected that a Florida trial judge would dismiss charges of attempted manslaughter against a prostitute who engaged in sex at a time when she knew that she tested positive for the AIDS virus, under circumstances where the alleged victims were not informed of this fact.[12] As the judge reasoned:

> Defendant may have certainly acted in a culpably negligent fashion; however, there is no evidence from which a jury could find that her alleged conduct evidenced an intent to kill.

The analysis is conventional, the tone dispassionate, the tradition familiar.

GROUPING ISSUES

In my view, the basic legal issues that the AIDS phenomenon resolves into are these: First, when, if at all, it is proper to attempt to identify people with AIDS or HIV carriers? Second, once they are identified, who is entitled to know about it? Third, once they are identified, what can be properly done with those who have an AIDS-related condition? Can they be segregated? Can they be otherwise treated differently from everyone else in a way that most would agree is unfavorable to them? On the other hand, are they entitled to be treated differently in a way that is favorable from their standpoint?

My perspective is that we are judges. It is not our inquiry to determine what *should* be done in all these categories. For the most part, this is a public policy question to be answered by legislative bodies. Our task is to determine whether, once the policy decisions are made, they properly conform to such constitutional considerations as the legitimate exercise of police power, due process and equal protection of law and the right to privacy. As far as statutes are concerned, we are called upon to determine whether AIDS fits within statutory definitions that confer rights or impose duties or disabilities. That is the context in which we must view AIDS issues.

Having said this, when, if at all, is it proper to attempt to identify AIDS virus carriers? The battleground here is mandatory testing. The first question, of course, is whether testing is ever appropriate. If so, what populations should be tested? Food handlers? Health care workers? Members of the military? Prisoners? A substantial number of jurisdictions have enacted or are close to enacting mandatory testing for prisoners.[13] But while testing involving prisoners may well survive legal challenge,[14] decisions remain to be made as to other populations.

Second, who is entitled to know about the test results? Some may say no one but the person tested and his or her physician. But what about law enforcement personnel? A recently enacted Maryland law requires treating doctors in certain circumstances to advise law enforcement officials that a person treated after being assisted by these officials tested positive for HIV.[15] What about judges? Court personnel? Jurors? Victims of crime? Public health authorities? Spouses or sexual partners? Co-workers?

Third, once the AIDS status of an individual is known, *e.g.* full-blown AIDS or simply seropositivity on tests, what can properly be done about it? In terms of segregation, is quarantine permissible?[16] Can a person with AIDS be excluded from the country?[17] From housing?[18] From custody or visitation?[19] From public schools?[20] From employment?[21] From certain kinds of jobs?[22] Can an inmate be segregated within the prisons?[23]

Further, can places where high-risk groups congregate be shut down, *e.g.* as with New York City's attempt to outlaw bath houses?[24] In apprehending criminal suspects, can unconventional means be used, *e.g.* moon suits or stun guns? In receiving individuals in public places, including the courtroom, can they be treated differently from other members of the public?

Yet, some persons with AIDS seek to be treated differently in a positive way. Are they entitled to medical treatment, either generally or in prisons?[25] Are they entitled to special benefits, such as workers', unemployment or disability compensation?[26] In the criminal process, are they entitled to special consideration in charging? Prosecutors say no, but experience may be saying yes.[27] Easier bail? At least one New York Court has said yes.[28] Expedited trials? A recent case also out of New York, giving trial calendar preference to an AIDS litigant in a civil case, may be a straw in the wind.[29] Shorter sentences and earlier probation? The *New York Times* last year reported on the discretionary policy of New York courts that allows early release for AIDS patients based on humanitarian grounds, pursuant to which some 50 inmates were granted release.[30] The New York City Bar Association has expressed concern that a lengthy jail sentence for an AIDS sufferer may be tantamount to a death sentence or a cruel and unusual punishment.[31]

Again, it is worth noting that in conventional sentencing and probation practice, medical considerations have always been appropriate in terms of the sentence or probationary conditions to be imposed.[32] Requiring medical treatment has been upheld as appropriate to probationary status.[33] Many jurisdictions have begun to use electronic monitoring of persons under house arrest or curfew, especially in drunken driving cases.[34] Use of electronic monitoring in AIDS cases does not seem especially problematic, at least where non-violent offenders are concerned. Certainly, given the exorbitant cost of treating AIDS prisoners, the electronic monitoring option becomes attractive.

All of this is to say again that the courts' inquiry into the AIDS field is not so novel or forbidding. Whether it is a burden or a benefit imposed by reason of an AIDS-related status, judges must still inquire whether our accumulated wisdom—as embodied in constitutional, statutory or case law—permits a given arrangement.

At the risk of oversimplifying, I would observe that even the policy considerations as to these essentially straightforward AIDS questions tend to be alike. Those who favor testing, segregating or otherwise isolating persons with AIDS fear the spread of contagion. They cite the legitimate exercise of the police power and specific precedents involving other diseases such as typhoid, TB, hepatitis B, herpes and venereal diseases. Those who oppose testing, segregating and isolation fear unwarranted intrusion into personal matters and cite general principles of equal protection, due process and right to privacy.

On both sides there is some measure of fear and uncertainty. In part, this arises out of a concern over how dependable the current state of medical knowledge is regarding AIDS. Are the three routes of transmission initially described—blood, shared IV needles and sexual fluids—the only ones to be taken into account? There has been a rapid increase in reported heterosexual cases as well as a questioning by at least a few in the scientific community of whether transmission by the three initially described routes is exclusive.[35] How reliable is the testing anyway? The ELISA (Enzyme-Linked ImmunoSorbent Assay) test does *not* show the presence of the virus, but only the presence of HIV antibodies. Some false negatives and false positives occur.[36]

There is also the fear of hidden agendas. Gay groups fear wholesale discrimination. Other groups see the entire visitation as a sort of divine retribution for the sins of some or all of us. Through it all, however, there is weighing and balancing for us to do, typical of the judicial craft. Even in our own backyards, time-tested judicial techniques will be brought to bear. Let us consider the matter of AIDS in the courtroom setting, because here one is tempted to say that AIDS presents new and different problems.

AIDS IN THE COURTROOM

As the problem is defined, familiarities emerge. Are there circumstances under which a defendant with a disease should either not be permitted in a courtroom or should appear only subject to certain modified arrangements? Does it depend on whether the defendant is unruly and likely to pose a physical threat to people present in the courtroom, particularly to law enforcement personnel? *Illinois v. Allen*,[37] involving the defendant who continues to be disruptive after warning, comes to mind.

Again, familiar policy arguments are put forth. On the one hand is the perceived public health/safety factor; on the other, the right of the defendants to a fair trial, due process, equal protection and privacy.

Courts that have addressed this issue have reached different conclusions. A bankruptcy court in Florida, confronted with an apparently non-violent AIDS litigant, said no special precautions were necessary.[38] A trial court in Minnesota held that gloves and leg irons were appropriate for an AIDS prisoner.[39] The Maryland Court of Special Appeals in *Wiggins v. State* decided that the wearing of gloves during a trial did not deny a fair hearing to a defendant with AIDS.[40]

Recently the State of New York Office of Court Administration issued guidelines for the handling of a court appearance involving a person afflicted with infectious disease, particularly AIDS.[41] As the guidelines observe:

> [t]he handling of a case involving a person afflicted with an infectious disease, particularly a case involving an AIDS-infected person, calls for a proper balance between concern for the safety of court personnel who have contact with an afflicted person and the basic right of all people to appear in a courtroom atmosphere of fairness and tranquility that assures due process, as well as freedom from bias and notoriety.

The Office of Court Administration therefore concludes that "[t]o the extent reasonably possible, each case involving a person afflicted with an infectious disease should be treated in a routine manner, no differently from any ordinary judicial proceeding." However, it suggests that certain measures may be taken with judicial approval, after notifying the judge that a litigant is believed to be infected with AIDS. This includes the possibility of seeking the consent of both parties to waive the person's presence at the hearing; reasonable modifications in seating arrangements; special positioning or stationing of court personnel; and the removal or securing of potentially injurious objects. Surgical gloves and surgical masks, as well as restraining bars, may be made readily available, if kept out of view. "[H]owever," the guidelines continue, "surgical gloves may be worn at all times provided they are worn under dress white gloves and with the uniform blouse." Antiseptics and disinfectants should be readily accessible, but maintained out of view. Potentially infected evidence is to be placed in a sealed transparent envelope, not to be removed or circulated except as the judge directs. Unusual incident reports are to be filed in all cases involving a person afflicted with an infectious disease. The guidelines end with a call for continuing educational programs for court personnel regarding AIDS and other infectious diseases.

On the other hand, consider that New York City's Health Commissioner said that key portions of the guidelines, especially the distancing rule and the wearing of surgical gloves, convey "a very inappropriate message" about transmission of the disease.[42] A New York lawyer said that judges informing court personnel about the medical condition of a defendant "may violate the defendant's right to medical confidentiality and may have serious prejudicial effects on the case."[43] She also objected to any judge routinely seeking waiver of the defendant's presence in the courtroom, adding "Defendants have a right to be present in all material aspects of their trial."[44]

Where does that leave us? The answer, of course, is we are where we have always been—faced with hard choices but possessed of a fairly well-developed body of precedent to draw upon.

CONFRONTING CHALLENGES

I believe judges are well up to the task of dealing sensibly with AIDS in the legal setting, on the case-by-case basis that is the hallmark of our common law system. Equally important is the deliberative approach that we will bring to our task, taking care that evidence is solidly grounded and that everyone entitled to be heard in a given situation is in fact heard. If there is room for optimism in a matter as grim as this, there is no reason not be sanguine about our future.

But this is a subject which perhaps ends better with a question than an answer. Here is a problem case which raises most of the issues surrounding AIDS in the administration of justice—fairness, due process, confidentiality and possible stigmatization of a defendant. It was asked recently of participants in a seminar on AIDS that took place in New York City.[45]

As jury selection begins, extra court officers appear, some wearing gloves and some wearing surgical masks. Defense counsel objects. The court requests that the gear be removed. The officers refuse. The judge orders a hearing. Defense counsel objects on the ground that the defendant's medical condition, if any, cannot interfere with courtroom conditions affecting the right to a fair trial.

Defense counsel also informs the court that defendant's medical condition is covered by the medical confidentiality privilege and the attorney/client privilege and any public testimony on his condition will result in objection. Defense counsel then files contempt motions against the court officers and the commissioner of the Department of Corrections. The question is, "Judge, what do you do?" That is a fundamental challenge of AIDS in our courtrooms today.

NOTES

This article is adapted from a speech to the Maryland Judicial Conference, Greenbelt, MD, May 6, 1988.

1. Quoted in Zane, *The Five Ages of the Bench and Bar in England*, in Vanderbilt, ed., STUDYING LAW 42 (New York: Washington Square Publishing Co., 1945).
2. *E.g.* Bourn v. Hinsey, 134 Fla. 404, 183 So. 614 (1938) (granting custody to third party over mother with TB); A.K.P. v. J.A.P., 684 S. W.2d 762 (Tex. Civ. App. 1984) (granting father expanded access to child, despite fact that he and second wife had herpes).
3. *See* Dornette, AIDS and the Law, Section 4.15 (New York: John Wiley and Sons, Inc., 1987).
4. *See* School Board of Nassau Co., Florida v. Arline, 107 S.Ct. 1123 (1987) (terminating employment of teacher due to relapse of TB not permitted simply because of fear of contagion, unless she is found to be otherwise unqualified; contagious disease is "handicap" protected from discrimination by Sec. 504 of Rehabilitation Act of 1973, 29 U.S.C. Section 794).
5. *Ann. Code of Md.*, Health General Article, Section 18–601, 18–602.
6. B.N. v. K.K., 312 Md. 135, 538 A.2d 1175 (1988); *see generally* Annot., *Tort Liability for Infliction of Venereal Disease*, 40 A.L.R. 4th 1089 (1985).
7. State v. Lankford, 102 A. 63 (Del. 1917).
8. *See* LaReau v. Manson, 651 F.2d 96 (2d Cir. 1981) (affirming, with minor modification, lower court's order requiring screening of new inmates for communicable disease); Heitman v. Gabriel, 524 F.Supp. 622 (W.D. Mo. 1981) (prison must screen inmates to prevent spread of disease and provide prompt medical treatment.
9. *Ann. Code of Md.*, Health General Article, Title 4.
10. *Ann. Code of Md.*, Article 27, Section 698.
11. State of Indiana v. Haines, Superior Court of Tippecanoe Co., Ind., Cause No. S-5585 (Opinion filed 2/25/88); *see also* Blackstone, 4 COMMENTARIES ON THE LAWS OF ENGLAND 197 ("year and a day rule").
12. State of Florida v. Sherouse, Cir. Ct. of North Jud. Cir. in and for Orange Co., Fla., Cr. No. 87–7057 (Opinion filed 3/18/88).
13. "As of November 1987, twelve state correctional systems (Alabama, Colorado, Idaho, Iowa, Missouri, Nebraska, Nevada, New Hampshire, Oklahoma, South Dakota, Utah, and West Virginia) have implemented or are planning to implement mass screening programs. The Federal Bureau of Prisons (FBP) reassessed its earlier policy of mass screening and now tests inmates: prior to release; who exhibit clinical indications of the virus; who request to be tested; who are released for community activity purposes; and who have exhibited predatory and promiscuous behavior. In addition, for study purposes, FBP tests a 10 percent sampling of incoming inmates who are retested at 3, 6, 12, and 18 month intervals." *Report of the Presidential Commission on the Human Immunodeficiency Virus Epidemic* (June, 1988), pp. 134–135. *See also* Lewis, *Acquired Immunodeficiency Syndrome: State Legislative Activity*, 258 JAMA, 2410 *et. seq.* (November 6, 1987). "A number of correctional administrators believe that mandatory mass screening legislation will probably pass in some states in 1988." National Institute of Justice, *AIDS in Correctional Facilities: Issues and Options* 191–192 (3d Edition 1987).
14. A class action suit brought by state prisoners in Alabama, apparently the first of its kind, challenges the recently established program of the Alabama Department of Corrections compelling all state prisoners to submit to HIV antibody testing. Harris, et al. v. Thigpen, Commissioner, C.A. 87-V-1109-N (M.D. Ala. N.D. 1987). Suits brought by non-AIDS inmates and others to compel AIDS testing in prisons have been uniformly unsuccessful. *See e.g.* Larocca v. Dalsheim, 467 N.Y.S. 2d 302 (Sup. Ct. Duchess Co. 1983). (no procedural regimen will be judicially mandated given scientific uncertainty of testing concerning AIDS and reluctance to intervene in prison management). For a more recent case, see Jarrett v. Faulkner, 662 F. Supp. 928 (S.D. Ind. 1987) (no constitutional claim implicated in suits by three prisoners seeking screening of all prisoners for AIDS: "The problem of protecting prisoners from AIDS is best left to the legislature and prison administrators," 662 F.Supp. at 929).
15. Chapters 275 and 276 of Maryland Laws of 1988, amending *Ann. Code of Md.*, Health General Article, Section 10–213.
16. *See* Compagnie Francaise v. State Board of Health, 186 U.S. 380 (1902); (statute excluding healthy persons from locality where contagious disease is present is constitutional); *see also* People ex rel Barmore v. Robertson, 302 Ill. 422, 134 N.E. 815 (1922) (typhoid); Ex Parte Shepard, 51 Cal. App. 49, 195 P. 1077 (1921) (suspected syphilis); Kirk v. Wyman, 83 S.C. 372, 65 S.E. 387 (1909) (leprosy).

[17] *See* Section 518 of Pub. L. 100–7 (requiring President on or before 8/31/87 to add HIV infection to list of dangerous diseases set forth in 42 C.F.R. Section 342(b) that make alien inadmissible to U.S. under Immigration and Nationality Act).

[18] *See generally* Lambda Legal Defense and Education Fund, Inc., *Housing and Real Estate Issues*, AIDS LEGAL GUIDE Ch. 8 (Second Edition, 1987).

[19] *See* Jane W. v. John W., 519 N.Y.S.2d 603 (N.Y. Sup. Ct. Kings Co. 1987). (father not precluded from visiting pendente lite with 1-1/2 year old daughter because he had AIDS). *See also* Stewart v. Stewart, 521 N.E.2d 956 (Ct. App. Ind. 4th Dist.). (AIDS seropositivity did not support complete termination of father's visitation rights).

[20] *E.g.* Chalk v. U.S. District Court Central District of California. 832 F.2d 1158 (9th Cir. 1987), 840 F.2d 701 (9th Cir. 1988); (preliminary injunction ordering that teacher with AIDS be permitted to return to classroom); Ray D. v. School District of Desoto County, 666 F.Supp. 1524 (M.D. Fla. 1987); (preliminary injunction granted to seropositive, but asymptomatic children to return to school); Thomas v. Atascadero Unified School District, 662 F.Supp. 376 (C.D. Cal. 1987); (preliminary injunction granted to student with HIV status to return to school, despite his having bitten another student); *see generally* Annot. *AIDS Infection Affecting Right to Attend Public School*, 60 A.L.R. 4th 15 (1988).

[21] The Supreme Court in *Arline, supra* n. 4, expressly did not reach "the questions whether a carrier of a contagious disease such as AIDS could be considered to have a physical impairment, or whether such a person could be considered, solely on the basis of contagiousness, a handicapped person under the [Rehabilitation] Act [of 1973]." 107 S.Ct. at 1128, n.7. The *Report of the Presidential Commission, supra* n. 13, at 121–123, citing lower court cases in the wake of *Arline*, supports the position that Section 504 of the Rehabilitation Act applies to persons who are HIV positive yet asymptomatic.

[22] *E.g.* Maryland administrative regulations provide that "a person may not work in a food service facility in an area and capacity in which there is a likelihood of transmission of disease to patrons or fellow employees." COMAR Section 10.15.03.04(A)(1).

[23] *See* Cordero v. Coughlin, 607 F.Supp. 9 (S.D.N.Y. 1984) (segregation of AIDS sufferers does not violate rights of equal protection, due process, privacy, free expression or free association, nor does it constitute cruel and unusual punishment); *see also* Larocca v. Dalsheim, 467 N.Y.S.2d 302 (Sup. Ct., Duchess Co., 1983) (segregation amounts to reasonable means of preventing transmission of AIDS by forced sex); Judd v. Packard, 669 F.Supp. 741 (D.Md. 1987); (no discrimination on basis of handicap where prisoner who tested seropositive for AIDS was kept in isolation pursuant to medical order); Cf. Doe v. Coughlin, 71 N.Y.2d 48, 518 N.E.2d 536 (1987) (denial of conjugal visits to AIDS prisoner violates no constitutional or statutory rights).

On the other hand, the Federal Bureau of Prisons has adopted a protocol regarding HIV-infected prisoners, consistent with policies of public health services in general, which does not segregate prisons except where predatory or promiscuous behavior is present. *See* U.S. Dept. of Justice: Federal Bureau of Prisons, Program Statement re *Procedures for Handling of HIV Positive Inmates Who Pose Danger to Others*, 28 C.F.R. 541.60–541.68 (effective 10/9/87).

[24] *See* City of New York v. The New St. Mark's Baths, 497 N.Y.S.2d 979 (Sup. Ct. N.Y.: Special Term: Part I: 1986), aff'd 505 N.Y.S.2d 1015 (1986). (granting preliminary injunction shutting down bathhouse based on regulation empowering local health officials to close establishments where "high risk sexual activity" present).

[25] *See* Estelle v. Gamble, 429 U.S. 97 (1976); (deliberate indifference to serious illness of inmate amounts to cruel and unusual punishment); Vinnedge v. Gibbs, 550 F.2d 926 (4th Cir. 1977); (prisoners are entitled to reasonable medical care); Todaro v. Ward, 565 F.2d 48 (2d Cir. 1987); (constitutional claim stated when prison officials intentionally interfere with prescribed medical treatment or deny access to medical care; inadequate resources do not excuse the denial of constitutional rights); Ortiz v. Hoehler, Commissioner of Corrections, et al., Supreme Court, N.Y. County, No. 46492–87 (10/29/87). (Corrections Dept. ordered to immediately provide experimental drug to AIDS prisoner).

[26] Compare Cambridge Mfg. Co. v. Johnson, 160 Md. 248, 153 A. 248 (1931); (workers' compensation not available for TB contracted as result of inhaling dust at work, since not an "accidental injury"); Union Mining Co. v. Blank, 181 Md. 623, 28 A.2d 568 (1942). (workers' compensation due for typhoid fever resulting from consumption of contaminated well water at work; held an "accidental injury").

[27] People v. Camargo, 516 N.Y.S.2d 1004 (Sup. Ct. for Bronx Co. 1986); (dismissing indictment for drug possession for reasons of justice, citing prognosis of three to four months for AIDS defendant to live); People v. Jacobs (N.Y. Sup. Ct., 8/22/86), reported in NEW YORK LAW JOURNAL, August 22, 1986, at

CHAPTER 5

14, col. 2 and in 1 *AIDS Policy and Law* 4 (9/10/86) (dismissing charges of third degree burglary against defendant in advanced stages of AIDS whose confinement to hospital bed posed no threat to public safety).

[28] People v. Gray (Queens Co., N.Y. Sup. Ct. 6/26/86), reported in NEW YORK LAW JOURNAL, June 26, 1986, at 18, col. 3, and in 1 *AIDS Policy and Law* 5 (7/2/86).

[29] Cf. Schneider v. Flowers, 521 N.Y.S.2d 647 (Sup. Ct. for Bronx Co. 1987).

[30] N.Y. TIMES, March 7, 1987, at 1. *Compare* New Jersey v. Wright, 221 N.J. Super. 123, 534 A.2d 31 (1987) (denying sentence reduction to AIDS inmate, citing violence of crime and prior record).

[31] *See* Joint Subcommittee on AIDS in the Criminal Justice System of the Committee on Corrections and the Committee on Criminal Justice Operations and Budget, *AIDS and the Criminal Justice System: A Preliminary Report and Recommendations*, THE RECORD OF THE ASSOCIATION OF THE BAR OF THE CITY OF NEW YORK, Nov. 1987, at 901, 909.

[32] *See generally* National Conference of Commissioners on Uniform State Laws, *Model Sentencing and Corrections Act*, Section 3–108(9) (1979); (ill health can reduce culpability and be a mitigating factor); *see also* Cohen & Gobert, THE LAW OF PROBATION AND PAROLE SECTION 2.16. (McGraw-Hill, Inc. 1983).

[33] Reese v. State, 320 S.W.2d 149 (Ct. Crim. App. Texas 1959).

[34] *See* Schmidt, *Electronic Monitoring: Who Uses It/How Much Does It Cost/Does It Work?* CORRECTIONS TODAY, December, 1987, at 28.

[35] *See generally* Masters, Johnson and Kolodny, CRISIS: HETEROSEXUAL BEHAVIOR IN THE AGE OF AIDS, (New York: Grove Press, 1988). This work, widely reported in the popular press, *see e.g.* NEWSWEEK, *The AIDS Threat: Who's At Risk*, March 14, 1988, at 42–52, provoked considerable criticism, particularly from the scientific community, for alleged deficiencies of method. *See e.g.* NEWSWEEK, *The Storm Over Masters and Johnson*, March 21, 1988, at 78–79. Right or wrong, appropriately scientific or not, Masters et al. still seem to make the relevant point as far as many judges will be concerned: "...(I)f there are lingering uncertainties about the transmission of a deadly infection, shouldn't we be adopting precautions against the worst-case possibility rather than making the most optimistic assumption?" *Masters* et al., at 26.

[36] *See Washington Post* article entitled *Study Faults Labs, Accuracy in Testing for AIDS Infection* in WEEKLY JOURNAL OF MEDICINE AND HEALTH, 10/27/87, at 5.

[37] 397 U.S. 337, reh. den. 398 U.S. 915 (1970); *see also* Fed. Rule Crim. Proc. 43(b)(2).

[38] In re Peacock, 59 B.R. 568 (Bankruptcy. S.D. Fla. 1986).

[39] State of Minnesota v. Santos, St. Louis Co. District Ct., 6th Jud. Dist. Minn. No. 17447 (Opinion filed 1/25/88).

[40] 76 Md. App. 188, 544 A.2d 8 (1988). The Maryland Court of Appeals has granted certiorari in this case, Petition Docket No. 319, September Term, 1988, 314 Md. 95 (1988).

[41] State of New York Office of Court Administration, *Guidelines for the Handling of a Court Appearance Involving a Person Afflicted With An Infectious Disease*, issued 1/88.

[42] N.Y. TIMES, January 23, 1988, at 31.

[43] *Id.*

[44] *Id.*

[45] *See*, N.Y. TIMES, February 7, 1988, at 56.

6

AIDS
in the Courtroom

Donald H. Wallace

AIDS has become an increasingly known fact of life in many American court-rooms. Courtroom personnel have been concerned that a range of situations could place them at risk of becoming infected with the human immunodeficiency virus (HIV) that causes AIDS (Hammett, 1988). Troubling questions arose in trials when judges were faced with criminal defendants infected with the AIDS virus. What precautions, if any, could court personnel (guards, attorneys, prosecutors, judges and others) use? Should defendants be required to use protective devices? Could a defendant's presence at various hearings, even at trial, be waived? Under what circumstances should a trial be delayed when the defendant showed symptoms of HIV infection, either AIDS-related complex (ARC) or full-blown AIDS? What questions can be put to potential jurors about a defendant who is seropositive? Should cases involving defendants with AIDS be dismissed?

The issues raised by the AIDS epidemic in the courtroom were not entirely novel (Messitte, 1989). Related legal precedents, though not explicitly dealing with HIV-infected defendants, have helped guide trial courts in assessing the appropriateness of various measures. Research has confirmed that *no* protective measures are necessary or appropriate for the routine presence of a defendant (or court personnel or visitor) with AIDS. While the extreme steps taken in some courts now seem ridiculous, it is reassuring to note that legal precedent tends to reach the same conclusions that public health experts now endorse. The following discussion

The author would like to express his appreciation to Mark Blumberg, who provided valuable editorial assistance.

examines how courts and policy makers have addressed some of the measures that have been used in American courtrooms.

PRECAUTIONS AND "PROTECTIVE" DEVICES DEMANDED BY COURT PERSONNEL

Defendants believed to be infected with the AIDS virus have been required to wear protective devices in some courtrooms. Certain judges in Broward County, Florida, reportedly required HIV-infected defendants to wear surgical face masks during courtroom proceedings (*In Re Peacock*, 1986). It has also been reported that some judges required asymptomatic infected litigants to wear gloves and full surgical garb in addition to masks (Nichols, 1987). Courts in New York City have kept seropositive defendants in segregated court pens (Joint Subcommittee, 1987) and have required them to wear special disposable plastic handcuffs that identified the infected prisoners (Hevesi, 1988). In *Minnesota v. Santos* (Sinkfield and Houser, 1987), the trial court ordered an infected inmate who had attempted to escape to be shackled during his trial.

Courts also permitted courtroom security personnel to wear gloves (*Wiggins v. Maryland*, 1988), as well as protective masks and winter coats in summer (Simon, 1988) while escorting a criminal defendant believed to have AIDS. In New York, the State Office of Court Administration established guidelines for handling infected inmates that allowed guards to stand up to ten feet behind an infected prisoner. Court personnel were also permitted, under this policy, to wear surgical gloves, if they were covered by dress white gloves (Rosenblatt, 1988). Although these guidelines were considered discretionary with the judge, the president of the State Association for New York Court Officers indicated that court officers would wear gloves and masks at all times, regardless of the judge's instructions (Hevesi, 1988).

An assessment of the legality of requiring a defendant to use these protective devices requires review of the U.S. Supreme Court decision in *Estelle v. Williams* (1976). In that case, the Court held that compelling a defendant to stand trial before a jury while dressed in identifiable prison clothes violates the Fourteenth Amendment. The Court determined that prison garb is likely to have an adverse effect upon the jury, and that compelling an accused person to wear such clothing furthers no essential state policy, other than convenience for the jailers.

The Supreme Court has not always forbidden inherently prejudicial practices used by trial court judges with defendants. In *Illinois v. Allen* (1970), the Court, while recognizing that the sight of shackles and gags on a defendant may have a significant effect on the jury's feelings toward the accused, nonetheless allowed the practice when it was found to be necessary to control a disruptive defendant. In these two cases, the Court suggests that prejudicial practices may be allowed when there is an essential need that goes beyond mere convenience for jail and court personnel.

It is unlikely that such an "essential need" will be found in most cases to justify the use of protective devices for seropositive defendants or court personnel. The Medical Epidemiologist of the AIDS Program for the Centers for Disease Control (CDC) advised a court that no special precautions are recommended for courtroom proceedings where one or more of the participants is infected with HIV (*In Re Peacock*, 1986). It was noted that there is no evidence that this virus can be transmitted through air, food, water, inanimate objects, or casual contact (see also Friedland and Klein, 1987). The CDC official knew of no routine courtroom procedure that could result in the transmission of HIV.

Court personnel often express concern about spitting or biting incidents. However, there have been no documented cases of HIV infection or AIDS traced to human bites or the exchange of saliva (American Bar Association, 1989; Hammett, 1988). HIV appears in such minute quantities in the saliva of infected persons that transmission is highly unlikely (Blumberg, 1989). Human bites cannot transmit the virus unless the perpetrator has blood in his or her mouth, which then comes into contact with the victim's blood. The improbability of infection through biting is underscored by a study of thirty health workers who had been bitten by infected patients. None of these workers became infected (Gostin, 1989).

One U.S. Supreme Court decision that may be supportive of the concerns of court personnel involves the use of innocuous security measures in a criminal trial. In *Holbrook v. Flynn* (1986), a unanimous Court found that the presence of four uniformed and armed state troopers seated in the first row of the spectator section to supplement the customary courtroom security force did not deny a fair trial to six co-defendants. The Justices determined that the four troopers were unlikely to have been taken as a sign of anything other than a normal official concern for the safety and order of the proceedings. The Court expressed the view that even had the jurors been aware that deployment of troopers at trials was not a common practice, the use of the four troopers did not tend to brand the defendants with a mark of guilt. The Court seems willing to approve of obvious yet innocuous security measures to maintain custody of defendants; because of the negligible risk of transmission, the use of obvious measures that are designed to protect court personnel from HIV infection may not be as readily justifiable. In addition, these measures may have prejudicial effects which go beyond security precautions. Protective devices used by defendants or court personnel raise the specter of AIDS, and can lead jurors to consider the defendant's case through prejudices connected with drug abuse or homosexual activity (Schechter, 1988).

The required use of protective devices by HIV-infected defendants in the presence of jurors may well be prejudicial. Public opinion data indicate that a sizeable proportion of the population is prejudiced against seropositive persons.

A substantial minority of individuals questioned favor isolating people with AIDS from the general community and from public places (Blendon and Donelan, 1988). In a survey conducted by the *Los Angeles Times* during July, 1987, a sizeable minority (29 percent—an increase from 15 percent in 1985), also favored tattooing those who are seropositive (Albert, Stewart, and Vermeulen, 1988). Such attitudes reflect a serious disregard for the rights of infected individuals. Blendon and Donelan (1988) suggest that intolerant attitudes may persist even when people understand that there is little risk of becoming infected themselves.

The question of prejudice has arisen in a Maryland case. Recently, the Court of Appeals overturned a conviction because the trial judge allowed security personnel to wear gloves in the presence of jurors while escorting the defendant (*Wiggins v. Maryland*, 1989). The Maryland appellate court considered the likelihood of prejudice arising because of the suggestion that the defendant might be infected with HIV. Even if the jurors had not put much weight on the evidence indicating guilt, the Court of Appeals stated, it was not "far-fetched that the jury, observing the gloves, thought it better, in any event, that Wiggins be withdrawn from public circulation and confined in an institution with others of his ilk" (*Wiggins v. Maryland*, 1989, p. 362).

The Maryland appellate court's dissatisfaction seems directed at the trial judge for proceeding on mere conjecture that the defendant was infected. Thus, the Court of Appeals suggested that a medical opinion that a defendant has AIDS or carries HIV could be treated differently. As an additional prerequisite, a trial judge should indicate in the record the prevailing expert view as to whether a particular protective device is necessary for the well-being of court personnel. Because medical experts view these precautions as unnecessary, this will be a difficult practice to sustain.

ABSENTING DEFENDANT FROM COURT PROCEEDINGS

Some judges have refused to allow people who are believed to be infected with the AIDS virus to stand trial (Nichols, 1987). In Birmingham, Alabama, three county district court judges required seropositive defendants to enter guilty pleas and hear their sentences by telephone ("3 Judges," 1989). In Indiana, a judge gave a defendant with AIDS twenty dollars from his own pocket and requested that deputies put him on a bus for Cleveland (Dornette, 1989:181). The State of New York Office of Court Administration guidelines allow for the possibility of seeking the consent of both the state and the defendant to waive the defendant's presence in the courtroom (Rosenblatt, 1988).

There have also been reports that court personnel in certain jurisdictions are simply refusing to interact with infected defendants. In New York City, incarcerated defendants with AIDS are taken to court in special vans and sometimes have been left in the vans all day without ever being escorted into the courtroom (Hevesi, 1988; Joint Subcommittee, 1987). There have also been instances of court-appointed attorneys in New York City refusing to represent HIV-infected defendants. Defense counsel rarely visit those defendants who are incarcerated in the AIDS unit of Rikers Island Hospital (Joint Subcommittee, 1987).

Suggestions have been made to substitute the use of closed circuit television for the presence of infected defendants in the courtroom (Raburn, 1988). This suggestion would minimize physical contact with infected defendants that is a source of anxiety for some persons working in the criminal justice system.

The constitutionality of closed circuit television must be evaluated in light of concerns expressed by the U.S. Supreme Court in *Iowa v. Coy* (1988). In this case, a defendant's right to confront adverse witnesses was deemed to have been violated by the use of a screen placed in front of him so that a child witness did not have to see the defendant. Despite the fact that the defendant could still see the witness and was physically present in the courtroom, the Supreme Court found this procedure to be a violation of the Sixth Amendment right to confront witnesses. However, this right is not absolute. The Court suggested that an individualized finding that a particular witness needs special protection may override the defendant's right to confrontation. Applying this principle to AIDS-related cases, it would seem that a finding of dangerous behavior which posed a risk of transmission to others would be required to justify the use of closed circuit television. However, the Supreme Court has already authorized, in *Illinois v. Allen* (1970), the outright removal of disruptive defendants from the courtroom, without requiring the use of closed circuit television. Therefore, in the case of violent seropositive defendants, it would not be necessary even to consider the question of infectiousness; the use of closed circuit television could be justified by the assaultive behavior alone.

JURY PREJUDICE TOWARDS DEFENDANT

The defense attorney may desire to explore the effects of the jury's suspicion or knowledge that the defendant is infected with HIV. The possibility of adverse jury verdicts raises concerns about the focus of questions about AIDS that are allowed on voir dire (Albert, et al., 1988).

The primary method of guaranteeing the Sixth Amendment right to a trial by an "impartial" jury is through the voir dire process (i.e., the questioning of prospective jurors). State and federal courts permit the voir dire to be exercised in various ways (Israel and LaFave, 1988). In some jurisdictions the latitude given to defense counsel to explore the attitudes of jurors is quite narrow. However, when extensive voir dire is allowed, it may be advisable for defense attorneys to explore areas of bias which are susceptible to challenges for cause (Albert, et al., 1988). Open-ended questions that require prospective jurors to formulate answers in their own words, rather than closed-ended questions which communicate to jurors the "correct" or "desired" response, have also been recommended for defense attorneys (Albert, et al., 1988).

An example of the closed-ended voir dire question that should be avoided is found in *Wiggins v. Maryland* (1989). The trial judge had informed the jury that "[t]his case has touches of homosexuality in it," and asked:

> "Would that prejudice any member of the jury so that they could not fairly and impartially decide the case based solely on the evidence they are going to hear in this courtroom? If that applies to anybody, come up and tell me about it here" (*Wiggins v. Maryland*, 1989, p. 360).

There was no response from the jurors to this question. The Maryland Court of Appeals found this question to be inadequate for the purpose of determining whether any jurors harbored prejudices that might have arisen from suspicion that the defendant was infected with HIV. The American Bar Association policy regarding AIDS states that the trial court should permit or conduct a full voir dire on the issue of the defendant's HIV status whenever this is a source of concern (American Bar Association, 1989).

DELAYS AND DISMISSALS OF CASES OF HIV-INFECTED DEFENDANTS

A defendant's ability to present a defense may be impaired by lengthy delays before trial. If an infected defendant becomes increasingly ill, or develops symptoms of dementia accompanied by memory problems, the case may become difficult to try (Albert, et al., 1988). Furthermore, because there have been instances in some jurisdictions where defendants dying of AIDS have had charges dismissed, delays may become part of the trial strategy. In one borough of New York City (Bronx), a number of cases involving HIV-infected defendants have been delayed repeatedly in anticipation of the death of the defendant, thus making prosecution unnecessary (Sullivan, 1987). Minor criminal cases involving physically disabled defendants who are not in custody have also been delayed in San Francisco; many never go to trial (Albert, et al., 1988).,

Delays in bringing an infected defendant to trial may result in a violation of the Sixth Amendment right to a speedy trial. In determining whether this right has been violated, flexibility appears to be the governing principle (Israel and LaFave, 1988). The Supreme Court has rejected a specific time limitation in favor of a balancing test that examines the conduct of both the prosecution and the defense (*Barker v. Wingo*, 1972). The absence of a defense demand for a speedy trial can work strongly against a defendant who has counsel, as delay can be a defense tactic (Israel and LaFave, 1988). In *Barker v. Wingo*, a five-year delay did not result in a violation of the defendant's right to a speedy trial. However, a violation was found in *Smith v. Hooey* (1969) when the state failed to respond to the trial demand of a defendant who was serving a federal sentence. The failure of the state in the latter case to respond to the defendant's demand for a speedy trial on pending state charges was not justified by the fact that the state would have been forced to bear the cost of transporting the prisoner. Thus, the expense of transporting seropositive defendants will not excuse states from providing a speedy trial for those individuals who make this demand. Furthermore, state statutes often place more restrictive limitations upon the time allowed to bring a case to trial than those found in U.S. Supreme Court decisions interpreting the Sixth Amendment.

When defendants with AIDS develop symptoms of dementia and accompanying memory problems, the question of their competence to stand trial is raised. According to this standard, competence requires a "sufficient present ability to consult [a] lawyer with a reasonable degree of rational understanding," and "a rational as well as factual understanding of the proceedings" (*Dusky v. U.S.*, 1960, p. 402). It is the first part of the standard where the loss of memory may adversely affect competence to stand trial. However, courts that have addressed claims of memory loss unrelated to AIDS have indicated that amnesia or general memory loss does not by itself render one incompetent to stand trial (Weiner, 1985). In the leading case in this area, *Wilson v. U.S.* (1968), the U.S. Court of Appeals for the District of Columbia Circuit set forth several factors to guide the trial court in deciding whether the amnesia affected the defendant's competence. Among the factors to be considered are the extent to which the evidence could be extrinsically reconstructed in view of the amnesia and the extent to which the government assisted the defendant and his or her counsel in reconstructing the evidence. Thus, loss of memory in defendants with AIDS will not necessarily prevent a trial on grounds of incompetence.

Given the physical and mental deterioration of defendants who are dying of AIDS, the use of limited judicial resources to prosecute such cases may be unwarranted. In a number of jurisdictions, the dismissal of criminal charges is allowed in cases of special and compelling circumstances (American Bar Association, 1989). The fact that AIDS is often fatal would seem to be one of these compelling circumstances.

CONCLUSION

The issues raised by the AIDS epidemic demand some new applications of established legal precedents. Questions such as the extent of voir dire, whether trials should be postponed, and the competence of a defendant to stand trial can all be answered by reference to fairly well established case law and statutes.

Other issues, including whether protective measures should be employed by court personnel, whether these should be required for infected defendants, and the question of the defendant's physical presence in the courtroom during the proceedings, present issues that require a balancing of the defendant's rights and those of court personnel. The courts' duty to protect the safety of court personnel, jurors, and counsel cannot interfere with the defendant's right to a fair trial under the Sixth and Fourteenth Amendments. The Supreme Court has decided cases in which the safety of court personnel has been balanced against a defendant's constitutional rights; though these cases did not involve HIV-infected defendants, the Court has provided ample precedent to guide us in this area.

Guidelines such as those issued by the New York State Office of Court Administration inappropriately equate courtroom violence and HIV infection, thereby rationalizing the use of altered courtroom procedures (Schechter, 1988). As a consequence, measures deemed allowable under *Illinois v. Allen* for violent defendants would, under these guidelines, be permitted for the HIV-infected defendant, without a specific finding that the individual poses a threat of violence. The resolutions recently adopted by the American Bar Association are more appropriate. They discourage courts from employing unusual precautions unless the infected inmate is violent, poses a demonstrated risk of escape, or is seriously ill (American Bar Association, 1989). These ABA guidelines also encourage all criminal justice agencies to develop and implement appropriate policies with respect to AIDS that reduce fear on the part of staff and avoid responses based on misinformation.

The most important fact regarding persons with AIDS and seropositive defendants in the courtroom is that the human immunodeficiency virus is not spread through casual contact. Nor are there reported cases in which HIV has been transmitted as a result of a bite or spitting incident. Therefore, most, if not all, protective measures in the courtroom are unnecessary and unfairly prejudicial to the defendant.

REFERENCES

American Bar Association. (1989). *Policy on AIDS and the criminal justice system*. Chicago, IL: American Bar Association.

Albert, P., Stewart, C., and Vermeulen, M. (1988). Criminal law and procedure. In Albert, P., Graff, L., & Schatz, B. (Eds.), *AIDS practice manual: A legal and educational guide*. (Chapter VI, 2nd ed.). San Francisco, CA: National Gay Rights Advocates and National Lawyers Guild AIDS Network.

Blendon, R. and Donelan, K. (1988). Discrimination against people with AIDS: The public's perspective. *New England Journal of Medicine, 319*, 1022–1026.

Blumberg, M. (1989). Transmission of the AIDS virus through criminal activity. *Criminal Law Bulletin, 25*, (September–October).

Dornette, W. H. L. (1987). *AIDS and the law*. New York: John Wiley and Sons.

Friedland, G. H. and Klein, R. S. (1987). Transmission of the human immunodeficiency virus. *New England Journal of Medicine, 317*, 1125–1135.

Gostin, L. (1989). The politics of AIDS: Compulsory state powers, public health and civil liberties. *Ohio State Law Journal, 49*, 1017–1058.

Hammett, T. (1988). *Precautionary measures and protective equipment: Developing a reasonable response*. Washington, DC: National Institute of Justice, February.

Hevesi, D. (1988). "New York health chief faults new courtroom guidelines on AIDS," *New York Times* (January 23), A-31.

Hevesi, D. (1988). "AIDS in justice system: Searching for fairness," *New York Times* (February 7), A-56.

Israel, J. H., and LaFave, W. R. (1988). *Criminal procedure: Constitutional limitations* (4th Ed.). St. Paul, MN: West Publishing.

Joint Subcommittee. (1987). AIDS and the criminal justice system: A preliminary report and recommendations. *Record of the Association of the Bar of the City of New York, 42,* 901–923.

Messitte, P. J. (1989). AIDS: A judicial perspective. *Judicature, 72,* 205–209.

Nichols, J. (1987). Can judges quarantine courtrooms? *Human Rights, 14,* 20–21, 52.

Raburn, P. (1988). Prisoners with AIDS: The use of electronic processing. *Criminal Law Bulletin, 24,* 213–238.

Rosenblatt, A. (1988). AIDS guidelines. *New York Law Journal* (January 14), 3.

Shechter, M. E. (1988). AIDS: How the disease is being criminalized. *Criminal Justice, 3,* 6–11, 41–42.

Simon, D. (1988). AIDS in prison: A first-hand view. *Criminal Justice, 3,* 10–11.

Sinkfield, R. and Houser, T. (1987). AIDS and the criminal justice system. *Journal of Legal Medicine 10,* 103–125.

Sullivan, R. (1987). "AIDS in prison: Hard questions for justice system," *New York Times* (March 5), B-1.

3 judges excluded AIDS defendants. (1989, January). *AIDS Law and Litigation Reporter, 9.*

CASES

Barker v. Wingo (1972), 407 U.S. 514.

Dusky v. U.S. (1960), 362 U.S. 402.

Estelle v. Williams (1976), 425 U.S. 501.

Holbrook v. Flynn (1986), 106 S. Ct. 1340 (U.S. Sup. Ct.).

Illinois v. Allen (1970), 397 U.S. 337.

In Re Peacock (1986), 59 Bankruptcy Reporter 369 (S. Dis. Florida).

Iowa v. Coy (1988), 108 S. Ct. 2798 (U.S. Sup. Ct.).

Smith v. Hooey (1969), 393 U.S. 374.

Wiggins v. Maryland (1988), 544 A. 2d 8, (Ct. of Special Appeals).

Wiggins v. Maryland (1989), 554 A. 2d 356, (Ct. of Appeals).

Wilson v. U.S. (1968), 391 F. 2d 460 (D.C. Circuit).

SECTION THREE

AIDS
and Rape Survivors

Thousands of persons are sexually assaulted in the United States each year, raising fears that these individuals face a significant risk of becoming infected with HIV. Discussion has centered on whether offenders should be required to undergo HIV testing and, if so, at what point in the criminal justice process. Eleven states currently authorize mandatory HIV testing either for persons charged with or convicted for rape. Relatively little attention has been paid to the realistic risk of HIV transmission in sexual assaults.

The chapters in this section approach this issue from different perspectives. The first reading is an excerpt from the Report of the Presidential Commission on the Human Immunodeficiency Virus Epidemic. The report acknowledged that no data were available on the number of sexual assault survivors who have become infected with HIV, and that the level of risk was also unknown. Nevertheless, the Commission recommended that offenders be required to "submit to an HIV test at the earliest possible juncture in the criminal justice process" (recommendation 9–63) and that the result be disclosed to the survivor.

The second reading by Mark Blumberg, "AIDS: Analyzing a New Dimension In Rape Victimization," takes a somewhat different view. The author notes that mandatory HIV testing of offenders poses legal and practical difficulties and asserts, contrary to the position of the Commission, that most female rape survivors face minimal risk of infection. Blumberg's conclusion is based on data on the proportion of rapists who are likely to be seropositive and the probability of transmitting the virus through a single heterosexual assault. Not a single case of AIDS has been linked to the crime of rape, despite thousands of sexual assaults in the

United States each year. Nonetheless, the author cautions that some rape survivors are likely to be at higher risk (especially those who are anally sodomized or repeatedly raped) and concurs with the Commission that HIV screening and counseling should be offered for all survivors on a voluntary basis.

7

Sexual Assault and HIV Transmission

The Presidential Commission on the Human Immunodeficiency Virus Epidemic

The HIV epidemic has added a new and disturbing specter to the problems of sexual assault victims. Witnesses have testified before the Commission about the increase in the numbers of victims of sexual assaults and their growing concern over the possibility of exposure to the HIV virus as a result.

Victims of sexual assault deserve consideration and must be given attention and support so that they will not be forgotten in the tragedy surrounding the HIV epidemic. The Commission believes that it is important to plan an approach which will take into consideration both the emotional impact of an assault and the possible exposure to HIV. This approach must balance the rights of the victims to be treated with fairness and dignity with the due process rights of the perpetrators.

In 1985, the FBI recorded 87,340 rapes in the United States, or approximately 239 rapes per day. This number greatly underestimates the true scope of rape since it includes only female victims 16 years and older and only instances that were reported to police. Government estimates suggest that for every rape reported to police, three to 10 rapes are not reported, making rape one of the most underreported crimes. In addition, the American Humane Association estimates that 110,878 children were reported as victims of sexual maltreatment in 1984, a 54 percent increase from 1983.

The risk level for HIV transmission to sexual assault victims is as yet unestablished. However, the physical trauma associated with sexual assault increases

---

"Sexual Assault and HIV Transmission" is Section V of Chapter 9: Legal and Ethical Issues of the *Report of the Presidential Commission on the HIV Epidemic*, submitted June 24, 1988.

the vulnerability of body tissue and must be factored into assessments of risk of viral transmission. In addition, the high-risk behavior of many sexual offenders (the term sexual offender refers to the perpetrator of a sexual assault), in turn, increases the risk level of their victims. Children who are sexually molested are potentially at elevated risk of infection if the sexual offender is HIV-infected, since many cases involving children have patterns of repeated contacts over long periods of time. The Surgeon General has stated that all child sexual assault victims must be considered at risk for exposure to HIV.

Studies of sexual offenders and child molesters indicate that many often have large numbers of victims and high rates of recidivism. Therefore, even a small number of infected sexual offenders have the potential for infecting large numbers of people.

Victims or their immediate family members are aware of their risk of exposure to sexually transmitted diseases, including HIV, and are beginning to ask questions about, and exhibit anxiety over, possible exposure to HIV. Many are requesting to be tested. Even in cases where the sexual offender is apprehended, the issues of testing perpetrators who refuse to be tested voluntarily without their consent and state laws governing confidentiality of all HIV test results may obstruct the victim's ability to get information on HIV status. This restriction on access to information can cause the victim anxiety added to the trauma of the crime itself. If HIV status information is available, it should be provided to the victim in the context of a support and counseling system which can help the victim understand the information and make decisions about testing or personal conduct.

The complexity of establishing HIV exposure and subsequent seroconversion requires follow-up over time. The presence of antibodies may take weeks or months to determine, and follow-up of sexual assault victims will be necessary. Unfortunately, success of past programs which included follow-up counseling have not been impressive for a variety of reasons.

Obstacles to Progress

The Commission has identified the following obstacles to assisting victims of sexual assault crimes in light of possible exposure to HIV:

- HIV testing is not currently included in the routine tests for sexually transmitted diseases offered to sexual assault victims. Where testing is requested, it may be expensive. Since routine tests are usually performed as soon as the assault is known, an HIV antibody test of the victim would not reveal exposure as a consequence of the rape.
- There are no published studies available on the incidence of HIV infection as a result of sexual assault or among perpetrators.
- The criminal justice system and most state laws have not addressed fully how to approach the HIV-infected sexual offender.

- Mandatory testing of accused sexual offenders is not widely available.
- In some states, laws prohibit release of information on a sexual offender's HIV status to victims.
- There is no mechanism for reporting cases of HIV-infected sexual offenders once apprehended and subsequent notification of victims.
- Most current counseling programs for victims of violent crimes do not include a component on HIV, and counselors are not currently trained to provide such services.
- Children typically experience problems in coming forward and making adults believe their accounts of molestation.

RECOMMENDATIONS*

Monitoring and Data Collection

9–52 Public health officials, criminal justice systems, and various organizations that deal with victims and perpetrators of sexual abuse must collect and compile data so that the scope of HIV prevalence and transmission associated with sexual assault can be determined.

9–53 The Centers for Disease Control should monitor and publish the number of reported cases where HIV transmission occurs through sexual assault including geographic breakdowns.

9–54 Criminal justice and victim service organizations should collect data on the frequency of sexual assault victims' requests for HIV testing and the frequency of positive results for both victims and perpetrators.

9–55 Support for incidence and prevalence studies of HIV among the sexual assault population, such as those currently funded by the National Institute of Mental Health, should continue with increased funding.

Testing and Counseling

9–56 Programs which provide medical and counseling services to sexual assault victims should make voluntary HIV testing a part of the sexually transmitted disease screening process free of charge and make appropriate counseling about assaults and HIV available by trained staff.

9–57 Training programs for HIV blood test counseling and partner notification techniques should include components focusing on the sexual assault population.

9–58 Federal and state public health authorities should provide service providers and counselors who assist child and adult victims of sexual crime with the most current information and training on HIV, along with in-

---

*We have retained the Commission's numbering of the recommendations for the reader's convenient reference.

formation on the location of confidential and anonymous testing sites and funding and training for the performance of tests.

9–59 Model programs for the long-term follow-up care of victims who do and do not test positive initially should be developed and funded. If a victim converts to positive infection status, there should be counseling and health care intervention provided throughout the various stages of HIV infection. These individuals should receive highest priority for participation in clinical drug trials.

9–60 Social services, law enforcement, mental health, medicine and community-based services should cooperate to provide effective response to child sexual abuse by a well-coordinated, multidisciplinary team which protects and treats victims and their families and deals effectively with perpetrators, incorporating concerns related to HIV exposure.

9–61 Basic curricula/training programs for health, counseling, and criminal justice professionals should include identification of undisclosed sexual trauma, dynamics of victimization, and patterns of trauma and recovery as well as HIV transmission.

9–62 Victim advocacy programs should increase public awareness concerning the potential impact of HIV on victims of crime through education.

Testing of Offenders and the Victims' Access to Results

9–63 Criminal justice authorities, under the guidance of public health officials, should develop a mechanism to order that a sexual offender submit to an HIV test at the earliest possible juncture in the criminal justice process. The results of such a test should remain confidential and be disclosed only to the victims, if they so desire, and public health officials. Where the victim of the sexual assault is a minor, the test results should be disclosed to the minor's parents and/or caretakers.

9–64 The criminal justice system should periodically conduct follow-up testing of convicted offenders who test HIV negative to monitor for possible development of antibodies or other evidence of infection at a later time, with notification of victims as appropriate.

9–65 In the cases where a sexual offender is not apprehended, or where apprehended and there is a possibility of HIV infection even though current test results are negative, victims should at least be offered testing over time and counseling as to the potential for transmitting the disease and as to proper precautions.

9–66 Adult victims who choose not to know of the sexual offender's HIV status should be informed of the possibility of infection and offered testing and counseling so that they can take appropriate precautions.

Criminal Justice System Approaches to Sexual Offenders

9–67 Courts should utilize restitution orders whenever possible so that sexual offenders are held directly accountable for the financial effects of their crimes.

9–68 State laws and federal laws (in the limited areas where federal laws preside over criminal actions, such as on Indian reservations) should include provisions for enhanced sentencing in cases where sexual offenders commit sexual crimes knowing they are HIV-infected.

9–69 Criminal justice facilities should test all convicted sexual offenders for HIV prior to a parole hearing or release from prison. If parole is granted, a positive test result should affect the degree of supervision the sexual offender receives following release.

9–70 If a convicted sexual offender is HIV-infected, this information should be included in the sexual offender's criminal record and used in sentencing hearings for subsequent sexual assault convictions as a basis to further enhance sentencing. The criminal justice system should restrict availability of information on HIV status to those individuals within the criminal justice system with a need to know. Under no circumstances should this information be released as general public information.

9–71 The criminal justice system should develop and implement sound treatment programs for sexual offenders which include an HIV prevention component.

8

AIDS: Analyzing a New Dimension in Rape Victimization

Mark Blumberg

INTRODUCTION

The trauma that results from sexual assault takes a number of forms. Many rape survivors[1] receive serious physical injuries. All confront the long-term psychological consequences that result from being sexually assaulted. In some cases, family members or friends do not provide the kind of emotional support that is desperately required. Finally, the survivor may be faced with the necessity of repeating her harrowing story over and over, both to police officers and in the courtroom.

The crime of rape has always inflicted pain upon the victim. In addition to the violence and the psychological trauma that are associated with this crime, females must be concerned about the possibility of being infected with a sexually transmitted disease (STD). Syphilis, gonorrhea, herpes, genital warts, and other diseases have long been a major source of concern for rape survivors.

The specter of Acquired Immunodeficiency Syndrome (AIDS) adds a frightening new aspect to this offense, which is explored in this article. Because it is impossible to understand the potential impact of AIDS on female[2] rape survivors without a full understanding of the nature of this disease, the discussion begins with a review of the medical and social facts surrounding AIDS. This is followed by an evaluation of the risk of infection that female rape survivors currently face.

This is a substantially revised version of a paper that was presented to the Annual Meeting of the Academy of Criminal Justice Sciences, San Francisco, CA, April 7, 1988. It also appeared in the Fall 1989 edition of *The Justice Professional*.

The author would like to express his gratitude to Dr. Allen Sapp, who reviewed this paper and provided a number of important suggestions which have been incorporated.

By examining both the medical and the criminal justice literature, it is possible to arrive at a crude estimate of the number of female rape survivors who are likely to become infected with the AIDS virus (HIV) through sexual assault. After assessing the actual level of danger that victims confront, the discussion focuses on the implications of these findings for rape survivor counseling. Finally, the issue of HIV testing as it relates to female survivors of sexual assault will be examined.

MEDICAL AND SOCIAL ASPECTS OF AIDS

The first reported case of AIDS in the United States was diagnosed in June 1981 (Morgan and Curran, 1986:459). During the next eight years, more than 100,000 additional cases were reported to the U.S. Public Health Service (Centers for Disease Control, August 1989) and approximately 1.5 million Americans became infected with the human immunodeficiency virus (HIV) (Centers for Disease Control, 12/18/87). By 1991, approximately 270,000 Americans will develop full-blown AIDS and 179,000 people will have died from this disease (Morgan and Curran, 1986:461). At present, there is neither a known cure nor vaccines to prevent AIDS. A comprehensive study released in 1987 indicated that the average life-expectancy for such individuals was only one year (Rothenberg, Woelfel, and Stoneburner, 1987:1298). Since that time, the release of the drug azidothymidine (AZT) has extended this limit for many persons with AIDS.

The number of diagnosed AIDS cases is only the tip of the iceberg. For every person with full-blown AIDS, there are many times that number who have become infected with the AIDS virus (HIV). Although these individuals show no symptoms of illness, they are able to transmit the virus to others through the exchange of body fluids, most notably semen or blood. Because the incubation period for AIDS is so long (between seven and eight years on the average—Lui, Darrow and Rutherford, 6/3/88:1334), it is not yet known what proportions of infected persons will eventually develop AIDS. Current data indicate that 20 to 30 percent of such persons will progress to the final stage (full-blown AIDS) of this disease within five years (Koop, 1986:5). However, a more recent study suggests that 99 percent of seropositive[3] individuals may eventually develop AIDS (Lui et al., 6/3/88:1334). In the absence of a scientific breakthrough, the long-term prognosis for these individuals is not encouraging.

In the United States, AIDS has been transmitted primarily in two ways: through sexual contact and through the sharing of infected needles by IV drug abusers. In fact, over 90 percent of the reported cases have occurred among two high-risk groups (homosexual/bisexual males and intravenous drug users—Centers for Disease Control, 12/26/88). Despite exaggerated claims to the contrary (Masters and Johnson with Kolodny, 1988), there is little evidence to suggest that the epidemic is breaking out of these high-risk groups and spreading into the general population. To date, only 4 percent of the cases have been linked to heterosexual transmission (Centers for Disease Control, 12/26/88:1), and the great majority of these have occurred among the female sex partners of IV drug addicts (Friedland and Klein, 10/29/87:1129).

ASSESSING THE RISK FOR FEMALE RAPE SURVIVORS

Based on interviews with households across the United States, it is estimated that 45,640 cases of rape occurred during 1986 (Bureau of Justice Statistics, 1988).[4] (This number is significantly lower than that reported by the FBI, because the latter includes attempted, as well as completed, rapes. Since attempted rape presents no risk of HIV transmission, that crime has been excluded from the analysis.) What is the risk of HIV infection for female rape survivors? In order to arrive at a definitive determination, answers to three questions are necessary:

1. What are the proportions of various forms of sexual assault that are committed by rapists?
2. What are the risks of HIV infection associated with various forms of sexual activity?
3. What proportion of offenders are infected with HIV?

Because tentative data regarding the latter two issues are now available, it is possible to estimate the risks associated with HIV infection that female rape survivors actually confront.

Researchers concerned with AIDS have devoted a great deal of attention to the risks associated with various sexual practices. Because the impact of this disease has been felt most heavily in the gay community,[5] it is not surprising that much of this research has attempted to learn the reasons why HIV has been transmitted with such efficiency among gay and bisexual males. Despite early theories about secondary precipitating factors that focused on practices such as the use of "poppers" (amyl or butyl nitrate inhalants) by gay men (Altman, 1987:33), epidemiological research (Winkelstein, Lyman, Padian et al., 1987) strongly suggests that two major risk-factors are associated with the rapid transmission of HIV in the gay community: the practice of anal intercourse[6] and a large number of sex partners. Other sexual practices, such as oral sex, while theoretically risky, have not been demonstrated to be associated with an increased risk of HIV transmission (Winkelstein, Asher, et al., 1986).

In order to assess thoroughly the risk of AIDS transmission for female rape survivors, empirical data regarding the number of females who are anally sodomized should be considered. Unfortunately, these data are not available. However, anecdotal evidence based on conversations with a number of counselors at rape crisis centers suggests that the proportion is rather small. It is therefore plausible to assume that the great majority of rape survivors suffer forced vaginal intercourse.[7] Assuming that this is the case, the following questions must be addressed:

1. What is the risk of a female becoming infected with HIV from a single act of forced vaginal intercourse?
2. What proportion of offenders are likely to be infected with the AIDS virus?

The answers to both questions give us cause to be hopeful that very few, if any, females are likely to become infected with this lethal disease as a result of forced vaginal intercourse.

In an important study reported in the *Journal of the American Medical Association*, Hearst and Hullen (4/22/88:2429) note that the likelihood of a female seroconverting[8] (i.e., becoming infected with the AIDS virus) as a result of a single act of unprotected heterosexual intercourse with an infected male is about 1 in 500.[9] From a biological standpoint, whether the act is consensual or forced, the risk of HIV infection appears to be similar.[10] As Friedland and Klein (1987) have noted,

> The available data indicate that HIV transmission is not highly efficient in a single or a few exposures, unless one receives a very large inoculum. The widespread dissemination of HIV is more likely the result of multiple repeated exposures over time. (1133).

Clearly, the risk of HIV transmission associated with a single heterosexual encounter is small.[11] In fact, the medical literature reports that the majority of heterosexual persons who have engaged in vaginal intercourse on a continuing basis with infected partners have not become seropositive (Friedland and Klein, 1987).[12]

As previously noted, the number of rape survivors who can be expected to become infected with HIV is a function not only of the risks inherent in a single assault, but also of the proportion of offenders who are seropositive. Unfortunately, this information is not currently available. However, as more states begin to require HIV testing for convicted rapists, we should gain some notion as to the prevalence of the AIDS virus among offenders. In the interim, it is possible to estimate the proportion of infected offenders using other epidemiological data that are available.

Since a blood test to detect antibodies to the AIDS virus (HIV) became available in 1985, it has been possible to test various populations to determine their rate of seroprevalence.[13] Hospital patients, blood donors, patient at clinics that treat sexually transmitted diseases (STDs), newborn infants, applicants for the armed forces and others have been tested for HIV. The Centers for Disease Control (12/18/87) have summarized the rates of seroprevalence for each of these groups. The critical question for our purposes is: Which group is most likely to approximate the rate of HIV infection to be found among rapists who assault females?

It is the view of this researcher that the most appropriate epidemiological data are the results of HIV tests given to all prospective recruits for the armed forces since October 1985. As noted earlier, gay males and IV drug users account for approximately 90 percent of the AIDS cases in the U.S. However, it is unlikely that gay males are, to any large extent, participants in sexual assaults directed at females. IV drug addicts are also unlikely to engage in this type of behavior. Generally, alcohol is far more likely to be a precipitating factor in the crime of rape than heroin addiction. Because the military attempts to exclude members of both these risk groups from its ranks, the process of self-selection[14] probably results in far fewer gay males and IV drug users being included in this data set than would be the case for an epidemiological survey that examined the entire general population.[15]

The military data are appropriate for other reasons as well. Because applicants for the armed services are largely male, at an age when they are likely to be sexually active, and disproportionately drawn from minority backgrounds, they share some of the same demographic characteristics as apprehended[16] rape offenders, who are most often young males and, disproportionately, members of minority groups.

The findings from tests that have been given to prospective military recruits over a two year period indicate that 1.5 out of 1,000 (0.15%) are infected with HIV (Centers for Disease Control, 12/18/87:5). Data from the National Crime Survey (NCS) indicate that 45,640 completed rape victimizations were committed in the U.S. during 1986 (Bureau of Justice Statistics, 1988). Assuming that 0.15% of these offenders are seropositive[17] (the rate found among military recruits), then 68 of these individuals have the capacity to infect their victims with HIV through forced vaginal intercourse. However, because the risk of infection from a single heterosexual exposure is slight (0.02%), we would expect less than one case of AIDS resulting from this type of sexual assault per annum in the U.S. among female rape survivors.

For victims of anal sodomy, the odds of infection are greater. The medical literature notes that the receptive partner in anal-genital intercourse has a substantial risk of exposure to the AIDS virus (Friedland and Klein, 1987). Therefore, individuals assaulted in this manner are likely to be alarmed by the possibility of contracting a life-threatening disease. Although it is true that the risk of infection is greater for these females, the odds are still against it. This is true for two reasons:

1. HIV has a low rate of infectivity, compared to other sexually transmitted diseases. With the exception of a contaminated blood transfusion, the virus is not likely to be transmitted by a single exposure of any kind. (Friedland and Klein, 1987:1133).

2. The rate of HIV infection outside the two groups at high risk for AIDS (gay males and IV drug users) is still exceedingly low in the U.S. As previously noted, few persons in these risk groups are likely to be involved in sexual assaults directed at females.

Our confidence in this conclusion is buttressed by the fact that not a single case has come to light in which a female rape survivor has become infected as a result of a sexual assault,[18] despite the fact that thousands of cases of forcible rape occur each year in the United States.

PSYCHOLOGICAL IMPACT ON THE VICTIM

Counselors have noted a growing concern among female survivors of rape that they have been infected with AIDS (Burnley, 1988). Indeed, the psychological trauma that generally accompanies a rape is exacerbated by a number of factors unique to this disease. For one thing, females who have been sexually assaulted in the 1980s are concerned about their long-term physical well-being because AIDS is almost always fatal. Second, there is the fear of passing the virus along to her spouse or lover. Although a single heterosexual encounter is highly unlikely to transmit HIV, the risks in an ongoing heterosexual relationship with an infected person are considerable (Hearst and Hullen, 4/22/88). The survivor must also be concerned that if she becomes pregnant, she may pass the virus on to her child. Third, it is not easy for a survivor to find out whether she has been infected. Not only is the incubation period for AIDS relatively long, but antibodies to the virus do not develop for at least 6 to 12 weeks after infection (Petricciani and Epstein, 1988:236) and in some cases, considerably longer. Finally, persons infected with this virus face enormous social stigma and discrimination.

Medical personnel and those who counsel survivors of sexual assault can assure the female that it is highly improbable that she has contracted AIDS. Survivors must be provided with accurate information that makes clear just how remote the risk is and informed that to date, not a single female has become infected as a result of being sexually assaulted in the U.S. This knowledge should go a long way toward comforting the victim. Rape survivors must be able to put the threat of AIDS in perspective and deal with the other tragic consequences of the assault. Proper counseling after the assault will enable the survivors to reassure their spouse or lovers that they, too, have little reason to be concerned about contracting HIV.

HIV TESTING OF OFFENDERS AND/OR VICTIMS

Much of the discussion surrounding the issue of AIDS as it relates to rape survivors has been focused on whether suspects should be required to undergo mandatory HIV testing in order that the victim may be informed of the results. Understandably, survivors of sexual assault are concerned that they may have been infected with an incurable disease that will eventually kill them. Unfortunately, both from a legal and a practical standpoint, a number of difficulties limit the utility of the HIV blood test as a means of providing reassurance to the victim.

The biggest hurdle is legal: only six states have passed statutes[19] requiring that convicted rapists be tested for HIV. In many states, the law does not allow for the testing of offenders without their consent. Recently, a Connecticut court ruled that a rape survivor is not entitled to have the suspect tested for HIV (Hevesi, 1988:30). Some jurisdictions permit the offender to be tested, but because of confidentiality provisions in the statute, the court is forbidden to share the results with the victim.

Statutes that mandate HIV testing of convicted rape offenders are ineffective for other reasons. For one thing, most rapists are never apprehended. In cases where the perpetrator is taken into custody, a great deal of time may pass before a conviction is obtained. To compensate for this delay, the President's Commission on the Human Immunodeficiency Virus Epidemic recommended in Standard 9–63 that offenders be tested "at the earliest possible juncture in the criminal justice process" (*National Organization For Victim Assistance Newsletter*, 1988:7). In fact, two states (Texas and Colorado) now allow HIV testing to be conducted prior to conviction (Hevesi, 1988:30). However, under our system of justice, suspects are presumed innocent until proven guilty. Mandatory testing prior to conviction raises a number of legal and constitutional questions.

Problems also arise due to the nature of the HIV blood test. As previously noted, the current test detects not the AIDS virus, but antibodies to HIV. Therefore, the test will result in a false negative outcome until the body has had an opportunity to develop antibodies to the virus. Consequently, negative test outcomes obtained before seroconversion takes place will not be conclusive. Until a more effective method of screening is available, courts that allow the HIV blood test before conviction should repeat testing at periodic intervals for at least one year, in order to be confident that the results are indeed reliable.

Given all the problems that surround mandatory testing of offenders, the best way for victims to ascertain whether they have contracted HIV is to get themselves tested. However, the same problem of repeated tests over many months to get a conclusive result applies. Victim compensation programs should reimburse rape survivors for medical expenses incurred in learning their HIV antibody status. Although the current ELISA test is relatively inexpensive,[20] costs can mount as the procedure is repeated.

It is imperative that counselors at rape crisis centers and medical personnel put the threat of AIDS infection in perspective. Although the risk of HIV infection may be negligible, rape survivors may wish to undergo testing for their own peace of mind. Rape survivors should be counseled that even if the offender were seropositive (which is highly unlikely), they are not automatically destined to contract HIV.

CONCLUSION

The AIDS epidemic has brought death and despair to many people in the U.S. Despite the suffering wrought by this disease, it appears that most rape survivors currently have little reason to despair. However, the risk is likely to be greater for those individuals who are anally sodomized and for those who are repeatedly raped. Although the risk for female survivors of sexual assault would increase were the virus to break out of the current high-risk groups into the general population, there is no evidence that this is occurring. Since the beginning of the AIDS epidemic in the U.S., heterosexual transmission has been confined primarily to the female sex partners of IV drug users (Friedland and Klein, 1987). Even if the rate of sero-prevalence were to increase among the heterosexual population, the fact that AIDS has a low rate of infectivity (i.e., a single exposure is unlikely to transmit the virus) means that even then, few rape survivors would be likely to become infected with HIV.

REFERENCES

Altman, Dennis. (1987). *AIDS in the mind of America*. Anchor Books, Garden City, N.Y.
Bureau of Justice Statistics. (1988). *Criminal victimization in the U.S., 1986*, U.S. Department of Justice (August).
Burnley, Jane Nady. (1988). "HIV commission" considers sex offenders, victims, in report; Recommendations on victims offered. *National Organization For Victim Assistance Newsletter*. Vol. 12, No. 5 (May), pp. 5–7.
Centers for Disease Control. (1987). Human immunodeficiency virus infection in the United States: A review of current knowledge. *Morbidity and Mortality Weekly Report*. Vol. 36, No. 49 (December 18), pp. 1–20.
———. (1988). *AIDS weekly surveillance report*. Atlanta, GA (December 26).
———. (1989). HIV/AIDS surveillance. U.S. Department of Health and Human Services, August.
Flanagan, Timothy and Ed McGarrell. (1986). *Sourcebook of criminal justice statistics*. Michael J. Hindelang Research Center, Albany, NY.
Friedland, Gerald H. and Robert S. Klein. (1987). Transmission of the human immunodeficiency virus. *New England Journal of Medicine*. Vol. 317, No. 18 (Oct. 29), pp. 1125–1135.
Grady, Denise. (1988). Just how does AIDS spread? *Newsweek*. March 21, pp. 60–61.
Hearst, Norman and Stephen B. Hulley. (1988). Preventing the heterosexual spread of AIDS: Are we giving our patients the best advice? *Journal of the American Medical Association*. Vol. 259, No. 16 (April 22–29), pp. 2428–2432.
Hevesi, Dennis. (1988). AIDS test for suspect splits experts. *New York Times*. October 16, p. 30.
Koop, C. Everett. (1986). *From the Surgeon General*. U.S. Public Health Service, Washington, D.C.
Lui, Kung-Jong, William W. Darrow and George W. Rutherford, III. (1988). A model-based estimate of the mean incubation period for AIDS in homosexual men. *Science*. Vol. 240 (June 3), pp. 1333–1335.
Masters, William and Virginia Johnson with Robert Kolodny. (1988). *Crisis: Heterosexual behavior in the age of AIDS*. Grove Press.
Morgan, W. Meade and James W. Curran. (1986). Acquired immunodeficiency syndrome: Current and future trends. *Public Health Reports*. Vol. 101, No. 5 (Sept.–Oct.), pp. 459–465.
Newsweek. (1987). No escaping the dilemma of kids in school. September 9, p. 52.

Petricciani, John C. and Jay S. Epstein. (1988). The effects of the AIDS epidemic on the safety of the nation's blood supply. *Public Health Reports.* Vol. 103, No. 3 (May–June), pp. 236–241.

Rothenberg, Richard, Mary Woelfel, Rand Stoneburner, et al. (1987). Survival with the acquired immunodeficiency syndrome. *The New England Journal of Medicine.* Vol. 317, No. 21 (Nov. 19), pp. 1297–1302.

Stengel, Richard. (1987). The changing face of AIDS: More and more victims are black or Hispanic. *Time.* August 17, pp. 12–14.

Time. (1987) Testing dilemma: Washington prepares a controversial new policy to fight AIDS. June 8, pp. 70–72.

Winkelstein, Warren Jr., David M. Lyman, Nancy Padian, et al. (1987). Sexual practices and risk of infection by the human immunodeficiency virus: The San Francisco men's health study. *Journal of the American Medical Association.* Vol. 257, No. 3 (Jan. 16), pp. 321–325.

———, M. Ascher, et al. (1986). Minimal risk of AIDS-associated retrovirus infection by oral-genital contact. *Journal of the American Medical Association.* Vol. 255, p. 1703.

———, Michael Samuel, Nancy S. Padian, et al. (1987). The San Francisco men's health study: Reduction in human immunodeficiency virus transmission among homosexual/bisexual men, 1982/1986. *American Journal of Public Health.* Vol. 76, No. 9 (June), pp. 685–689.

NOTES

[1] This article is concerned solely with the issue of AIDS as it pertains to female victims of rape. Much of the analysis undertaken is inapplicable to male victims of sexual assault.

[2] The term "female" is used throughout this paper because some rape victims are adults and others are juveniles. As a consequence, using the term "women" to refer to victims would not be inclusive.

[3] The term "seropositive" refers to individuals whose blood test indicates that they have been exposed to the human immunodeficiency virus (HIV), regardless of whether they exhibit symptoms of illness.

[4] The National Crime Survey (NCS) is based on data collected by interviews with persons 12 years of age or older in a stratified random sample of households across the nation. It excludes assaults that victims may not define as rape, e.g., date rapes. This fact has little bearing on the analysis undertaken in this study.

[5] Epidemiological surveys indicate that almost half the gay men in San Francisco are infected with HIV (Winkelstein, Samuel, Padian, et al., 1987:685).

[6] In order for a person to become seropositive, it is necessary for infected blood or semen to enter the bloodstream. Anal intercourse is extremely risky because of the danger that it may result in tears to tissue, thus facilitating the entry of infected semen into the bloodstream.

[7] The statistical analysis in this paper is based on the assumption that each of these rape victimizations involved forced vaginal intercourse. However, our findings must be tempered by the fact that there is a small, but unknown, number of victims who are anally sodomized. For these individuals, the risk of HIV infection is undoubtedly greater.

[8] In medical parlance, this term refers to a positive HIV antibody status on the part of a person who was not previously infected with the virus.

[9] These researchers note that this probability is a group average and that the likelihood of any particular individual becoming infected as a result of a single encounter with a seropositive partner may vary (Hearst and Hullen, 1988:2429).

[10] Because of the violence that often accompanies rape, the President's Commission on the Human Immunodeficiency Virus Epidemic suggests that female victims of sexual assault may be at high risk of HIV infection. (*National Organization For Victim Assistance Newsletter*, 1988:6). This fear is based on the belief that the violent nature of this crime makes it more probable that it will result in the

tearing of vaginal tissue. If this were to happen, it would allow the AIDS virus to enter the bloodstream. However, the lack of any cases to date of HIV infection among female rape victims would appear to belie this concern.

[11] Likewise, research on medical personnel indicates that the risk of becoming infected with HIV as a result of a single needle-stick is also minimal (less than 1 percent—Friedland and Klein, 1987:1127).

[12] However, the risk of infection does increase dramatically for persons who have an ongoing sexual relationship with an infected partner. Even if the likelihood of viral transmission for a single encounter is only 1 in 500, there is still a significant risk to the noninfected partner as the number of contacts increases.

[13] The term "seroprevalence" refers to the proportion of individuals in a specific group who are seropositive.

[14] There is little doubt that some members of these groups still attempt to enlist in the military. This is not problematic for our analysis because it is likely that some rapists have also engaged in bisexual activities or shared needles during intravenous drug use. Unfortunately, there are no data on the proportion of high-risk individuals in either population. By utilizing the armed forces' epidemiological data, we make the assumption (plausible, we hope) that these proportions are comparable.

[15] Epidemiological data that examine the rate of HIV seroprevalence among a random sample of persons in the general population are not yet available.

[16] The F.B.I. reports that 46 percent of the persons arrested for rape in 1984 were black and that 43 percent were below the age of 25 (Flanagan and McGarrell:1986).

[17] Clearly, not all these assaults were committed by different offenders. However, this fact has no bearing on the statistical analysis being undertaken.

[18] In telephone conversations with the National Institute of Justice AIDS Clearinghouse on Jan. 5, 1989 and the Centers for Disease Control (CDC) on Jan. 12, 1989, staff persons indicated that no cases of AIDS among female rape victims had come to their attention. Although neither agency has compiled data that specifically address this issue, the spokesperson at CDC noted that the agency had undertaken an analysis of cases in which females with no known risk factor (i.e., no history of IV drug use, no record of receiving a possibly contaminated blood transfusion, and no identifiable sex partner in a high-risk group) had become infected with AIDS. The agency did not find any of these cases attributable to sexual assault.

[19] Illinois, Oregon, Washington, Indiana, Georgia, and South Carolina (Hevesi, 1988:30).

[20] In many communities, the test is available at certain sites without charge. Otherwise, the cost is generally less than fifty dollars.

SECTION FOUR

Female Prostitution
and AIDS

The AIDS crisis has focused public attention on whether or not female prostitutes are a source of viral transmission to the general population. Many questions have been asked, such as:

1. What proportion of female prostitutes is infected with HIV?
2. Are these individuals transmitting the virus to their male customers?
3. Should prostitutes undergo mandatory HIV testing?
4. Should infected women who are convicted of prostitution be placed in quarantine or face heavy criminal penalties?

The first reading, "Prostitutes and AIDS: Public Policy Issues" by Cohen, Alexander, and Wofsy examines many of these issues. Their research shows that the rate of seroprevalence among female prostitutes varies substantially across communities; and that this rate relates strongly to how many IVDUs in the region are infected with HIV. Almost all cases of AIDS or seropositivity among female prostitutes are the result of IVDU. Many prostitutes take precautionary measures to avoid exposure to the virus, and there is little evidence that prostitutes are transmitting HIV to their customers in significant numbers. Thus the authors believe that mandatory HIV screening or heavy criminal penalties for infected persons convicted of prostitution are measures that are not likely to be effective in controlling the epidemic.

The authors conclude by recommending that additional resources be directed to three key areas:

1. educational efforts that teach prostitutes how to reduce their risk of exposure
2. expanded drug treatment facilities
3. programs that help prostitutes find work in other occupations

The second reading in this section is the policy statement of the American Civil Liberties Union (ACLU) on the mandatory testing of female prostitutes. Despite the fact that certain jurisdictions have adopted mandatory testing for arrested or convicted prostitutes, the ACLU policy statement offers a number of compelling arguments that suggest this course of action is unwise. The policy statement notes that the likelihood of viral transmission as a result of a single heterosexual contact is minimal and that there is no evidence that female prostitutes are infecting their male customers with HIV.

Notice that public concern has focused almost exclusively on the threat that female prostitutes pose for men. There has been little attention directed to the dangers that these sex workers may face as a result of contact with their clients.

Likewise, there has been little discussion of the possible dangers posed by male prostitution. To date, no systematic research has been conducted that examines the sexual practices of male prostitutes and relatively little public discussion has taken place regarding the risks of viral transmission that may be associated with male prostitution.

Future research must be directed at assessing the role, if any, of these sex workers in the transmission of the AIDS virus. Among the questions needing to be answered:

1. Do male prostitutes (and their clients) view themselves as gay? If they do not, they are unlikely to be reached by the intensive "safer sex" educational campaign that has been undertaken by the gay community.
2. Are these individuals and their customers avoiding the types of sexual acts that have a high risk of spreading the AIDS virus (i.e., unprotected anal sex)?
3. Are the customers of male prostitutes mostly gay men or are they likely to have heterosexual relationships with women?
4. To what extent are these sex workers transmitting the virus to their customers?

9

Prostitutes and AIDS: Public Policy Issues

Judith Cohen, Priscilla Alexander, and Constance Wofsy

INTRODUCTION

Prostitutes have often been held responsible for the spread of AIDS into the heterosexual population in this country, and various policy recommendations and enforcement procedures have been based on this assumption about transmission.[1] However, these actions have often been taken without direct evidence of such transmission and without assessing the feasibility or effects of the proposed programs. This article will review available evidence concerning prostitution as a means of human immunodeficiency virus (HIV) transmission and will discuss policy recommendations and their effects.

What are current rates of HIV infection among prostitutes in the U.S.? What kinds of prostitutes and what geographic areas show increased rates of infection? What is known about how infected sex workers acquired HIV? What is the likelihood that an HIV-infected prostitute will transmit the virus to customers? Finally, how have past policies and sexually transmitted disease (STD) prevention programs directed at prostitutes affected STD rates in the areas of enforcement?

For the purpose of this discussion, prostitution will be defined as the exchange of sexual services for money. Furthermore, although male, transsexual, and transvestite prostitution clearly occur and carry the risk of HIV transmission, information on these kinds of prostitution is nearly nonexistent; therefore, we will stay within the conventional boundaries of female prostitution. The most familiar

Reprinted from *AIDS and Public Policy Journal*, Vol. 3, No. 2 (1988), pp. 16–22. University Publishing Group, Inc., Frederick, MD 21701.

form of prostitution, and the one that draws the most attention, is street prostitution, although this form represents only about 20 percent of all prostitution in this country. Primarily an urban phenomenon, it is also the form most likely to be associated with intravenous drug use. The remaining 80 percent of prostitution is fairly evenly spread among four other types of sex work, namely, massage parlors, bar and cafe prostitution, outcall and escort services, and, in some areas, brothels. These latter categories of prostitution are much less likely to involve intravenous drug abuse.[2]

WHAT IS THE PREVALENCE OF HIV INFECTION AMONG PROSTITUTES IN THE U.S.?

The Centers for Disease Control (CDC) does not record the number of prostitutes who have been diagnosed with AIDS. If HIV seroprevalence studies of prostitutes and/or IVDUs are accurate, diagnosed prostitutes would be counted under the intravenous drug user category, which includes 1,485 female cases reported since 1981 and 470 female cases reported since January 1, 1987.[3]

Several studies have attempted to determine HIV seroprevalence among U.S. prostitutes and IVDUs. These investigations suggest that seropositivity among prostitutes is more common on the east coast than on the west coast or in the center of the country, a difference that directly correlates with HIV seroprevalence among IVDUs in each area. In New York City, 50 to 60 percent of IVDUs are seropositive,[4] while the prevalence of infection among San Francisco IVDUs is currently about 10 percent.[5,6] The results of U.S. seroprevalence studies involving prostitutes are summarized in Table 1.

Los Angeles: As part of the CDC Collaborative Study, Gill *et al.* found that eight of 184 (4.3 percent) women in the Sybil Brand Correctional Institute tested positive.[1] All those with evidence of infection had histories of intravenous drug use.

Orange County: Tom Prendergast of the Orange County Department of Public Health tested 400 women in jail in October 1985; 10 (2.5 percent) tested positive.[7] Virtually all of these women were street prostitutes, many of whom had a history of intravenous drug use.

San Francisco: In another aspect of the CDC Collaborative Study, Cohen and Wofsy of Project AWARE found nine seropositive women among 146 tested (6.2 percent).[1] Study participants were recruited by word of mouth, street outreach, and publicity in mainstream, gay, feminist, and heterosexual sex-related media. All of those who tested positive had a history of intravenous drug use. In a related study of more than 500 sexually active non-prostitutes, a similar percentage were found to be antibody positive, although the association with intravenous drug use was not as strong in this group.[8]

Seattle: In 1985, Handsfield *et al.* reported the results of mandatory testing of 92 women arrested for prostitution in Seattle. Using only an enzyme-linked

TABLE 1
Seroprevalence Studies Involving U.S. Prostitutes

	Prostitution			Prostitutes	
Location	Site	Type	No.	Antibody Positive (%)	% IVDU
Los Angeles	Jail	Street	184	8 (4.3)	
Orange County, CA	Jail	Street	400	10 (2.5)	
San Francisco	Mixed	Mixed	146	9 (6.2)	
Seattle	Jail	Street	92	0 (0)	
	STD Clinic	Mixed	33	0 (0)	
Las Vegas	STD Clinic	Brothel	34	0 (0)	
Colorado Springs	STD Clinic	Street	71	1 (1.4)	
Atlanta	Mixed	Mixed	92	1 (1.1)	
Miami	Middle-Class	Escort	25	0 (0)	0
	Inner-City	Street	90	37 (41)	70
	Jail	Street	252	47 (18.7)	
	AIDS Clinic	Unknown	25	10 (40)	
New Jersey	Methadone Clinic	Street	56	32 (57.1)	100
New York City	Jail	Street	95	25 (25)	50*

*Estimated

immunosorbent assay, five (5.5 percent) were seropositive, but retesting with a more sensitive Western blot test failed to confirm infection in any of these women.[9] A 1986 study of 35 women, all but two of them prostitutes, found that none were seropositive.[10] Participants were recruited from an STD clinic.

Las Vegas: Participating in the CDC Collaborative Study, Ravenholt and co-workers at the Clark County Health Department found that none of 34 women working in legal brothels tested positive for antibody to HIV.[1] Women who use or have used intravenous drugs are barred from such employment in Nevada.

Colorado Springs: Potterat and Phillips found that one of 71 women (1.4 percent) recruited from an STD clinic was HIV antibody positive.[1]

Atlanta: Sykes and Leonard recruited 92 women through word of mouth, street outreach teams, and publicity in the mainstream, gay, feminist, and hetero-sexual sex-related media and found one woman (1.1 percent) who was antibody positive.[1] Because of the broad recruitment effort, this study represents the range of prostitutes in the Atlanta area.

Miami: Witte and Bigler discovered that 47 of 252 women (18.7 percent) tested in jail were seropositive.[1] All of the women either had histories of intravenous drug use or were in long-term sexual relationships with men who were IVDUs. Again, these figures estimate the rate for street prostitutes, because all study subjects were tested in jail.

At the Third International Conference on AIDS, Fischl and colleagues reported a study in which they compared the incidence of HIV infection among 90 prostitutes from inner-city south Florida and 25 women who worked for escort services in a middle-class urban area.[11] Of the working class prostitutes, all of whom had arrest records and had worked on the street, 41 percent were HIV antibody positive. Of the 63 who used intravenous drugs, 46 percent were antibody positive, while 30 percent of the non-drug users were infected. All of the women who worked for escort services were seronegative for HIV. Fischl *et al.* concluded that the major risk factors for HIV infection were intravenous drug use and multiple heterosexual partners who came from an area with a high incidence of AIDS. On the other hand, the investigators pointed out that the escort service prostitutes had had greater numbers of sex partners than the street prostitutes, suggesting that number of sex partners was not, per se, a significant factor.[11]

In an earlier, widely publicized study, 10 of 25 prostitutes (40 percent) visiting an HIV screening clinic were seropositive; eight of the 10 admitted intravenous drug use.[12] Because the study was conducted at a screening clinic, the results are not reflective of the prostitute population in Miami.

New Jersey: French *et al.* found that 32 of 56 women (57.1 percent) tested at a methadone maintenance program had antibodies to HIV.[1] Participants in methadone maintenance programs must have a recent history of serious intravenous drug addiction to be eligible for treatment. No studies of off-street prostitutes in the Jersey City area have yet been reported, although the investigators are in the process of broadening the scope of their original study to include women who do not use intravenous drugs.

New York: In various voluntary testing studies conducted in Manhattan, approximately half of all intravenous drug-using women were seropositive.[4] In a companion study involving interviews with 95 women jailed for prostitution, half had histories of intravenous drug use.[4] Des Jarlais assumed that half of the drug-using women would be seropositive, although he did not test any of the women because of the invasive nature of the test. This estimate implies that up to a quarter of street prostitutes in New York may have been infected through intravenous drug use.

IS THERE EVIDENCE OF TRANSMISSION FROM PROSTITUTES TO THEIR CLIENTS?

In the U.S., as of October 19, 1987, 218 of the men and 710 of the women diagnosed with AIDS had heterosexual contact with a person with AIDS or at risk for AIDS as their only known risk factor. Thus, 2 percent of the 43,533 cases diagnosed since June 1981 have been attributed to heterosexual contact. An additional 990 men and 333 women (3 percent) are heterosexuals with no identified risk factors.[3] This last group includes a few men who claim contact with prostitutes as their only risk factor. In terms of contact tracing, there have been no documented cases of men becoming infected through contact with a specific prostitute.

If prostitutes were effectively transmitting the AIDS virus to their customers, there would be far more cases of white, heterosexual males diagnosed with AIDS than are reflected in the current statistics, because some IVDUs in New York, including some prostitutes, have been infected with the AIDS virus since at least 1978. The average street prostitute sees 1,500 customers a year. If even 5 percent of female street prostitutes in New York City were infected by 1981, the year AIDS was first identified, even moderately efficient transmission of the virus from prostitutes to clients would have resulted in the diagnosis of at least 100,000 white, heterosexual men by now.

One justification for prohibiting prostitution is the alleged correlation of prostitution with the prevalence of STDs in this country. Legal and regulated prostitution systems often require that prostitutes have regular check-ups for STDs. Such programs have had minimal effect on the STD rates, however, because infection rates are low. When the "Chicken Ranch," in Fayette County, Texas, was closed, the number of local gonorrhea cases rose substantially.[13] This is consistent with the rise in venereal disease following the closing of brothels from 1917 to 1920.[14] The U.S. Public Health Service estimates that only about 5 percent of the venereal disease in this country is related to prostitution.[15]

There has been only one U.S. study of seropositivity among clients of prostitutes. Wallace tested 300 volunteer clients of prostitutes in New York City.[16] Six (2 percent) tested positive; of these, two admitted to other risk behavior, and two did not return for test results and further interviewing. A possible connection between prostitution and heterosexual males who deny known risk factors was reported by Redfield et al.[17] They found that of 10 heterosexual men at Walter Reed Army Hospital who had been diagnosed with AIDS or ARC, eight reported sexual contact with prostitutes in various parts of the world, one had had multiple female sex partners in New York City, and one had had sex with a woman from Haiti. The authors concluded that these cases were evidence of female-to-male transmission. After the publication of Redfield's article, the journal published a series of letters disputing his findings. Some of the correspondents argued that Redfield's reliance on self-reported behavior was unacceptable because of the serious negative consequences of admitting to homosexual activity and/or intravenous drug use in the military.[17]

WHAT ARE PROSTITUTES DOING TO PREVENT AIDS?

Prostitutes have always been cautious about STDs, out of concern for their own health and their ability to work. Therefore, they have tended to be more responsible about preventing transmission in order to protect themselves as well as others. They learn to recognize symptoms in men and refuse to have sexual contact with those they believe to be infected. Most have made use of whatever preventive measures were available, including soap and water, condoms, and spermicides. This caution has increased with their awareness of AIDS. Brothels and outcall services, which in the past discouraged women from demanding condoms, and charged more for unprotected sex, are now changing to an all-condom policy.

Des Jarlais in New York[4] and studies conducted in all seven test cities participating in the CDC Collaborative Study[1] found that most of the prostitutes interviewed used condoms. In the CDC study, more than 80 percent of the prostitutes reported at least occasional use of condoms.[8] However, they were more likely to use condoms with clients (78 percent) than with their husbands or boyfriends (16 percent), a fact that increased their risk of exposure, especially if their regular partners were IVDUs. Four percent, none of whom were antibody positive, used condoms with all sexual contacts.

At Project AWARE in San Francisco, more than two-thirds of 134 female sex workers reported condom use at initial interviews in 1985 and 1986.[1] In follow-up interviews in 1987, we found that more than 80 percent were using condoms, suggesting that education about condom use in the Bay Area has been effective. In contrast, 525 sexually active non-prostitutes in the companion study were much less likely to use condoms, although condom use had also increased among this group.[8]

In general, sex workers who are seriously addicted and need the income to pay for illegal drugs are less likely to protect themselves. It is this relatively small group of prostitutes (approximately 5 to 10 percent of prostitutes) who are the key subjects of public health policy concerns.

POLICY RECOMMENDATIONS

There are two basic approaches to limiting the potential for virus spread through prostitution. The first, which we endorse, is to develop educational strategies for reaching prostitutes, giving them accurate information about the most effective ways of preventing transmission and supporting them in their efforts to utilize these measures consistently. The other, which we believe would be ineffective, involves testing all prostitutes, and particularly those who have been arrested, for evidence of HIV infection and increasing the charge and/or the penalty for convicted prostitutes who are antibody positive.

The U.S. expends a great deal of money to arrest, prosecute, and incarcerate women and men involved in prostitution. In 1985, there were 113,800 prostitution arrests, with an average cost of nearly $2,000 per arrest, including court and jail costs, for an estimated total of $227,600,000 per year.[19] Intense enforcement of the prostitution laws since the 1920s has not eliminated, or even reduced, the amount of prostitution in this country. Furthermore, the closing of brothels and other prostitution businesses has often been accompanied by a local rise, not a reduction, in the incidence of STDs.[14] Removing experienced prostitutes from the street, or barring them from working in licensed massage parlors and escort services, has encouraged the continual recruitment of younger, inexperienced sex workers who are more likely to engage in practices that put them at risk for HIV and other sexually transmitted infections.

We are concerned about both the feasibility and the effects of the U.S. Public Health Service's recommendation that prostitutes be "routinely" tested for evidence of HIV infection and that "local or state jurisdictions should adopt procedures to assure that" prostitutes who are antibody positive "discontinue the practice of prostitution."[20] Routine or mandatory testing of prostitutes, with or without increased enforcement of the law or longer jail sentences, will be far less effective in preventing the transmission of the AIDS virus than education programs to help prostitutes avoid high-risk activities. For one thing, it is not feasible to test or to identify, arrest, and incarcerate *all* infected prostitutes. Moreover, such policies would create the illusion that all infected prostitutes had been identified and isolated. Customers, believing that prostitutes who had not been tested and/or jailed were not infected, would be less likely to adopt safer sex practices. Moreover, mandatory testing of convicted prostitutes, and particularly increased penalties, would discourage those who had not been arrested from voluntary testing or participation in preventive education programs.

Instead of increasing funding for existing police programs, jurisdictions would do better to allocate these funds for outreach programs to help working prostitutes reduce, if not eliminate, the risk of HIV transmission to themselves and their sex partners. Outreach programs have already been implemented in California, New Jersey, and New York, at a much lower cost per staff member. Such programs would most effectively be staffed by people who have worked as prostitutes, preferably at the same level as those they are trying to reach. Educational programs should be conducted in language appropriate to the target group and should contain explicit information about condoms and spermicides and about strategies for convincing customers and, more importantly, regular partners, to use condoms. Participation in such education programs should be voluntary; that is, it should not be a condition of probation or in any way be perceived as "punishment." It would, however, be appropriate for outreach workers to meet with prostitutes in jail, as long as it is on a voluntary basis. Jails and other facilities (e.g., hospitals) are also effective distribution points for condoms and spermicides on the day of release.

Since the primary risk of HIV transmission to prostitutes is intravenous drug use, it is important that educational programs include explicit information on cleaning needles and other drug paraphernalia to avoid sharing contaminated injection equipment. Several community outreach programs in San Francisco have been distributing one-ounce bottles of bleach, with great effect.

On-going prevention education is best accomplished through a combination of street outreach programs, involving teams of community health workers who have worked as prostitutes, and voluntary support groups and/or workshops led by the same workers, where risk-reduction information can be given in more detail and participants can discuss their problems and use role-play and other strategies to improve their negotiation skills. In cities where there are several "stroll districts," the use of vans could be a cost-effective means of bringing the support group to street prostitutes.

Resources should also be allocated for programs to help prostitutes who want to pursue other occupations. Certainly, any prostitute who finds that she is infected should immediately qualify for financial assistance so that she can stop working as a prostitute. Women should be eligible for immediate entry into drug or alcohol treatment programs, where necessary, and should have access to job retraining that would enable them to earn a reasonable living. Given the seriousness of AIDS, it would be even more effective to make such programs available to all prostitutes who want them, irrespective of HIV antibody status.

Transition programs should be staffed by ex-prostitutes. In addition to the vocational counseling and job development training usually included in transition programs involving other ex-offenders, programs for prostitutes must deal with sexual stigmatization and the sexual and physical abuse tolerated in prohibited prostitution. In addition, ex-prostitutes provide unique role models for women who have felt they had no alternative to working as prostitutes.

There are not nearly enough drug and alcohol treatment slots available in this country for all those at risk for AIDS who would like help in dealing with their addictions. As bad as the situation is for men, it is worse for women, because there are few drug treatment slots for women, especially in residential programs and particularly for women with children.[21]

CONCLUSION

Prostitutes in the U.S. are not and have not been significant vectors for the transmission of STDs, including AIDS. To the extent that prostitutes have become infected, their rate of infection has parallelled the rate among IVDUs in their communities, and almost all prostitutes who have tested positive in seroprevalence studies or who have been diagnosed with AIDS have had a history of intravenous drug use. Evidence to date suggests that HIV is much more likely to be transmitted to prostitutes than from them.

We recommend that local, state, and federal funds be allocated for education programs directed at prostitutes—particularly street prostitutes, because of the higher prevalence of intravenous drug use at that level of the industry. We also recommend that funding be provided for increased drug and alcohol treatment slots for women, especially women with children, and for job training and other transitional programs for those who no longer want to work as prostitutes. On the other hand, there is ample evidence that mandatory testing of prostitutes and increased penalties for those who test positive would be ineffective, costly, and have dangerous consequences for the further spread of HIV.

NOTES

1   Centers for Disease Control, "Antibody to Human Immunodeficiency Virus in Female Prostitutes," *Morbidity and Mortality Weekly Report* 36 (1987): 157–61.
2   For a more complete discussion of prostitution, see Priscilla Alexander, "Prostitution: A Difficult Issue for Feminists," in *Sex Work: Writings by Women in the Sex Industry* (F. Delacoste and P. Alexander, eds.), Pittsburgh, Cleis Press, 1987, pp. 184–214.
3   Centers for Disease Control, "AIDS Weekly Surveillance Report," October 19, 1987.
4   Personal communications with Don Des Jarlais, New York State Division of Substance Abuse Services, in 1985, 1986, and 1988.
5   R. E. Chaisson, A. R. Moss, R. Onishi, *et al.*, "Human Immunodeficiency Virus Infection in Heterosexual Intravenous Drug Users in San Francisco," *American Journal of Public Health* 77 (1987): 169–72.
6   R. E. Chaisson, D. Osmond, A. R. Moss, *et al.*, "HIV, Bleach, and Needle Sharing," *Lancet* 1 (June 20, 1987): 1430.
7   The Orange County, CA, study was conducted among jailed prostitutes. The women were invited, but not required, to participate, although "voluntary" participation in an institutional setting, particularly in a prison, is questionable. Personal communication with Roseann Lowery, Orange County Department of Public Health, October 25, 1985.
8   J. B. Cohen, L. Poole, L. Hauer, *et al.*, "Risk of HIV Infection in Sex Industry Women: AIDS Research and Education in a Unique Population in the San Francisco Bay Area," presented at the Annual Meeting of the American Public Health Association, New Orleans, LA, October 21, 1987.
9   The initial results of the first Seattle study were reported in a number of publications, including the December 6, 1985, *Morbidity and Mortality Weekly Report*. Although Hunter Handsfield, Director of Public Health, has been urged to publish the results of the more accurate Western blot test, he has declined to do so. Personal communications with Debra Boyer, Seattle AIDS Advisory Task Force (September 27, 1986, and November 8, 1986) and Ann Collier (December 20, 1986).
10 Personal communication with Ann Collier, December 30, 1986.
11 M. A. Fischl, G. M. Dickinson, S. Flanagan, and M. A. Fletcher, "Human Immunodeficiency Virus (HIV) Among Female Prostitutes in South Florida," presented at the Third International Conference on AIDS, Washington, DC, 1987.
12 *Los Angeles Times*, December 8, 1985. The women were voluntarily tested in an HIV screening clinic.
13 G. L. Conrad, G. S. Kleris, B. Rush, and W. W. Darrow, "Sexually Transmitted Diseases Among Prostitutes and Other Sexual Offenders," *Sexually Transmitted Diseases* (1981): 241–4.
14 A. M. Brandt, "A Historical Perspective," in *AIDS and the Law: A Guide for the Public* (H. L. Dalton and S. Burris, eds.), New Haven, Yale University Press, 1987, p. 40. See also A. M. Brandt, *No Magic Bullet: A Social History of Venereal Disease in the United States Since 1880*, New York, Oxford University Press, 1985.
15 J. S. Millard, *Basic Statistics on Venereal Disease Problems in the United States*, Centers for Disease Control, 1971.
16 Personal communication between Joyce Wallace, MD, and Priscilla Alexander at the Third International Conference on AIDS, Washington, DC. Beth Bergman, in an article slated for publication later this year, writes that both Rand Stoneburner, director of the AIDS Surveillance Unit in New York City, and a social worker who interviews people with AIDS report difficulty in determining risk factors using the standard questionnaire. Both professionals said that when they departed from the questionnaire to discuss risk factors with patients, most of those who had initially reported contact with prostitutes admitted to homosexual activity or intravenous drug use and needle sharing. Bergman also reports that 154 of 156 cases of heterosexually acquired AIDS in New York City were females. See also K. G. Castro, A. R. Lifson, C. R. White, *et al.*, "Investigations of AIDS Patients With No Previously Identified Risk Factors," *Journal of the American Medical Association* 259 (1988): 1338–42.
17 R. R. Redfield, P. D. Markham, S. Z. Salahuddin, *et al.*, "Heterosexually Acquired HTLV-III/LAV Disease (AIDS-Related Complex and AIDS): Epidemiologic Evidence for Female-to-Male Transmission," *Journal of the American Medical Association* 254 (1985): 2094–6. Letters disagreeing with Redfield's conclusions were published in *Journal of the American Medical Association* 255 (1986): 1702–6.
18 J. B. Cohen, L. Hauer, L. Poole, *et al.*, "Risk Factors for HIV Infection in 500 Sexually Active Women in San Francisco," presented at the Annual Meeting of the American Public Health Association, New Orleans, LA, October 18–22, 1987.

[19] J. Pearl, "The Highest Paying Customers: America's Cities and the Costs of Prostitution Control," *Hastings Law Journal* 38 (1987): 769–800.

[20] Centers for Disease Control, "Public Health Service Guidelines for Counseling and Antibody Testing to Prevent HIV Infection and AIDS," *Morbidity and Mortality Weekly Report* 36 (1987): 509–15. See especially page 512, where the Public Health Service describes prostitutes, whether or not they are IVDUs, as a high-risk group, and page 513, where they recommend routine testing of prostitutes and coercive measures to ensure that antibody-positive sex workers discontinue prostitution, without consideration of whether the individual prostitute's practices involve any risk of virus transmission.

[21] *A Federal Response to a Hidden Epidemic: Alcohol and Other Drug Problems Among Women*, New York, National Council on Alcoholism, 1984.

10

Mandatory HIV Testing of Female Prostitutes: Policy Statement of the American Civil Liberties Union

AIDS and Civil Liberties Project, American Civil Liberties Union Foundation

ISSUES

A common policy proposal is the mandatory HIV antibody testing of persons arrested for, or convicted of, prostitution. Such proposals generally provide that a positive test result becomes part of the individual's court record and forms the basis for a longer sentence in the event of a second arrest.

The ACLU opposes laws which single out any group for mandatory testing, but also supports widespread voluntary access to HIV testing as an important part of counseling and educational efforts. Laws in Georgia and in Newark, NJ which compel HIV testing of persons convicted of prostitution are currently being challenged by ACLU affiliates in those places.

BEST ARGUMENTS AGAINST TESTING OF PROSTITUTES

1. Proposals to single out prostitutes for mandatory testing rest upon the belief that female prostitutes are spreading the human immunodeficiency virus into the "general population."* In fact, there are virtually no reliably reported cases of

---

*The discussion in this memorandum has been based on the model of a female prostitute and a male customer. Most of the policy discussion centers on that situation, and virtually all arrests of prostitutes who would be subject to forced testing or longer sentences are of female prostitutes. Male prostitutes may present different issues. We know of no studies, however, which reliably report activities of male prostitutes (e.g., frequency of oral sex) or analyze male prostitution as creating a heightened risk of HIV transmission to gay and bisexual men. To our knowledge, no health department has developed special outreach or HIV counseling programs for male prostitutes.

customers contracting the AIDS virus from prostitutes. (See generally, Decker, "Prostitution as a Public Health Issue," in *AIDS and the Law*, (Dalton, ed.) 81, 83–84 (1987).) If prostitutes were actively spreading the AIDS virus, one would expect many more cases by now of both AIDS and HIV infection attributable to that source. As Decker writes:

> By conservative estimate, there are more than 200,000 female professional prostitutes in the United States, who engage in more than 300 million acts of prostitution annually. Yet, of the thousands of AIDS cases in the United States, not a single one has been definitively traced to prostitution. *Id.* at 84–5.

For example, in New York City as of January 1988, there have been only six cases of AIDS attributed to female-to-male transmission, out of more than 11,000 cases to date of AIDS in men. The data published by the city do not indicate whether any of these six cases involved prostitutes. (New York City Department of Health, "AIDS Surveillance Update: Jan. 27, 1988.") Further, the number of cases in the female-to-male transmission category is increasing at a slower rate than the number in other categories. If transmission by prostitutes was happening in New York City, one would expect exactly the opposite.

A 1987 study of 2,700 men who attended a Baltimore clinic for treatment of sexually transmitted diseases found no statistically significant association between a history of sex with prostitutes and positive HIV antibody status. (Quinn et al., "Human Immunodeficiency Virus Infection Among Patients Attending Clinics for Sexually Transmitted Diseases," 318 *New England Journal of Medicine* (Jan. 28, 1988) 197, 199.) Seropositivity was significantly associated with homosexual or bisexual activity, use of intravenous drugs and a history of other STDs such as syphilis, but not with prostitutes.

Early reports which suggested prostitutes as a source of infection came largely from HIV-positive servicemen who were interviewed by military doctors and asked how they had been exposed to HIV. When a group of those servicemen were re-interviewed by civilian public health investigators, virtually all of the men who previously had claimed contact with prostitutes reported either same-sex contact or drug use. (See Potterat et al., "Lying to Military Physicians About Risk Factors for HIV Infections," 257 *Journal of American Medical Association* 1727 (Apr. 3, 1987). This experience confirms the suspicion that military personnel are more likely to claim having seen prostitutes (which is not punishable) than to acknowledge to military health officials that they have engaged in drug use or homosexual acts, which can form the basis for expulsion from the military.

In short, the epidemiological data do not support the belief that prostitutes are spreading the AIDS virus.

2. There are several reasons why the activities of female prostitutes pose less risk of transmission than is often thought. When one analyzes the *activities* involved in prostitute-customer encounters, rather than focusing on the *group*, the risk can be put in better perspective:

(a) First, the frequency with which female-to-male transmission occurs during vaginal intercourse "remains controversial." (Friedland and Klein, "Transmission of the Human Immunodeficiency Virus," 317 *New England Journal of Medicine* (Oct. 29, 1987) 1125, 1129.) Female-to-male transmission is believed to be less efficient than male-to-female transmission because there is usually no female-to-male passage of bodily fluids into the bloodstream. (Guinan and Hardy, "Epidemiology of AIDS in Women in the United States," 257 *Journal of American Medical Association* (Apr. 17, 1987) 2039.)

(b) Second, most sex with prostitutes is *not* vaginal intercourse, but rather oral sex. (Decker, *supra* at 85.) As many as 75% of patrons seek only oral sex. The risk of transmission of the virus from a female prostitute during oral sex with a male customer is minute. (*Id.*)

(c) Third, virtually all prostitute-customer encounters are single episodes. The likelihood of female-to-male transmission in a single encounter is extremely remote. By comparison, the likelihood of male-to-female transmission in a single episode of vaginal intercourse has been estimated at one in 1,000. ("Study Sees Low AIDS Risk for Women in Single Episode," *New York Times*, June 6, 1987.)

(d) However small the risk of female-to-male transmission in a single episode, it is further reduced by the use of condoms. The Centers for Disease Control, which is studying HIV infection among prostitutes, found that more than 80% of prostitutes reported at least some condom use by partners, although regular boyfriends (rather than customers) were much less likely to have used condoms. (U.S. Centers for Disease Control, "Antibody to Human Immunodeficiency Virus in Female Prostitutes," 257 *Journal of American Medical Association* (Apr. 17, 1987) 2011; hereafter, "CDC Study." See also Mann et al., "Condom Use and HIV Infection Among Prostitutes in Zaire," 316 *New England Journal of Medicine* (1987) 354; Miller, "Prostitutes Make Appeal for AIDS Prevention," *New York Times*, Oct. 5, 1986; and Decker, *supra* at 84.) Used properly, condoms are considered to be highly effective in preventing transmission of HIV. (Reitmeijer et al., "Condoms as Physical and Chemical Barriers Against Human Immunodeficiency Virus," 259 *Journal of American Medical Association* (Mar. 25, 1988) 1851.)

(e) Lastly, the data do not indicate that prostitutes themselves are likely to harbor the AIDS virus, and thus be capable under any circumstances of transmitting it, unless they exhibit the same risk factors as other women: either being users of intravenous drugs or being the sex partners of men who use drugs. The Centers for Disease Control study found that HIV infection among prostitutes correlated almost entirely with those two factors. (CDC Study, *supra*.) In Nevada, none of the women working as legal prostitutes reported intravenous drug use and none were positive for the

AIDS virus. ("Infection Not Reported Among Legal Prostitutes," *AIDS Policy and Law*, Nov. 18, 1987 at 2–3.) Similar results were found among prostitutes in West Germany. (Smith and Smith, "Lack of HIV Infection and Condom Use in Licensed Prostitutes," 5 *The Lancet* (Dec. 13, 1986) 1392.) Because drug use is the critical risk factor, prevention strategies should be focused on that issue and directed to women—whether they work as prostitutes or not—who use drugs or are the partners of male drug users.

In sum, proponents of mandatory testing of prostitutes generally fail to make the distinction between what is illegal and what is unsafe. The momentum for testing prostitutes is driven in part by the fact that criminal laws against prostitution exist almost everywhere, thus making it easier to carry out street sweeps and to impose mandatory testing, even if these actions are misdirected from a public health perspective. Politicians, faced in many places with pressure to propose some mandatory testing, may select the most politically powerless and socially stigmatized group and require that they be tested, even though the epidemiological evidence does not support it. The result is bad public health policy.

3. The absence of medical support for compulsory testing of prostitutes means that such testing programs may not survive legal scrutiny. Such a policy may be invalid under any of several theories:

(a) A law which singles out one group for forced testing and/or longer incarceration without data indicating that the group is more likely to be spreading the virus is constitutionally suspect on equal protection grounds. When policies originate from "an evil eye and an unequal hand," rather than from the medical evidence, they may be stricken as unconstitutional. In *Jew Ho v. Williamson*, 103 F. 10, 22 (N.D. Cal. 1900), the federal court ruled unconstitutional the quarantine of the Chinese community in San Francisco when the evidence of outbreak of bubonic plague was slight and the law operated exclusively against that neighborhood.

(b) Standards for searches and seizures under the Fourth Amendment may require probable cause to believe that an individual is infected before an involuntary blood test is permitted; the fact that the person belongs to a certain group (in which infection has not been shown to be probable) would be an insufficient basis for ordering a test. (See Decker, *supra*, at 86–7; compare, *Railway Labor Executives' Association v. Burnley*, F.2d (9th Cir. 1988); *National Treasury Employees Union v. Von Raab*, 808 F.2d. 1057 (5th Cir. 1987), cert. granted 56 U.S.L.W. 3582 (Mar. 1, 1988) (drug testing cases).) Similarly, the due process clause of the Fifth and Fourteenth Amendments may require a stronger and more individualized basis for involuntary testing than mere membership in a group. (See e.g., *Capua v. Plainfield*, 643 F. Supp. 1507 (D.N.J. 1986) (drug testing case).)

(c) Subjecting prostitutes—and not others—to longer sentences without regard to whether the behavior in fact does create a significant risk of transmission amounts to a punishment based on status. In *Robinson v. California*, 370 U.S. 660 (1962), the Supreme Court distinguished between criminal laws prohibiting drug use behavior and those outlawing the status of being an addict. Statutes which impose testing or punishment based on the status of working as a prostitute could be found unconstitutional on this basis.

(d) Most of the proposals concerning prostitutes are open to challenge on the grounds of sex discrimination. They are almost always aimed at testing only the female prostitute, implicitly functioning as protection for the actions of male customers, who may be as likely or more likely (depending on their use of drugs) than the woman to be HIV-positive. Laws which punish only the female prostitute may be stricken as discrimination against women.

4. As a practical matter, targeting prostitutes for forced testing simply won't work as a prevention strategy. If there is any group which will be driven underground by such a policy, it is prostitutes. The history of law enforcement is replete with examples of crackdowns which had no effect except to move this activity from one neighborhood to another. Indeed, there is no evidence that criminalization has decreased prostitution. "The laws and general strategy of repression seem to have had remarkably little effect on the prostitution economy." (Hobson, *Uneasy Virtue: The Politics of Prostitution and the American Reform Tradition* (1988) at 156.) Like episodic police crackdowns, forced HIV testing will produce dislocation and further secrecy, but not less activity.

Moreover, the public health efforts geared to educating prostitutes about the need to avoid high-risk activities and about the risks to the prostitutes themselves will fail if public health agents are perceived as police. In New York City, the health department has been involved for several years in a voluntary STD education and testing program which has done outreach to prostitutes by making regular, informal visits to brothels. (Testimony of New York City Department of Health before the New York State Bar Association, Hearings on Prostitution (Oct. 30, 1985).) If police round-ups were initiated, this much more effective program would be destroyed. Similar programs, although unpublicized, may exist in other cities.

5. Finally, we should learn from history. The results of efforts to control sexually transmitted diseases (STDs) during the two world wars are instructive. During World War I, concern about syphilis and the infection rates among American soldiers reached new heights. The military embarked on a massive campaign to eradicate STDs, with an emphasis on curtailing prostitution. More than 20,000 prostitutes were quarantined during the war under federally funded programs, and thousands more were incarcerated by local initiative. Despite these efforts, rates of disease remained high. "The war tested the basic assumptions of the social

hygiene movement: rigorous education promoting sexual abstinence coupled with vigorous repression of prostitution would conquer the problem. The war revealed the limits of this approach." (Brandt, "The Syphilis Epidemic and Its Relation to AIDS," 239 *Science* (Jan. 22, 1988) 375, 377.) By contrast, in World War II, the military opted for a program which provided free condoms to soldiers and de-emphasized the suppression of prostitution. "The military program, which combined a massive education program, prophylaxis, and rapid treatment without punitive measures proved to be highly successful as rates of disease were controlled." (*Id.* at 379.) The work of Professor Brandt, an historian who teaches at the Harvard Medical School, demonstrates that police action against prostitutes has never been effective in the past to decrease STDs. There is no reason to believe that it will be any more effective now in fighting AIDS.

ALTERNATIVE PROPOSALS

The ACLU has long supported decriminalization of prostitution, which we believe would substantially decrease the problems of furtiveness and auxiliary criminal activity associated with prostitution.

An alternative to mandatory testing of prostitutes would be a program of required AIDS counseling (which would offer testing on a voluntary basis) for anyone working as a prostitute or for anyone convicted of prostitution, similar to the programs required for persons convicted of driving while intoxicated. As with any counseling and testing program, confidentiality and anti-discrimination protections should be enforced.

REFERENCES (In order of discussion in article)

Decker, "Prostitution as a Public Health Issue." In *AIDS and the Law* (Dalton, ed.) (1987), 81.
Brandt, "The Syphilis Epidemic and Its Relation to AIDS," 239 *Science* (Jan. 22, 1988), 375.
  Brandt, *No Magic Bullet: A Social History of Venereal Disease in the United States Since 1880* (1985).
On the history of prostitution: Hobson, *Uneasy Virtue: The Politics of Prostitution and the American Reform Tradition* (1988); Rosen, *The Lost Sisterhood: Prostitution in America, 1900–1918* (1982); and Walkowitz, *Prostitution and Victorian Society: Women, Class and the State* (1980).
U.S. Centers for Disease Control, "Antibody to Human Immunodeficiency Virus in Female Prostitutes," 257 *Journal of American Medical Association* (Apr. 17, 1987), 2011.
"HIV Antibody Prevalence in Female Prostitutes," 36 *Morbidity and Mortality Weekly Report* (Dec. 18, 1987), 34.
Potterat et al., "Lying to Military Physicians About Risk Factors for HIV Infections," 257 *Journal of American Medical Association* (Apr. 3, 1987), 1727.
Mann et al., "Condom Use and HIV Infection Among Prostitutes in Zaire," 316 *New England Journal of Medicine* (1987), 354.

Smith and Smith, "Lack of HIV Infection and Condom Use in Licensed Prostitutes," 5 *The Lancet* (Dec. 13, 1986), 1392.

Quinn et al., "Human Immunodeficiency Virus Infection Among Patients Attending Clinics for Sexually Transmitted Diseases," 318 *New England Journal of Medicine* (Jan. 28, 1988), 197.

Miller, "Prostitutes Make Appeal for AIDS Prevention," *New York Times*, Oct. 5, 1986.

Guinan and Hardy, "Epidemiology of AIDS in Women in the United States," 257 *Journal of American Medical Association* (Apr. 17, 1987), 2039.

Reitmeijer et al., "Condoms as Physical and Chemical Barriers Against Human Immunodeficiency Virus," 259 *Journal of American Medical Association* (Mar. 25, 1988), 1851.

SECTION FIVE

AIDS
and the Law

Harmonious ow can the state modify the behavior of persons infected with the AIDS virus? One method is to provide education to encourage individuals to reduce high-risk behavior.

Another method is to restrain or coerce these individuals. For example, the state could enact a criminal statute that proscribes certain conduct. It could impose a quarantine of certain infected individuals. These strategies may be broad-based (restrict the liberty of a whole class of individuals) or narrow (i.e., applied only to specific individuals whose conduct jeopardizes the well-being of others).

The first article in Section V, "AIDS and the Criminal Law" by Martha A. Field and Kathleen M. Sullivan examines possible uses of the criminal law in the battle to control AIDS. The authors discuss what can happen when criminal laws are applied to AIDS carriers. Because of the limitations of laws already in effect, Field and Sullivan suggest that states could avoid these problems by enacting AIDS-specific statutes. However, they believe that it would be unwise to do so because the deterrent impact of these statutes would be outweighed by the costs that such an approach would entail. They believe that these statutes would jeopardize sexual privacy, be used to harass gay men, and discourage infected persons from cooperating with public health officials.

Twenty states already have enacted AIDS-specific statutes that make it a crime to knowingly or intentionally expose another person to HIV (Gostin, 1989:1622–23). Most of these laws are aimed at sexual conduct but some also encompass needlesharing and/or the donation of infected blood as well. Gostin (1989:1627) observes that although 50–100 prosecutions of HIV-infected individuals have been brought in the United States, most of the civilian cases were later dropped or unsuccessful.

The second article, "The Limits of Quarantine as a Measure for Controlling the Spread of AIDS" by Mark Blumberg, examines the practical, ethical, and legal problems of quarantine. The author discusses the difficulties of forced isolation and its lack of effectiveness in slowing such an epidemic.

No state has seriously considered any form of broad-based isolation for members of high-risk groups, either for seropositives or for individuals diagnosed with full-blown AIDS. However, 15 states authorize the forced isolation of seropositive persons whose behavior constitutes a threat to the health of the community (Gostin, 1989:1622–23). These laws have been invoked in cases where an infected individual has refused to refrain from a pattern of high-risk behavior.

Gostin, Larry O. (1989). "Public Health Strategies for Confronting AIDS: Legislative and Regulatory Policy in the United States," *Journal of the American Medical Association*. Vol. 261, No. 11, pp. 1621–1630.

11

AIDS and
the Criminal Law

Martha A. Field and Kathleen M. Sullivan

AIDS is spread by acts, not by casual exposure. As AIDS spreads further, some are urging that those acts, including sexual acts, be treated as crimes.[1] Indeed, two AIDS carriers have already been charged with crimes for risking sexual transmission of AIDS to others. In one case, the United States Army has court-martialed an infected soldier, Pfc. Adrian Morris, Jr., charging that when he had sex with two other soldiers, he committed the crime of "aggravated assault." Aggravated assault requires use of a "dangerous weapon or other means of force likely to produce death or grievous bodily harm."[2] What was the "weapon" in his case? The sexually transmittable AIDS virus itself. In the other case, the Los Angeles district attorney has charged an AIDS carrier, Joseph Markowski, with attempted murder for selling his blood and for having sex with another man while infected.[3]

Should the transmission of AIDS be treated as a crime? If so, under what circumstances? In this paper we explore these issues. We first describe ways that traditional criminal laws and public health offenses might be found to cover AIDS transmission, and describe why those laws are ill suited to this context. We then describe what the most appropriate form of criminal proscription would be, if the criminal law were to intervene. But we conclude that the criminal law should not intervene. The social costs of criminalizing AIDS transmission would far outweigh the benefits of deterrence such a law might have. Serious and well-funded

Reprinted from *Law, Medicine and Health Care*, Vol. 15:1-2 (Summer 1987), pp. 46-60. A publication of the American Society of Law and Medicine.

public education about AIDS prevention is a far preferable means of influencing behavior.

APPLYING TRADITIONAL CRIMINAL LAW TO AIDS TRANSMISSION

The criminal law punishes a culpable act in order to incapacitate and reform the offender while deterring others from committing similar acts. The principal purpose of criminalizing AIDS transmission would be to deter persons with AIDS and AIDS carriers[4] from infecting others.

The best argument for criminalizing AIDS transmission is, perhaps, that it would be far preferable to quarantine, another form of regulation frequently advocated for preventing the spread of AIDS.[5] The criminal law would focus on culpable acts of AIDS transmission; quarantine would punish persons with AIDS or AIDS carriers for the mere status or condition of being infected or ill. The criminal law would punish actual offenders; quarantine would sequester a far larger group of people on the basis that they might infect others. Quarantine of persons with AIDS and AIDS carriers would presume that they cannot control their own behavior; the criminal law would recognize that most people do act responsibly and would punish only those who do not.

For all these reasons, using the criminal law to regulate AIDS transmission would pose far less threat to civil rights and civil liberties than quarantine does, although we still believe that threat excessive, as discussed below.

What might count as a "crime" of AIDS transmission? The criminal law typically punishes an act, accompanied by a culpable state of mind, that causes or risks causing a serious harm. None of these requirements, however, is straightforward in the context of AIDS transmission. To be sure, AIDS transmission involves more of an "act" than does transmission of a disease that is communicable by breathing, coughing, sneezing, or other involuntary body functions. Indeed, it is that very fact that makes quarantine of persons with AIDS or AIDS carriers so inappropriate. But the acts most likely to transmit AIDS—the act of sexual intercourse, whether anal or vaginal, and the act of needle-sharing for intravenous injection of drugs[6]—will rarely be accompanied by a conscious choice or wish to transmit AIDS. Quite the contrary: in criminalizing AIDS transmission, we would typically be criminalizing not intentional harms but simply the taking of risks.

The traditional criminal law, to be sure, does sometimes punish risk-taking. For example, the American Law Institute's Model Penal Code, which has greatly influenced state criminal code reform over the past three decades,[7] defines four states of mind, in descending order of culpability, that might be required to accompany a crime: purposeful, knowing, reckless, and negligent. *Purposeful* is defined as wanting the prohibited result; *knowing* is defined as consciously aware that the result will occur, and proceeding anyway; *reckless* is defined as consciously aware of a substantial and unjustifiable risk that the result will occur, and proceeding anyway; *negligent* is defined as possessing knowledge that should cause a reasonable person to avoid such a risk, and proceeding anyway.[8]

The Model Penal Code requires for most crimes a culpability level of recklessness or higher. Since negligence can be the product of carelessness, inadvertence, or ignorance, it is generally considered an insufficiently culpable state of mind to support criminal sanctions, with the stigma and severe deprivation of liberty that they impose. In the rare instances when the Code does accept negligence as sufficient, it invariably reduces the severity of the offense. Moreover, for *both* recklessness and negligence, the Code requires more than mere carelessness; it requires a "gross deviation" from ordinary standards of care.[9] Lesser deviation from such standards may create civil but not criminal liability.

Criminal liability may sometimes be imposed without any showing of a culpable state of mind—not even negligence.[10] But such "strict" liability is a relative anomaly in the criminal law, and it has been confined mainly to areas of life that are highly regulated by government, such as food and drug manufacture and railway and highway safety.[11]

What state of mind, if any, should be required if the transmission of AIDS is to be treated as a crime? We examine this problem first with respect to the traditional crimes most likely to be invoked to punish transmission of AIDS: homicide and assault. We argue that the established laws of homicide and assault fit AIDS transmission too poorly to be useful in any effort to treat AIDS transmission as a crime. We next consider whether traditional public health offenses fit AIDS transmission any better, and conclude that they too are inappropriate in this context.

Murder

If a person with AIDS or an AIDS carrier were found to have transmitted the disease to another with the effect of causing that person's death, he might be charged with murder or manslaughter.[12] Murder is distinguished from the lesser offense of manslaughter by the more culpable state of mind murder requires. The Model Penal Code, for example, defines murder as the killing of another human being either purposely, knowingly, or recklessly under circumstances manifesting "extreme indifference to the value of human life."[13] Such a mental state is required with regard to every element of the offense.

To be guilty of *purposeful* murder, therefore, an AIDS transmitter would have to commit an AIDS-transmitting act with the *desire* to cause his partner to die of AIDS. An AIDS transmitter would have *knowingly* caused the death of another only if he was consciously aware that he had AIDS or carried the HIV virus, and that his conduct *would* infect and kill another. And for an AIDS transmitter to commit *reckless* murder, he would have to be consciously aware that he carried or might well carry the AIDS virus and that his conduct might well transmit it to another person and cause that person to die. Moreover, he would have to manifest some unusual disregard for human life in *addition* to that recklessness in order to be guilty of reckless murder, as distinct from the lesser offense of reckless manslaughter. Deaths resulting from some violent felonies, including rape, may be treated as murders under this reckless-plus-extreme-indifference standard.[14]

Cases of purposeful or knowing murder by AIDS transmission are conceivable but likely to be extremely rare. The AIDS transmitter will rarely if ever be certain that an act of sex or needle-sharing will transmit AIDS, as knowing murder requires. Having sex or sharing needles, moreover, is a highly indirect modus operandi for the person whose *purpose* is to kill.

In the unusual situation where purpose or knowledge could be shown, however, the person who deliberately used AIDS to kill would seem just as culpable as a person who deliberately injected a victim with a lethal poison in the hope of causing death. Nor is culpability much in doubt in other instances that are likely to count as murder under the Code: for example, the prostitute who knows he or she is contagious and nonetheless plies his or her trade without precautions, indifferent to the number of persons thus fatally infected,[15] or the person who, knowing he has AIDS, rapes another and so eventually causes his or her death.[16]

Manslaughter

Where criminal culpability becomes more doubtful—and the application of traditional murder rules more troubling—is in the realm of recklessness and negligence, the two mental states that are by far the likeliest to accompany AIDS transmission. Reckless killing can be either murder or manslaughter. When it does not reflect the "extreme indifference to the value of human life" that is the standard for reckless murder, the Model Penal Code treats it as the lesser offense of manslaughter.

Many instances of AIDS transmission might qualify as manslaughter under the Model Penal Code's definition. Recklessness means simply adverting to a known substantial and unjustifiable risk, and disregarding it anyway. For example, a lover carried away by passion who has intercourse with his friend or spouse without taking precautions against transmission could be guilty of manslaughter if he was aware that he might well be transmitting AIDS to his partner, who later dies.

What would count as awareness of a "substantial and unjustifiable risk" of AIDS transmission? Diagnosis of AIDS-related complex (ARC) might be enough, even though people with ARC symptoms do not always contract full-blown AIDS. Knowledge that one had tested positive on an HIV-antibody test might be enough. Although the test does generate a significant number of false positives and not all true positives develop AIDS, the medical presumption is that all true positives are contagious. Indeed, persons just developing the infection, although they seem healthy, may be as contagious as persons who have developed the full disease.[17] Knowledge that one had had high-risk sexual contacts in the past might be enough, even in the absence of any diagnosis or test. Thus, applying the manslaughter provisions to AIDS transmission might embrace many cases in which one knew of a risk but in which killing one's sexual partner was the last thing one *wanted* to do.

Negligent Homicide

The Model Penal Code treats grossly negligent killings as negligent homicide, a lesser offense than manslaughter, although many states continue to treat grossly negligent killings simply as manslaughter, as did the common law. Negligent homicide under the Model Penal Code does not require "conscious disregard" of risk, as the recklessness crimes do, but only that the actor disregard a risk of which he "should be aware"—even if he is not. As noted above, the Model Penal Code limits negligence for this crime, as for all negligence crimes, to "*gross* deviation from ordinary standards of conduct."[18]

It is possible that some prosecutors would treat many transmissions of AIDS as negligent homicide, even under this strict requirement. They might, for example, prosecute a person who did not actually know that he had AIDS, or that he carried the AIDS virus, or even that AIDS is deadly and transmittable by some sexual acts he engages in. And a jury could convict him so long as it believed that a "reasonable person" in his circumstances should have known those facts, even if the defendant genuinely did not. The crime of negligent homicide could thus cast a very wide net over AIDS transmitters, because the fears and prejudices of juries could greatly influence their judgments about what conduct is "reasonable."

Problems in Applying Homicide Law

There are many problems with using these traditional homicide provisions as a means of regulating the transmission of AIDS. To name two obvious ones, the victim may well have consented to expose himself or herself to the risk of contracting the disease from the defendant, and a long time usually elapses between exposure and death.

Under the law of both murder and manslaughter, consent of the victim is irrelevant to the crime—a homicide exists even if the victim has consented, or indeed requested, to be killed.[19] But the presence of "consent" to acts that can transmit AIDS may well affect the degree of culpability that should attach—at least in the context of sexual transmission. A person who transmitted AIDS after informing his sexual partner of everything he knew about his own condition and the contagious properties of AIDS seems far less blameworthy than someone who carefully hid from his sexual partner the fact that he was infected.

Under the law of murder and manslaughter, moreover, the transmitter cannot be convicted unless the victim has died, no matter how malicious the intent in exposing the victim to the disease. In the AIDS context, however, blameworthiness relates far more to factors like the defendant's knowledge and intent than to the timetable of the victim's life in relation to the defendant's. After all, the transmitter of AIDS will often die before the person to whom he has given the disease.

Even if the victim does pre-decease the defendant, proving that the defendant's act was the *cause* of the victim's death will be difficult. The victim may have had other relationships, prior or subsequent, that could have been the cause instead. Moreover, half of the states still follow the common-law rule that homicide can be charged only if death has occurred within a year and a day of the act.[20] In those states, given AIDS' long latency period, AIDS transmission will rarely be chargeable as murder or manslaughter.

Solutions to these problems might be reached along other avenues of traditional criminal law. Even when the victim does not die, so that homicide cannot be charged, an AIDS transmitter might be prosecuted for the crimes of attempted murder, or assault.[21] Both offenses, as their penalties reflect, are considered substantially less serious than criminal homicide.[22]

Attempted Murder

A finding of guilt of attempted murder would not require that the victim die; guilt for *attempt* turns principally upon the intent of the would-be perpetrator—the factor that seems most closely correlated with blameworthiness in the transmission of AIDS. Because attempt makes liability turn on intent while shifting the focus away from the timing of death, it may fit AIDS transmission better than the law of homicide. On the other hand, attempt may sometimes impose more liability than is desirable. It would potentially apply not only when the victim has not yet died from AIDS, but even when the victim does not become infected with the AIDS virus at all. As long as the would-be transmitter (1) had or carried AIDS or believed he did;[23] (2) engaged in conduct that could transmit it (or even attempted to engage in that conduct); and (3) did so with the requisite state of mind, he could be guilty of attempt to kill.

As a practical matter, however, attempt law could reach very few cases of AIDS transmission because it requires a purposeful or knowing state of mind. To be guilty of attempted murder for transmitting AIDS, a person would have to act "with the purpose of causing" his partner to be infected and die "or with the belief that it will cause such result."[24] While there may be the rare case in which a person with AIDS shared a needle or had sexual intercourse with a person out of a conscious desire that that person acquire AIDS and die, that certainly is not the paradigm case. Even if such a case could be proved, punishing it as attempted murder would have little effect on the overwhelming majority of AIDS transmissions, which are either reckless, negligent, or wholly accidental.

Assault

Assault may seem a more appropriate tool for reaching AIDS transmission than homicide or attempted murder. The victim need not die in order for the offense to be complete, and consent may be a defense in some circumstances. Under the Model Penal Code, a person can be guilty of assault if he "attempts to cause or purposely, knowingly or recklessly causes bodily injury to another."[25] Assault is a misdemeanor. A person can be guilty of aggravated assault—a second-degree felony—if he "attempts to cause serious bodily injury to another, or causes such injury purposely, knowingly or recklessly under circumstances manifesting extreme indifference to the value of human life."[26]

One reason assault may seem better suited than homicide or attempt to cases of AIDS transmission is that the consent of the victim may be relevant to guilt. An assault is an unwanted or offensive touching. Brain surgery is a touching but not an assault, because the patient consents; consensual sex is normally not an assault either. The common law regarded consent as a complete defense to otherwise offensive contact, as the consent vitiated the element of offensiveness. The Model Penal Code, by contrast, would treat consent as a defense in some cases but *not* in cases of serious bodily harm.[27]

Both these approaches to consent would have to be refined in the context of AIDS transmission. Consent to sexual activity itself should not constitute consent to contracting AIDS—or any other serious sexually transmittable disease—if one did not know that one's partner was infected. Rather, only *informed* consent should suffice. That is, unless the victim agreed to have sexual intercourse with the transmitter knowing that the transmitter had AIDS or had tested positive for HIV exposure, an assault prosecution might proceed.

English common law offers some support for this approach. In one case, for example, a defendant was found guilty of assault and battery for transmitting venereal disease to a woman who was held to have consented to sexual intercourse but who was not aware that the defendant had venereal disease. In *Regina v. Bennet*, Bennet had sex with his thirteen-year-old niece and infected her with gonorrhea. He was charged with indecent assault, the assault being the act of infecting the girl with gonorrhea. The court instructed the jury that it could find the defendant guilty if the girl did not know that her uncle had gonorrhea, even if she could be deemed to have consented to the act of sexual intercourse.[28]

The Model Penal Code might be read to reach the same result today, for a different reason: because it generally precludes consent to serious bodily harm as a defense.[29] No consent defense would be allowed even in cases of consensual sex where AIDS is transmitted, since one is legally precluded from "consenting" to the receipt of a deadly disease that is the real assault here.

Although assault law might thus be stretched to fit the AIDS transmission context, it has been developed with circumstances very different from AIDS transmission in mind. Indeed, we are using fictions when we label as "assault" sexual activity that is generally consensual but where the consent was obtained by fraud.[30] Assault law purports to punish unconsented contact, but in this context would in fact punish consented contacts that happened to transmit AIDS. Moreover, assault is often concerned with rather minor offenses—not with offenses associated with causing death. Finally, the possible reach of assault law in this context would be extremely broad, because the victim may not even have to become infected with AIDS for assault to be charged. While assault could provide a framework for prosecuting some AIDS transmission cases, therefore, it is ill suited to the context.

APPLYING TRADITIONAL PUBLIC HEALTH OFFENSE LAWS TO AIDS TRANSMISSION

Many states have long had statutes making it a criminal offense for a person with a contagious disease willfully or knowingly to expose another person to that disease.[31] Many states have specifically criminalized willfully or knowingly exposing another to sexually transmitted diseases, making having sex itself the crime so long as one is infectious.[32] Most of these statutes treat such willful communication of disease only as a misdemeanor punishable by fines or by imprisonment for no more than a year.

While such statutes are little enforced today, they might be resurrected as an alternative to using traditional crimes such as homicide, attempt, and assault to regulate and punish intentional or knowing transmission of AIDS. At least one state with such a statute has explicitly amended it to embrace the intentional transmission of AIDS;[33] others have bills pending to do so.[34] In other states, courts may treat AIDS as covered by the terms "infectious and contagious disease" or "venereal or sexually transmitted disease" even without explicit legislative amendment.

In one sense these statutes are well tailored to culpability in the AIDS context: most include within their purview only persons who know they have the disease and who willfully or knowingly expose another. But these enactments are not a proper vehicle for the prosecution of AIDS transmission. Unless the offenses are explicit in including AIDS within their purview, judges should not interpret them to do so. Nor should legislators expand these statutes to include the AIDS virus within their scope.

"Contagious" disease statutes are overinclusive with respect to AIDS because they appear to count as "exposure" casual contacts that pose no risk whatever of spreading the disease. And "venereal" disease statutes are underinclusive because AIDS can be spread by means other than sex—for example, by needle-sharing and blood transfusions. Neither sort of statute, of course, was originally conceived with AIDS in mind.

More important, these statutes do not take into account the fact that AIDS is incurable and fatal. On the one hand, these statutes thus may be too lenient: they impose only misdemeanor liability, in recognition of the fact that modern medicine can cure most if not all of the diseases they are meant to cover. They would not permit felony liability for the rare but highly culpable cases of purposeful, knowing, or reckless-and-indifferent AIDS transmission discussed above. On the other hand, it is the very deadliness of AIDS that make these statutes too harsh here. For most sexually transmittable diseases, these statutes impose merely temporary abstinence until one is cured by antibiotics;[35] for persons with AIDS and AIDS carriers, however, they would require abstinence for life.

We believe it would be better for any legislature that is contemplating making intentional AIDS transmission a crime to give more precise attention to the factors that make AIDS unique. If it is to criminalize AIDS transmission at all, it should enact an AIDS-specific statute. The next section describes what such a statute might look like. The section after that, however, argues that even though such a statute would be clearly preferable to using existing criminal laws to regulate AIDS transmission, it would still be undesirable to use the criminal law in the fight to control AIDS.

CREATING A NEW, AIDS-SPECIFIC OFFENSE

If the criminal law were to operate in this area at all, a statute specific to AIDS would be a better means of regulation than the use of general criminal prohibitions enacted with very different situations in mind. A statute specific to AIDS transmission would convey maximum warning and have maximum deterrent value. After all, deterrence, not punishment, is the chief purpose of applying the criminal law to AIDS transmission.[36]

A specific statute would be preferable primarily because it could be tailored to what we decide we really want to prevent. Use of traditional criminal law leaves many central issues unanswered. If a victim had full knowledge that he or she risked infection with AIDS, does that constitute a defense? If a transmitter thinks he *might* be an AIDS carrier but does not know and has not been tested, can he be guilty of crime? Can someone be guilty if he consciously risks infecting another even though the victim in fact never becomes infected with the AIDS virus? An AIDS-specific statute could explicitly resolve these and other important issues. In taking a position on these issues and embodying it in the criminal law, such legislation would announce a societal judgment about appropriate standards of behavior. The educative and normative functions of that announcement are likely to be more important than the actual prosecution rate.

The most basic point about an AIDS-specific criminal statute is that a great deal of what it would criminalize is intimate sexual activity[37]—activity that should normally not be regulated by government, and that if regulated at all should be regulated to the least extent possible. Although some activities that may transmit AIDS, such as needle-sharing or donation of infected blood, involve no similar privacy interest, the implications of regulating people's sex lives must be taken into account in any law that would regulate AIDS transmission.[38]

It is a familiar principle that government should use far greater restraint in policing our bedrooms than in policing our streets. Rights associated with intimate sexual conduct have in many contexts been given constitutional protection against state interference. While the right to make one's own decisions concerning intimate sexual relationships is not mentioned in the language of the United States Constitution, the United States Supreme Court has interpreted the Constitution to contain a right to privacy allowing individuals to make decisions about contraception, abortion, and family matters for themselves.[39] Protecting these decisions as private might be explained either on the ground that sexual activity is central to personality,[40] or on the ground that government has no business regulating matters that involve none of the tangible harms government was constituted to prevent.[41]

We do not claim it would be unconstitutional under these precedents for the state to regulate the sexual conduct of AIDS carriers or others, in an effort to contain the AIDS virus. It might not be unconstitutional even to order persons with AIDS or AIDS carriers not to engage in sex. The transmission of AIDS obviously implicates serious and tangible harm, both to the immediate victims and to the public at large. Thus even though regulating AIDS transmission entails intrusion by government into the bedroom, some intrusion may be necessary to protect the public health against an epidemic.[42]

The principle at the core of the right-to-privacy cases counsels, however, that even if a law criminalizing AIDS transmission would be constitutional, it should be carefully tailored so that it does not reach too far into the private sexual realm.[43] The following sections detail how an AIDS-specific criminal law might be so tailored.

What Behavior Should an AIDS-Specific Law Encourage or Discourage?

In deciding what to criminalize, it is important to consider how we would want a person with AIDS or an AIDS carrier to act. The answer to this question involves a balancing of sometimes conflicting interests. At one extreme, some might argue that persons with AIDS and AIDS carriers should abstain altogether from behavior with any risk of transmitting the virus to others. Under such a view, having sexual intercourse while knowing one was an AIDS carrier would be a crime no matter how much one disclosed about one's condition and no matter how many precautions one tried to take. Advocates of such a view would emphasize that condoms may break and that no one should be allowed to consent to engage in a risk that endangers the public. Under this "total-abstinence" view, the social interest in stopping the spread of AIDS would flatly outweigh any individual interest in continuing to engage in sex.[44]

At the opposite extreme, some might argue that decisions about what risks to undertake should be an entirely private matter. Such an approach would value the individual interest in pursuing intimate sexual relationships over the public interest in preventing transmission of AIDS. Under such a view, consent and precautions would be matters for individuals and not the state to regulate. The only AIDS transmission such a view might regard as criminal is that involving an unwitting victim—one to whom a knowing AIDS carrier did not disclose his condition. And even then, a "total-permissiveness" approach might regard such a victim as having assumed the risk by having engaged in sex.

We believe that both these extreme views are too simplistic, and we conclude that the most appropriate policy would fall somewhere in between. The "total-abstinence" view both overestimates the effectiveness of the criminal law and undervalues the individual interest in continuing intimate sexual relationships. But the "total-permissiveness" approach wrongly minimizes the public interest in stopping the spread of an escalating epidemic.

A "total-abstinence" policy would be unrealistic. Such a policy would in effect require persons with AIDS and AIDS carriers to give up sexual intercourse for what will amount to the rest of their lives. Because AIDS is lifelong—because it is not currently curable—a prohibition on sexual intercourse is of a different order than prohibitions that last during the period that a person is afflicted with curable venereal diseases like gonorrhea or syphilis. After all, many people who find out they have AIDS will be involved in long-term romantic relationships, homosexual or heterosexual. Love for the AIDS victim may make a partner unwilling either to discontinue the relationship or to alter it drastically by avoiding intercourse altogether. Moreover, if such a partner would consent to sex with someone he knows to be an AIDS carrier despite the plain risks it poses to his life and health, he would most likely ignore a criminal prohibition too. Thus if a law criminalized all sexual intercourse by persons with AIDS or AIDS carriers, some of these people and their partners would follow it, but more would not.[45]

Indeed, a "total-abstinence" policy might well be self-defeating. The goal of such a policy would be to stop the spread of the disease. But if sexual relationships are likely to continue despite such a ban—as sexual relationships long have in defiance of other laws that have tried to regulate them—the best way of preventing the spread of the disease is to create incentives for sexual partners both to disclose their condition and to use precautions. A flat ban on all sex by AIDS carriers, however, would create just the opposite incentive: if the sex is criminal no matter what one does to inform or protect one's partner, why bother with information or protection?

A flat ban on sex for AIDS carriers seems not only unrealistic but also inhumane. It adds to the already considerable burdens of persons who find out they are

AIDS carriers to require them to sever what may be long-term relationships, or to brand them as criminals unless they give up sexual intercourse for life. As well as being self-defeating, it seems wrong to so burden them for having sex with adults who know of their condition and who want nonetheless to continue a sexual relationship.

On the other hand, a "total-permissiveness" approach is likewise inadequate. First, it is not clear that people should always be permitted to endanger themselves as they see fit. Our general prohibition of euthanasia and suicide reflects the value of intervention to prevent even harms one would inflict upon oneself. Of course, consenting to sex with an AIDS-infected person is not the product of suicidal impulse; it is typically the product of love or sexual desire to which some risk is attached. But not all will assess the situation intelligently; some may not understand the risks, and love or desire may lead others to play them down. Accordingly, this may be an especially strong case for paternalistic intervention. Moreover, even apart from protecting the victim from him or herself, there is a strong public interest in containing the virus—in protecting the victim's potential future partners. Unlike suicide, contracting AIDS is a harm to the self that may tangibly harm others as well. In this way, the case for intervention here is stronger than it is with respect to suicide.

An appropriate regulation would give weight to *both* the individual's interest in sexual intimacy *and* the public interest in protecting the uninfected and stopping the spread of AIDS. Such a middle course would permit sex but encourage disclosure and safety. It would tell persons with AIDS and AIDS carriers that their sexual contacts are punishable only if they do not use precautions or if they do not disclose their condition to their sexual partners. Such an approach would have far more chance of actually influencing the behavior of both AIDS victims and their sexual partners than would the "total-abstinence" approach. But at the same time, unlike the "total-permissiveness" approach, it would contribute to community awareness of a societal judgment that AIDS carriers should both inform their partners and take precautions against transmission. If the criminal law were to increase disclosure and the use of precautions, it would have made as great a contribution as it can here.

How Might an AIDS-Specific Law Be Structured?

There are two basic approaches that might be taken to criminalizing AIDS transmission. One would be to legislate a general prohibition against purposely, knowingly, recklessly, or perhaps even negligently transmitting AIDS to another person, and would leave it to courts and juries to give meaning to those terms over time in particular cases. The other would be to legislate more particularly in order to impose specific affirmative duties on knowing AIDS carriers to disclose and to use precautions. This section discusses these two approaches and concludes that the second is plainly preferable, because it is the only one that gives clear and consistent guidance about what behavior is and is not desirable for persons with AIDS or AIDS carriers.

The Classical Culpability Approach. The first is the more classical criminal law approach. It would criminalize the act of AIDS transmission by any means, sexual or non-sexual, so long as it was accompanied by the requisite state of mind. The advantage of such an approach is that it focuses on acts, not persons; it would thus apply to all rather than singling out the group of persons with AIDS and AIDS carriers as such. The difficulty with this approach, however, is in defining a state of mind requirement that is both practical and fair.

As discussed above in connection with homicide and attempt, criminalizing only purposeful or knowing acts of AIDS transmission—that is, acts that a person intends or knows will transmit AIDS—would be quite fair but highly ineffectual, because such acts are likely to be very rare. If reckless or negligent AIDS transmission is criminalized, the law becomes more effective, but other problems arise.

AIDS transmission could be "reckless" if one was consciously aware of a substantial risk one might have or carry AIDS, and if one was consciously aware of a substantial risk that one's conduct might transmit it. AIDS transmission could be "negligent" if one took such a risk even if one was wholly unaware that one was infectious or that one's conduct might transmit the virus—as long as a jury finds one *should* have been aware of these risks.

Using either of these standards here would give far too much power to juries. In many contexts, criminal liability for recklessness and perhaps even negligence may be desirable.[46] But in this context, popular anxiety, irrationality, and even hysteria about AIDS are far too likely to cause vindictive or discriminatory verdicts, especially while AIDS is disproportionately concentrated in already unpopular groups such as gay men and intravenous drug abusers. Moreover, even the most rational jury may be confused by ever-evolving scientific understanding about the nature of the disease and its transmission. Where science is uncertain, some juries may wish to impose very strict norms of conduct.

For example, juries would be free under either a recklessness or a negligence standard to convict even those who did not know when they committed the charged act that they had AIDS or were AIDS carriers—so long as the jury deems them to have disregarded clues of which they were aware (recklessness) or should have been aware (negligence). But what would count as such a clue? Should it be enough that one is a member of a "high-risk" group such as gay men or intravenous drug abusers? That one had never been tested for HIV antibodies, and had never therefore obtained a negative result? If the former is enough, a recklessness or negligence standard would be a license to juries to discriminate against unpopular groups. If the latter is enough, it would be a license to juries to enforce mandatory AIDS testing even where the legislature has not, if and when they wish to do so.

If testing is to be required, it would be far fairer for such a decision to be made by the legislature, subject to usual processes of judicial review, rather than imposed selectively and in an ad hoc fashion by juries. We do not think, however, that even legislative enactment of mandatory testing is warranted at this time. One reason is that the tests now available are not sufficiently accurate bases for the enormous consequences that can attach to them. The antibody tests currently in use still generate a significant number of false positives and accordingly give uncertain guidance about one's ability to transmit the disease to others. Moreover, under current social conditions a person who tests positive risks severe hardship if that result becomes public: one may lose one's job, home, or insurance benefits, with little if any protection from current anti-discrimination law.[47] It would be far better for legislatures to do what they can to encourage voluntary testing by funding it, by guaranteeing the confidentiality of results,[48] and by passing anti-discrimination laws that would protect positive testers from becoming social pariahs overnight.[49]

Criminalizing the reckless or the negligent transmission of AIDS not only threatens to punish those who did not know they had it; it also threatens to punish those who did not know they were transmitting it. The reckless AIDS transmitter—because he was aware there was substantial risk—may seem sufficiently culpable for punishment to be appropriate, but negligence liability would be troubling. Negligence liability would punish any act a jury believes "unreasonably" risked transmission, regardless of the defendant's own knowledge or actual state of mind. It thus would risk branding an individual a criminal because of his ignorance or stupidity rather than because of any malice.

While negligent liability seems inappropriately strict, there is one respect in which requiring recklessness might treat the AIDS transmitter too leniently: if an AIDS carrier used precautions, such as wearing a condom during sexual intercourse, that might negate "conscious disregard" of risk.[50] While it is appropriate for the law to encourage precautions, we believe it would not be appropriate for a law to make precautions alone negate the offense. Rather, the AIDS carrier should also be obligated to disclose his condition to his partner before intercourse.[51]

Such disclosure is highly desirable. An AIDS carrier has no right to defraud others into taking deadly sexual risks by being silent about his condition. His sexual partner deserves to know the facts before consenting to sexual contact.[52] Even if the AIDS carrier believes he can shield his partner from risk by silently taking precautions, he should nonetheless disclose the truth and allow his partner to make the choice. If many people believe that safe sex with an AIDS carrier is possible, then a person who has tested positive will not have a problem finding sexual partners despite his disclosure of that fact. If the uninfected shun him, he may be able to find willing sexual partners among others who have tested positive.[53]

Full disclosure or informed consent might, therefore, constitute an affirmative defense to any crime of AIDS transmission. The difficulty with viewing full disclosure as a complete defense on its own, however, is that it would tend to undermine the incentive to use precautions. However imperfectly, criminalizing reckless or negligent transmission will tend to encourage the use of precautions. But if *either* precautions or disclosure could help negate liability, people who mold their behavior according to the criminal law would be less likely to do both. There is a strong case to be made for requiring both, and thus for not allowing informed consent to be a complete defense in the absence of precautions. For one thing, mistakes about consent here may have lethal consequences. For another, even if the sexual partner is genuinely informed and is willing to forego precautions, there may be an important public interest in denying him or her that choice in order to contain the spread of the disease. Finally, requiring available precautions to be used notwithstanding a sexual partner's consent might also serve as useful insurance for situations in which the sexual partner may not wholly understand the situation to which he or she consents.

The Affirmative Duty Approach. Many of the problems with the first, more traditional approach might be avoided by enacting instead a criminal law geared less to punishing culpable acts than to imposing affirmative duties of disclosure and precaution on persons with AIDS and AIDS carriers. Such a law might specify those duties, leaving less discretion to juries to import them as they pleased through determinations about state of mind. Such a law might punish AIDS transmission, for example, only when the defendant (1) actually knew from testing or diagnosis that he had AIDS or was an AIDS carrier; and (2) failed to disclose his condition to his partner or failed to use appropriate precautions. In other words, only the combination of disclosure and precautions could suffice as a defense.

Why require actual knowledge of one's infection with AIDS? The advantage of such a requirement over the more traditional recklessness or negligence liability discussed above is that it avoids imposing punishment for ignorance, while preventing the backdoor imposition of mandatory testing. True, it has some disadvantages. First, the knowledge requirement appears to single out a particular group; it thus makes the offense resemble quarantine more than a traditional criminal law applying equally to all. But singling out only knowing AIDS carriers is fairer than subjecting even unwitting ones to criminal sanctions, and the burden upon them is not unreasonable because even those singled out are still permitted to have sex. While perhaps it would be fairer and more logical to require *every* sexually active person—not just persons with AIDS and AIDS carriers—to disclose their health status and to use condoms as long as AIDS remains uncured, it would be quite harsh as well as politically impossible to do so through the criminal law.[54]

Second, an actual knowledge requirement may discourage voluntary testing. After all, as long as one does not "know" for sure that one is infected, can't one go on having sex with impunity? But this deterrent to voluntary testing should not be exaggerated. Many incentives exist to get tested, without adding the threat of criminal punishment to the list. One may wish to gain peace of mind from a negative result, or to learn that one is positive so that one can begin to treat oneself and to protect one's loved ones. Moreover, in cases where a person has clear enough reason to suspect he is infected, "conscious avoidance" of an AIDS test may not necessarily negate knowledge. In some other criminal contexts, knowledge of a key fact has been found despite similar attempts at "willful blindness."[55]

Why require that no culpable mental state accompany the act of transmission itself? The proposed law here would require knowledge that one carried AIDS, but nothing more except an act of transmission without disclosure or precautions. In this sense, it imposes a kind of strict liability. Like strict-liability crimes that help to enforce the affirmative duties of those who drive dangerous cargoes or ship dangerous drugs, the purpose here is to mold behavior, to induce people to take care with a dangerous disease when they alone are in a position to do so.

But strict in this context does not mean unfair. It seems that AIDS carriers would be more fairly treated by the proposed offense than by the classical criminal law approach. There are definite advantages to having legislatures rather than juries set the rules in this area. A law specifying that one will not be criminally liable if one discloses and uses appropriate precautions not only would clearly preserve AIDS carriers' right to engage in sexual intercourse but would also give them much clearer notice of what their obligations are than would the recklessness or negligence liability discussed above. Moreover, such a law would pose far less danger of jury arbitrariness and selectivity. And finally, there is little danger that the law in practice would unfairly sweep in many who transmit AIDS through complete ignorance of how it is transmitted. Because the law covers only those who have tested positive or been diagnosed as having AIDS, most will be informed at the time of the positive diagnosis of how an infected person might transmit the disease and what precautions he should take.[56]

Of course, the warning can only be as clear as the legislature is specific. If the legislature deems "appropriate precautions" a partial defense, considerable ambiguity about what is "appropriate" would be left for juries to resolve, with many of the attendant dangers discussed above. But if the legislature becomes too specific, it may intrude too far into private sexual decision-making. The specter of a legislative debate over which precautions are appropriate or which particular techniques should be used for "safer sex," is extremely disturbing. Could certain sexual practices themselves be banned under this rubric?

We would oppose any attempt to codify precautions by legislatively blacklisting specified sexual practices or contacts between specified body parts. In order to minimize legislative intrusion into intimate sexual activity, a precaution provision should be limited to a requirement that condoms or an equally safe substitute be used.[57] Of course, it can be problematic to be this specific; regular condoms may be widely thought adequate today, but perhaps only state-of-the-art germicidal condoms will seem appropriate tomorrow.[58] But such a specific provision would have the key virtue of leaving less to juries' imagination and prejudice than the classical culpability approach.

In sum, the second approach appears preferable to the first. It more clearly imposes on persons with AIDS and AIDS carriers an affirmative duty, as a condition of engaging in sexual intercourse, of fully disclosing their condition to their sexual partners and obtaining their partners' knowing consent, and also an affirmative duty of using precautions like condoms. Such a statute has a realistic chance of influencing behavior, because it permits a person to pursue a sexual relationship if he complies with these affirmative duties. And perhaps most important so long as an epidemic of prejudice accompanies the epidemic of AIDS, such a statute would minimize the risk that jury verdicts will be determined by fear and discrimination. Indeed, such a statute is probably the best the criminal law could do to stem the tide of AIDS while respecting conflicting interests. In the next section we argue, however, that even such a model criminal statute should be rejected.

ASSESSING THE DESIRABILITY OF CRIMINALIZING AIDS TRANSMISSION

Even if an AIDS-specific criminal statute could be closely tailored to the harms we wish to prevent, is criminalization a desirable means of fighting the spread of AIDS? We conclude that it is not.

The Benefits and Costs of Criminalization

Criminalizing forms of transmission other than sexual contact is not likely to provide major deterrent force but does impose little social cost. For example, it might increase existing incentives for intravenous drug abusers with AIDS not to share needles. Although the criminal law evidently does not deter intravenous drug abusers from using drugs, it might be marginally more successful in discouraging them from spreading the disease by sharing needles.[59] At the same time, there is no particular social value in the sharing of intravenous needles—whatever one might think of the morality of drug use generally. Accordingly, there is something to gain and little to lose by prohibiting persons who know they have AIDS or have tested positive from passing the needle.

With respect to the sexual transmission of AIDS, however, the balance is somewhat different. Criminalization of such transmission might well have a significant deterrent effect—at least if drawn along the lines suggested in the preceding section—by increasing both the amount of disclosure and the use of precautions against infection. The issue is whether these gains would be great enough to outweigh the costs of criminalization.

We conclude that the criminal law is not a desirable means of regulating sexual transmission of AIDS. The deterrent effect such an approach would have would not be great enough to be worth its costs: first, the threat of massive government intrusion into sexual privacy and second, the predictable danger of selective prosecution and misuse of the criminal law to harass particularly unpopular groups, especially gay men.

Sexual Privacy. The enactment of even a narrowly defined criminal law would create grave risks to sexual privacy throughout the population, heterosexual as well as homosexual. Enforcement of such a law would implicate not only the purposeful, knowing, and reckless AIDS transmitters who are the law's ultimate target but also a vast number of others who are or have been sexually involved with them. To be sure, if all it took to trigger such a law was a complaining witness' allegation against a named defendant—as is the case, for example, in date-rape cases—then it might seem that only the witness' and the named party's sexual privacy would be breached, the witness' voluntarily and the suspect's justifiably. But suppose that the complaining witness had recently had sex with more than one partner. Would the criminal law stop with the initial complaint? Or would the complainant's other sexual partners now be subject to investigation or surveillance? How else could potential sources other than the suspect be ruled out? And what about the defendant's other sexual partners, if any? Should the authorities seek them out if they have not come forward?

Nor can we assume that investigation and prosecution would be limited to cases where a complaining witness has come forward. Law enforcement authorities might well seek on their own to trace the sexual history of those persons they know to be infected with AIDS. In that event, would the victim's medical records and private papers be opened to police scrutiny as possible sources of leads? And would all the past sexual partners whom such sources might identify be subject to criminal investigation as well?

The possibilities are manifold. Wholesale sexual surveillance through the apparatus of the criminal law could clearly sweep in a great deal of sexual activity that involves no harm to others, in pursuit of the few instances of sexual activity that do. However laudable the end of preventing the intentional or reckless transmission of AIDS, using criminal enforcement as the means threatens to sweep too broadly.

Selective Prosecution and Harassment. Until AIDS spreads more deeply through the heterosexual population, gay men and intravenous drug abusers are the likeliest target for enforcement of an AIDS-specific criminal law, because they are the largest groups systematically and visibly at risk from AIDS. A parallel may be drawn with the criminal sodomy laws, which have been enforced against homosexuals more than heterosexuals even where they apply on their face to both groups.[60] An AIDS-specific offense could become a tool of official persecution—an outlet for irrational fear and hostility toward gay men or drug abusers independent of, though perhaps reinforced by, fear of AIDS.

A criminal law could provide a tool for harassment in the sexual context even if a defense of disclosure plus precautions were available. Victims angry with a person who may be the source of their infection could tip off the police, causing the suspect to be picked up and detained even if he would ultimately be able to establish his innocence. The criminal process can substantially restrict liberty and impose stigma long before any prosecution has begun, much less conviction been entered.[61] There is a risk in this context that gay men will be punished for their sexual orientation, apart from their guilt of any crime.[62]

The danger that a criminal law against AIDS transmission will furnish a new tool for harassment is greater for gay men than for intravenous drug abusers. Narcotics use is already criminal, and laws against it are enforced, however ineffectively. By contrast, being gay is not illegal, and in most states, the oral and anal sex acts in which many gay men engage have been decriminalized.[63] Moreover, sodomy is plainly not taken as seriously as a crime as drug abuse even in jurisdictions where it is still denominated criminal.[64] Thus an AIDS-specific statute would cast the shadow of the criminal law upon gay male sex even in those jurisdictions that have repealed or overturned their sodomy laws. And in those few places where sodomy is sometimes enforced as a criminal offense, harassment under the new AIDS-specific enactment might be easier, partly because the offense would be viewed as a more serious one.

To empower the state to investigate gay sexual contacts is to empower the state to harass and intimidate a group that is popularly disliked at best, and despised at worst. There is every reason to fear that popular irrationality and hysteria about AIDS would reinforce efforts to use an AIDS-specific law not just to track down "killers" but also to intimidate the entire gay male community, in places where the police were inclined to do so.

If used to intimidate, an AIDS-specific criminal law would be precisely counterproductive to the aim of fighting the spread of AIDS. Public health authorities have argued that even criminal laws against sodomy impede medical efforts to control the spread of AIDS. Some who suspect they may have AIDS will be deterred from seeking medical advice by a fear that doing so would result in criminal investigation.[65] If such fears seem speculative against the backdrop of the largely unenforced sodomy laws, they could become all too real if new AIDS crimes were placed on the books.

Alternatives to the Criminal Law

Civil remedies in tort for transmission of AIDS[66] may pose less of a threat than the criminal law to sexual privacy generally and to the gay community in particular. Civil remedies, unlike criminal ones, do not invoke the specter of state surveillance of a wide range of sexual partners and acts. Moreover, only a sexual partner or other transmission victim, not the state, could initiate suit, which may limit the range of cases actually brought. On the other hand, however, the intrusion into privacy entailed by civil discovery may be great in particular cases, and may touch many wholly innocent persons simply because of their past sexual contacts. Moreover, while the threat of monetary damages might provide some measure of deterrence, it would be limited to persons who have funds, unlike criminal law deterrence. Finally, enough stigma may be attached to such suits that both living victims and their estates will be discouraged from bringing them. And even if they do, a victory may not send out a clear message that spreading AIDS to unwitting victims is wrong—only that it is costly.

Notwithstanding these shortcomings, tort suits are preferable to criminal prosecutions as a means for influencing behavior in this context because they minimize the risk of state intrusion into a sensitive area of private life. The greatest advantage of civil over criminal enforcement is not that it would provide more deterrence but, rather, that it would impose less social cost.

Nor are tort suits the sole alternative to criminal remedies here. The point is less that civil remedies are superior to criminal than that all legal remedies for past wrongs have limited capacity to control the mounting AIDS epidemic. If we care as a society about containing the disease and protecting potential victims, we should pour funds into medical research about AIDS transmission and cure, and into public education and counseling about prevention until a medical solution can be found.

The surgeon general of the United States, for example, has recommended a vigorous expansion of public education efforts on AIDS prevention, beginning even in childhood.[67] Such a program would acknowledge that it is ignorance and not malice that puts people most at risk of contracting AIDS. Social services might also aid containment: providing shelter and welfare to infected prostitutes might do a better job of stopping them from transmitting AIDS to their clientele than would repeated arrests;[68] making the HIV-antibody test anonymous and free might drastically increase its use and accordingly change behavior; and providing free needles and high-quality, free condoms at public expense, controversial as that would be, might do more to stop the spread of AIDS than criminal or civil sanctions. If legal sanctions are to be used at all, they must only supplement, not substitute for, education and social services. It would be a huge misuse of effort and resources to criminalize transmission of AIDS while at the same time underfunding AIDS-related research, education, and social services.

In sum, we believe that criminal law, like civil law, can have some deterrent effect on AIDS transmission. If criminalization imposed no social cost, we would view it as a useful backstop to education and the dictates of individual conscience, and would urge adoption of AIDS-specific statutes. But there are real costs involved in regulating this area by criminal enactment—costs that threaten the sexual privacy of us all and that risk official harassment of gay men. The marginal deterrence that such an enactment might add to incentives that already exist is not worth the costs that criminal regulation would entail.

NOTES

The authors are grateful to Valerie Sanchez for invaluable research assistance.

[1] The call for criminalization is becoming more fashionable daily, across the political spectrum. See, e.g., Grady, A haunting issue for '88, *Boston Globe*, June 3, 1987: 19, col. 5 (noting that potential presidential candidate Mario Cuomo, the governor of New York, "would make it a crime to knowingly transmit AIDS"); Safire, Failing the tests, *New York Times*, June 4, 1987: A27, col. 5 ("Should states make it a crime to knowingly transmit [AIDS] with malice aforethought? You bet"); Tax change advocate suffering from AIDS, *New York Times*, June 10, 1987: A29, col. 4 (quoting California tax revolt leader Paul Gann, infected with AIDS through a blood transfusion, as saying that people who knowingly transmit AIDS "should be tried for murder, because if you give it to someone, it's a death sentence").

[2] See Turner, The military battles a new biological weapon: AIDS, *National Law Journal*, May 11, 1987: 6; AIDS-infected soldier faces trial for having sex, *Boston Globe*, June 4, 1987: 14, col. 3. In announcing the court-martial, Army officials called it the first such case in military or civilian courts. Civilian criminal codes likewise typically define aggravated assault as assault "with a deadly weapon." See, e.g., *Model Penal Code* §211.1(2)(b).

[3] See Cummings, Charges filed against blood donor in AIDS case, *New York Times*, June 30, 1987: A18, col. 1.

[4] In this paper we use the term "person with AIDS" as defined by the Centers for Disease Control: someone who has one of eight sorts of diseases that indicate the suppression of the immune system where there is no other explanation for that suppression. See Masur and Macher, Acquired immune deficiency syndrome (AIDS), in Mandell, Douglas, and Bennett, eds., *Principles and practice of infectious diseases*, 1985: 1670. We use the term "AIDS carrier" or "HIV carrier" to describe someone who is infected with the human immunodeficiency virus that is believed to be the cause of AIDS but who has not yet contracted any of the diseases. Some AIDS carriers exhibit symptoms of "AIDS-related complex." Others do not exhibit such symptoms, although they would test positive on the HIV-antibody test. See id.: 622; Weber et al., Three-year prospective study of HTLV-III/LAV infection in homosexual men, *Lancet*, May 24, 1986: 1179. Other infected individuals would not even be detected by the test, which yields negatives as well as a substantial number of false positives. See Counsel on Scientific Affairs, Status report on the acquired immunodeficiency syndrome: HTLV-III testing, *Journal of the American Medical Association* 1985, 245(10): 342–45.

[5] For example, calls for quarantine led in November 1986 to a California ballot measure that would have subjected those testing positive for HIV to reporting and isolation. The measure was defeated by a large margin. Proposition 65 on the California Ballot (November 4, 1986). But calls for quarantine persist today. See, e.g., Roberts, AIDS alert: Politicians awaken to the threat of a global epidemic, *New York Times*, June 7, 1987: sec. 4, p. 1 (noting that evangelist and presidential candidate Rev. Pat Robertson has advocated quarantine). When "quarantine" is mentioned in connection with AIDS, it might imply any of a range of possibilities, from public incarceration to confinement to one's home, from total isolation from others to prohibition only of sexual contacts, to name but a few possibilities. We regard all of these methods as grossly overbroad and possibly unconstitutional. The issue of quarantine is more fully discussed in Curran WJ, Clark ME, Gostin L, AIDS: Legal and policy implications of the application of traditional disease control measures, *Law, Medicine & Health Care* 1987, 15 (1–2): 27–35.

[6] Sexual acts of transmission apparently account for the overwhelming majority of AIDS cases today. Curran JW et al., The epidemiology of AIDS: Current status and future prospects, *Science* 1985, 229: 1352–57. Blood-to-blood contact through the sharing of needles for intravenous injection and blood transfusions have been the major other vehicles of transmission. Some unusual cases of blood-to-blood contact have also been documented, including one where a boy transmitted the AIDS virus to his brother by biting him, and others where hospital workers became infected when AIDS-infected blood splashed onto their broken skin or mucous membranes. Boy apparently gave AIDS to sibling, *Boston Globe*, Sept. 28, 1986: 28; 3 Health workers found infected by blood of patients with AIDS, *New York Times*, May 20, 1987: 1, col. 3. But such cases are exceedingly rare. Finally, transmission of AIDS from mothers to children during pregnancy or childbirth accounts for some cases.

This paper will focus on sexual acts of transmission, both because they are the most prevalent and because they raise especially grave questions about the limits of government power to regulate privacy. Regulating transmission by pregnancy would of course raise similar questions. To the extent that this paper touches on non-sexual acts of transmission, it will chiefly address needle-sharing, as transmission of AIDS through blood transfusions has by now been virtually eliminated by screening of the country's blood supply.

We do not discuss at any length non-sexual acts or threats of transmission that are just like conventional assaults or threats of assault. Such cases occasionally catch press attention. For example, police have charged a number of suspected AIDS carriers with such crimes as assault, reckless endangerment, and even attempted murder for trying to bite officers while in custody for other offenses. See Boorstin, Criminal and civil litigation on spread of AIDS appears, *New York Times*, June 19, 1987: 1, col. 3. It would be a great error, however, to use such cases as a guide to criminalizing AIDS transmission. They are exceedingly rare, and may in any event be treated as analogous to conventional assaults without raising the special problems that are our focus here.

[7] See *Model Penal Code* part 1, vol. 1, p. 233 n.4.

[8] See *Model Penal Code* §2.02(2). The degree of criminal intent required for a particular crime is central in determining whether criminal liability exists and, if so, how harshly it will be punished.

[9] See *Model Penal Code* §2.02(s)(c)–(d).

[10] The *Model Penal Code* acknowledges that legislatures may choose to impose such liability. *Model Penal Code* §2.05.

[11] See gen., *Morissette v. United States*, 342 U.S. 246 (1952). As Justice Jackson wrote in *Morissette*, strict liability crimes "do not fit neatly into . . . common-law offenses [for they] are not in the nature of positive aggressions or invasions . . . but are in the nature of neglect where the law requires care, or inaction where it imposes a duty. Many violations of such regulations result in no direct or immediate injury to person or property but merely create the danger or probabilty of it which the law seeks to minimize." Id.: 255–56.

[12] We generally use the pronoun "he" to refer to AIDS transmitters in this paper. We do so because male-to-male and male-to-female sexual transmission has been to date more prevalent than female-to-male. Female-to-female sexual transmission is virtually unknown though not impossible. Of course, non-sexual transmission is more symmetrical across gender lines. Where appropriate, our use of the pronoun "he" is intended to be generic.

[13] *Model Penal Code* §210.2(I)(b).

[14] The common law punished deaths caused in the course of such independent felonies as "felony murder." The *Model Penal Code* abandons the strict liability aspects of the felony murder rule but still gives some weight to the fact that the homicide was accompanied by a violent felony. It substitutes for the felony murder rule a presumption that the recklessness and the extreme-indifference-to-the-value-of-human-life requisite to murder exist when a homicide is committed during the course of certain enumerated felonies, one of which is rape. See *Model Penal Code* §210.2(I)(b). Recklessness and extreme indifference are presumed if the defendant "is engaged or is an accomplice in the commission of, or an attempt to commit, or flight after committing or attempting to commit robbery, rape, or deviate sexual intercourse by force or threat of force, arson, burglary, kidnapping or felonious escape." Id.

[15] By endangering many people for profit, the prostitute might well satisfy the standard of extreme indifference to the value of human life that separates reckless murder from reckless manslaughter.

[16] Such a rapist might well be guilty of felony murder as well as rape under the common law, or of reckless-plus-extreme-indifference murder under the *Model Penal Code* approach.

[17] See Barnes DM, Grim projections for AIDS epidemic, *Science* 1986, 232: 1589–90.

[18] *Model Penal Code* §210.4, comment #3, at p. 86. The defendant's failure to perceive a risk that he will cause death must involve a "gross deviation from the standard of care that a reasonable person would observe in the actor's situation." *Model Penal Code* §2.02(2)(d).

[19] The *Model Penal Code* explicitly makes it an offense purposely to help another to commit suicide. See *Model Penal Code* §210.5(2).

[20] See, e.g., *State v. Minster*, 486 A. 2d 1197, 1200 & n. 5 (Md. Ct. App. 1985) (listing states).

[21] The *Model Penal Code* also makes it a crime recklessly to endanger another person. See *Model Penal Code* §211.2. This crime is classified as less serious than negligent homicide. The reckless transmitter of AIDS might be liable under this provision, as well as for attempted murder or assault, without regard to whether the victim died.

[22] Homicide is always punished as a felony, with sentences ranging from one year to life in prison, or the death penalty in those states that retain it. Most states punish attempted murder less severely than they would punish the equivalent acts if the victim had died, and they never utilize the death penalty for attempt. Assault is normally a misdemeanor punishable by no more than one year in prison. If assault is "aggravated" by conduct manifesting extreme indifference to the value of human life (for example, by use of a deadly weapon), it may be punished for a longer term as a felony.

[23] The common-law doctrine of "factual impossibility" might provide a defense if one's belief that one was an AIDS carrier proved in fact to be mistaken, so that one's "attempt" proved futile. Many jurisdictions, however, have abandoned that defense because it makes liability of equally culpable persons turn on a fortuity. For example, the *Model Penal Code* provides for attempt liability where one "purposely engages in conduct which would constitute the crime if the attendant circumstances were as he believes them to be." §5.01(I)(a).

[24] *Model Penal Code* §5.01(I)(b)

[25] *Model Penal Code* §211.1 (I)(a). The common law labeled such crimes of physical injury "battery" and treated attempted battery as "assault." We here take the *Model Penal Code's* approach of labeling as "assault" what the common law would have called "battery."

[26] *Model Penal Code* §211.1(2)(a). Use of a deadly weapon is the typical conduct manifesting the required indifference. Aggravated assault was one of the crimes charged in the military court-martial case described at the beginning of this paper, on the theory that the AIDS virus itself is a deadly weapon.

[27] See *Model Penal Code* §2.11(2)(b)(permitting consent as a defense to serious bodily injury *only* where such injury is a "reasonably foreseeable hazard" of participation in sports or athletic contests).

[28] 176 Eng. Rep. 925 (W. Cir. Ct. 1866). The Army court-martial described at the beginning of this paper provides a modern analogue. In that case, the Army dropped the aggravated assault charge with respect to the defendant's sex acts with a soldier who was aware that the defendant had tested positive for AIDS. The Army pursued only the charges involving the defendant's sex acts with two other soldiers who had not known that fact. Army will try AIDS carrier, *National Law Journal*, June 15, 1987:7, col. 1.

[29] See *Model Penal Code* §2.11(2)(b)(2).

[30] Indeed, if lack of information about a sexual partner's disease vitiates consent, the same analysis would turn consensual sexual intercourse into rape where disease is transmitted in the process—a metamorphosis that shows that the point goes too far.

[31] See, e.g., Texas Rev. Civ. State Ann. §4419b-I, 6.01–6.07 (making it a third-degree felony for a person to knowingly conceal or attempt to conceal the fact that he or she has been exposed to or is a carrier of a communicable disease that constitutes a threat to the public health, and a misdemeanor for a person with such a disease to attend or attempt to attend a public or private place or gathering).

[32] See, e.g., Cal. Health & Safety Stat. §3198 (making it a misdemeanor for any person afflicted with a venereal disease to willfully expose himself to others, and for any person so to willfully expose another person afflicted with such disease); N.Y. State Sanitary Code, §§2307, 2309 (making it a misdemeanor for anyone who knows she/he has an infectious venereal disease to have sexual intercourse with another); Fla. Stat. Ann. §§384.01, 384.02 (making it a second-degree misdemeanor for any person infected with venereal disease to have sex with a person of the opposite sex or to expose another to infection); Colo. Rev. Stat. §25-4-401 (making it unlawful for any person who has knowledge or reasonable grounds to suspect tthat he is infected with a venereal disease to willfully expose or infect another, or to knowingly perform an act that exposes or infects another person with venereal disease).

[33] See Idaho Code §39-601 (classifying AIDS, ARC, or HIV as venereal diseases and prohibiting persons with these diseases from knowingly or willfully exposing another to the infection).

[34] See, e.g., Fla. House Bill 484 (would designate AIDS as a venereal disease and prohibit infected individuals from transmitting it to others); Fla. Senate Bill 576 (would make it a misdemeanor for anyone with a sexually transmitted disease to have sexual intercourse); Pa. House Bill 1787 (would make it a misdemeanor for a person who knows that he has AIDS to transmit the disease to another person through sexual contact; second or subsequent offenses would constitute a felony); Ga. House Bill 1187 (would define AIDS as a venereal disease).

[35] Under some of the definitions of the offenses, using precautions might constitute a defense; under others, even using precautions and obtaining the informed consent of one's partner could not exculpate one from the crime of having sex while infected.

[36] It would be difficult to make a priority of punishing persons already dying from AIDS. Some carriers, however, are symptomless.

[37] We define "intimate sexual activity" broadly to include all consensual sexual contacts. It does not include rape. How to treat prostitution is unclear. At first glance, the public interest appears unambiguous and the private interest minimal in the case of the prostitute who continues to ply his or her trade after a diagnosis of AIDS. Prostitution involves multiple sex partners by definition, and is premised on money, not love. On the other hand, people other than prostitutes also have sex with multiple partners, and prostitutes may be more likely than others to institutionalize the use of precautions against AIDS transmission as a business practice.

[38] The important interest in avoiding governmental regulation of intimate sexual activity of course applies no matter how the AIDS virus was acquired. The person who acquired it through intravenous drug abuse or through a blood transfusion has the same interest in a future intimate sex life as the person who acquired it initially through sexual intercourse.

[39] See *Griswold v. Connecticut*, 381 U.S. 479 (1965) (invalidating state criminal law barring even married couples from using contraceptives); *Eisenstadt v. Baird*, 405 U.S. 438 (1972) (extending to unmarried persons the right of access to contraceptives); *Carey v. Population Services, Inc.*, 431 U.S. 678 (1977) (same); *Roe v. Wade*, 410 U.S. 113 (1973) (invalidating state criminal law barring woman's choice of abortion). Laws burdening the right to privacy are subject to strict scrutiny and can be upheld only upon demonstration that the law is necessary to serve a compelling state interest.

To be sure, the Supreme Court has never held in such cases that the constitutional right to privacy protects consensual adult sex acts themselves, as opposed to access to contraception and abortion that may facilitate those sex acts. Indeed, the Court recently held that a law criminalizing oral and anal sexual contacts between consenting adults in private need not serve any compelling interest, but may be upheld simply because it expresses majority morality. *Bowers v. Hardwick*, 106 S. Ct. 2841 (1986); see id. at 2844 (asserting that the right to engage in oral or anal sex bears no "resemblance" to the right to use contraceptives). But we believe that any attempt to sever the contraception decisions from sexual activity is absurd; anti-contraception laws were no burden, after all, for the sexually celibate or abstinent.

[40] Justice Blackmun articulated such a theory in his dissent in *Bowers v. Hardwick*, joined by three other Justices. Id. at 2851. Choice concerning sexual activity might also be protected under the First Amendment as expression. The Court's decision in *Stanley v. Georgia*, 394 U.S. 557 (1969), lends indirect support to both these stories. *Stanley* held that it violated a person's right to privacy to convict him for possessing pornography in his own home. *Stanley* expressly linked the value of privacy to the liberty of conscience and self-expression protected by the First Amendment.

[41] Such a theory seems to underlie the Supreme Court's general efforts to locate the right to privacy in either the liberty clause of the Fourteenth Amendment or in the Ninth Amendment, which protects fundamental rights not explicitly enumerated in the Bill of Rights. The premise of either approach is that our society cannot be truly free if government interferes in such matters as whether and when we breed, see, e.g., *Skinner v. Oklahoma*, 316 U.S. 535 (1942) (striking down law providing for mandatory sterilization of recidivist felon), or how we choose to arrange our family household, see, e.g., *Moore v. City of East Cleveland*, 431 U.S. 494 (1977) (striking down conviction of grandmother for living with two non-sibling grandchildren, in violation of local zoning ordinance). Under a Fourteenth Amendment approach such interference would be incompatible with "ordered liberty;" under a Ninth Amendment approach, it would transgress the boundaries of a sphere we never ceded to government, such as the sphere of family and reproduction.

[42] Accordingly, even if such regulation did implicate a constitutionally protected right to privacy, it might still be upheld as closely serving a compelling state interest. The only time in the nation's history that the Supreme Court has upheld a severe deprivation of liberty on such a ground was in its decisions upholding the internment of Japanese-Americans during World War II. See *Korematsu v. United States*, 323 U.S. 214 (1944). There the compelling factor was war, and even so many have since considered the Supreme Court deeply wrong in its judgment that herding Japanese-Americans into camps was necessary to avert the danger of wartime espionage. See, e.g., Irons P, Justice at war, 1983; Grodzins M, Americans betrayed, 1974; Rostow, The Japanese-American cases—A disaster, *Yale Law Journal* 1945, 54: 489. But epidemics, like war, may be held to create compelling circumstances.

[43] In other words, the key question in assessing whether laws regulating AIDS transmission violate constitutionally protected liberty or privacy will concern means more than ends. It will ask not whether fighting AIDS is important but, rather, whether each law is closely tailored to the fight. See, gen., Note, The constitutional rights of AIDS carriers, *Harvard Law Review* 1986, 99: 1274, 1279–92.

[44] Those who hold such a view would presumably advocate also abstinence from drug use, at least illegal drug use. The problem is that such a prohibition would be without effect, given that the law already forbids such drug use.

[45] Such a law would be even more unrealistic and unjustifiable if it criminalized sexual acts other than vaginal and anal intercourse. AIDS is not transmittable by hand-to-genital contact. To date, there is likewise no evidence that AIDS is easily transmittable by kissing, even though experts have not excluded the possibility of such transmission. See, e.g., Altman, Health experts find no evidence to link AIDS to kissing, *New York Times*, June 8, 1987: B6, col. 2. Doubt similarly exists about the transmissibility of AIDS through oral sex. Curran et al., supra note 6. Fear of AIDS transmission may of course induce people to shift their sexual practices away from sexual intercourse and toward these other modes. Indeed, evidence of sharply reduced rectal gonorrhea rates among gay men suggests that many in that community have done just that. Centers for Disease Control, Self-reported behavior change among gay and bisexual men—San Francisco, *Morbidity and Mortality Weekly Report* 1985, 34(40): 613–15; Schecter MT et al., Changes in sexual behavior and fear of AIDS, *Lancet* 1984, 1: 1293; Centers for Disease Control, Declining rates of rectal and pharyngeal gonorrhea among males—NYC, *Morbidity and Mortality Weekly Report* 1984, 33: 295–97. But we believe the state should not seek to rule out sexual intercourse altogether for AIDS carriers for life.

[46] Some believe that criminal stigma should be reserved only for conscious wrongdoers, because those who fail to take care out of ignorance or carelessness cannot be deterred by the criminal law. See, e.g., Williams G, *Criminal law*, 1953: 120–25. The more plausible position, however, would seem to be that imposing criminal liability for negligence *can* deter by providing an additional motive to "take care before acting." *Model Penal Code* §2.02, comment at 126–27; see also Hart HLA, *Punishment and responsibility*, 1968: 152–54.

[47] The fact that these social consequences now attach to a positive AIDS test is the principal reason that mandatory AIDS testing is controversial. Public health officials widely fear that if mandatory testing is imposed, fear of these consequences will drive many of the infected "underground." See, e.g., Boffey, Health officials fear "sideshow" efforts will hurt AIDS fight, *New York Times*, June 8, 1987: B6, col. 2. If these consequences could be eliminated, much opposition to testing would disappear. It is not the invasion of bodily privacy itself that is objectionable; just as the Supreme Court long ago held that mandatory smallpox vaccination did not unconstitutionally invade liberty or privacy, so a blood test involves minimal intrusion. See *Jacobson v. Massachusetts*, 197 U.S. 11 (1905). What is feared is, rather, that the test will be a vehicle for discrimination, whether against currently unpopular groups at high risk, such as gay men and intravenous drug abusers, or against a new social underclass of AIDS carriers of all descriptions.

[48] Indeed, the most widely used voluntary test might be one that is entirely anonymous—for example, one that could be used at home, like a home pregnancy test. The problem with such an innovation might be, however, that it would be administered without the opportunity for immediate counseling about its meaning and about how a positive tester should now behave.

[49] Senator Ted Kennedy recently introduced such an anti-discrimination measure as part of a proposed Senate bill dealing with AIDS. 100th Cong. S.1220.

[50] By contrast, a jury might convict an AIDS carrier of negligent AIDS transmission even if he used a condom during sex. The statistics on pregnancy despite use of condoms as a contraceptive suggest that condoms break between 2 and 20 percent of the time. Fischl MA et al. Evaluation of heterosexual partners, children and household contacts of adults with AIDS, *Journal of the American Medical Association* 1987, 257: 640–44. A jury might deem the risk of sex even with a condom unreasonable.

[51] A requirement of disclosure seems more realistic as applied to sexual transmission in intimate relationships than to cases of transmission by needlesharing, where the parties may be strangers. Needlesharing is not an intimate act in the sense that sexual relations are. Accordingly, use of precautions alone might appropriately negate the offense of transmission by needlesharing.

[52] It is often suggested that failure to inform one's sexual partners of an AIDS risk is not blameworthy because they assume the risk by having sex at all. We do not think that approach is appropriate. Because only one party has access to the relevant information, it does not unduly burden him to have to disclose it. Having sex should no more mean one is assuming the risk of disease than going to a singles bar and having a drink should mean one is assuming the risk of date rape. See generally Estrich S, *Real rape*, Cambridge: Harvard University Press, 1987.

[53] The problem is that the chance of actually contracting AIDS after exposure to the virus increases with increased exposure. American College Health Association, *AIDS—What everyone should know*, Health Information Series, 1985: 2.

[54] A statute that *required* the use of condoms would in a sense be the inverse of state statutes *forbidding* contraceptive use, such as the one struck down in *Griswold v. Connecticut*, supra note 39. Surely an exception to a condom requirement would have to be made for persons trying to become pregnant. The precise scope of any such exception would no doubt be the subject of heated debate.

[55] See, e.g., *United States v. Cincotta*, 689 F.2d 238, 243 & n. 2 (1st Cir. 1982); *United States v. Jewell*, 532 F.2d 697 (9th Cir. 1976); see also *Model Penal Code* §2.02(7) ("knowledge [of a fact] is established if a person is aware of a high probability of its existence, unless he actually believes that it does not exist.") Of course, the "willful blindness" theory will tend to collapse knowledge into recklessness unless the defendant is shown to have known other facts suggesting a very high probability of the "fact" he was trying to avoid.

[56] To the extent this is not the case, the solution is not to broaden the category of persons covered by the criminal law here but, rather, to provide for adequate counseling in conjunction with voluntary tests.

[57] The best precaution for needle-users would be not reusing needles. But that is a requirement that only the wealthy addict may be able to meet. Unless free new needles were widely available at public expense, therefore, a reasonable attempt to sterilize a needle before reuse should be enough.

[58] If so, it would be better for the government to remove from the market the condoms that are thought inadequate, rather than to broaden the criminal law.

[59] The law elsewhere as well imposes separate penalties on those who cause harm to others while doing something that is already criminal—for example, one who kills while committing the crime of drunk driving may also be convicted of manslaughter.

[60] The Supreme Court's recent decision in *Bowers v. Hardwick*, 106 S. Ct. 2841 (1986), may be interpreted by police as legitimating such discrimination. In that case, the Supreme Court held that a statute criminalizing anal and oral sex violated no constitutional right to privacy when applied to same-sex contacts, while leaving open whether it would do so when people of opposite sexes commit precisely the same sex act.

[61] Indeed, the Supreme Court this term upheld as constitutional a federal statute providing for the pretrial detention of persons deemed likely to be dangerous to the community if freed on bail. *United States v. Salerno*, 107 S. Ct. 2095 (1987). The Court's tolerance of such a measure as permissibly "regulatory" rather than impermissibly "punitive" may arguably signal a willingness to tolerate the preventive incarceration of suspected AIDS carriers even in the absence of any conviction of guilt.

[62] Of course, the danger of such selectivity will diminish as AIDS spreads further through the heterosexual population. Moreover, such selectivity might be unconstitutional if it is sufficiently systematic. While it is doubtful that anti-gay discrimination in the application of the law would be strictly scrutinized, as would racially selective prosecution—see, e.g., *Yick Wo v. Hopkins*, 118 U.S. 356 (1886) (striking down the selective prosecution of Chinese-owned laundries under a facially neutral ordinance purporting to regulate all wooden laundries)—it might be struck down even under minimal scrutiny as arbitrary and irrational, provided the selection could be shown to be motivated by "mere negative attitudes [toward], or fear [of]" gay men. See *City of Cleburne v. Cleburne Living Center*, 105 S. Ct. 3249, 3259 (1985) (invalidating the exclusion of a group home for the mentally retarded from a residential neighborhood where no reason beyond irrational fear and hatred of the mentally retarded had been demonstrated).

[63] See *Bowers v. Hardwick*, 106 S. Ct. at 2848 n. 2 (Blackmun, J., dissenting) (listing states).

[64] While the plaintiff in *Hardwick* was arrested and jailed overnight, he was not ultimately prosecuted, convicted, and sentenced. See id. at 2848 (Powell, J., concurring). The very absence of convictions under the sodomy laws made it difficult for civil liberties lawyers to find any better test case than *Hardwick* with which to challenge the validity of those laws.

[65] See, e.g., Brief of Amici Curiae American Psychological Association and American Public Health Association at 19–27, *Bowers v. Hardwick*, 106 S. Ct. 2841 (1986) (arguing that sodomy laws disserve the public health by interfering with AIDS treatment, research, and education).

[66] See Hermann DHJ, Liability related to diagnosis and transmission of AIDS, *Law, Medicine & Health Care* 1987, 15(1–2): 36–45.

[67] See Top health official urges frank talks to young on AIDS, *New York Times*, Oct. 23, 1986: 1, col. 6.

[68] For example, Markowski, allegedly a prostitute, charged with attempted murder for selling his blood even though he knew he was infected with AIDS said he did so because "when you have to survive you'll do anything." Cummings, supra note 3.

12

The Limits of Quarantine as a Measure for Controlling the Spread of AIDS

Mark Blumberg

$\mathbf{T}$his article analyzes the limitations inherent in utilizing quarantine as a means of controlling the transmission of the human immunodeficiency virus (HIV).[1] The discussion focuses on several possible types of forced isolation which could be employed to slow the spread of the epidemic. In each case, the analysis examines whether the proposed measure achieves its intended public policy goal (i.e., controlling the epidemic) or whether the social costs of a particular course of action outweigh any benefits to be derived.

Quarantine is an attempt to protect the health of the community through the forced isolation of infected persons.[2] The courts have consistently ruled that state officials have the power to impose a quarantine when public health concerns make this necessary.[3] Historically, forced isolation has been used to control a variety of diseases (e.g., smallpox, bubonic plague, yellow fever, syphilis, etc.—Parmet, 1985). Despite a considerable degree of public support for such a policy (Blendon and Donelan, 1988:1025), quarantine has not been utilized in the battle against AIDS except in the case of a few infected individuals who have continued to engage in high-risk sexual behavior. Because HIV is not transmitted through casual contact

This is a revised version of a paper that was presented to the 1989 Annual Meeting of the Academy of Criminal Justice Sciences in Washington, D.C.

The author would like to express his appreciation to Harriet Frazier, Douglas Heckathorn, Allen Sapp, and Donald Wallace, who reviewed an earlier draft of this paper and contributed valuable comments. A debt of gratitude is also owed to Monica Weaver for her painstaking proofreading and typing assistance.

137

(Friedland, Saltzman, Rogers et al., 1986), nearly all public health officials oppose this measure with respect to the control of AIDS.

Several different forms of quarantine could conceivably be implemented to control HIV. The broadest approach would be the forced isolation of all seropositive individuals. Another possibility is a quarantine directed only at persons who actually have symptoms of AIDS. A third approach would be to quarantine only those infected individuals who continue to engage in the types of high-risk behaviors (unsafe sex or needlesharing) that jeopardize the health of others. Finally, a quarantine could be directed at members of certain groups that are at high risk of developing AIDS (i.e., gay males, intravenous drug users, and/or female prostitutes).[4] The social benefits and costs of each of these approaches are examined.

SEROPOSITIVES

The most extensive quarantine would be the forced isolation of all persons infected with HIV. Because such a policy would be misguided for practical, ethical, and financial reasons no jurisdiction has seriously contemplated this course of action. For one thing, the number of persons estimated to be infected may be as high as 1.4 million (Centers for Disease Control, 1987:15). Clearly, any quarantine that involved this many individuals would be extremely expensive. Not only would the government be faced with the costs of housing and feeding these individuals,[5] there would be the additional medical costs of providing AZT[6] and treating individuals who become ill.[7] Because the purpose of this detention would be civil in nature and not for punishment, the courts would require that isolated individuals be confined in humane facilities (Gostin and Curran, 1986:27). This would entail large expenditures of public funds.

Society would also be faced with the question of identifying all infected persons. Because no master list exists, it would be necessary to institute mandatory testing of the entire population. In addition to the costs of testing, police and public health officials would be required to spend a substantial amount of time apprehending those who refused to be tested. Clearly, these resources could be more effectively utilized for education, research and treatment.

Quarantining all infected persons would be problematic for other reasons as well. Such a policy would entail depriving of their liberty many individuals who do not engage in high-risk behavior and thus pose no threat to the health of others. In addition, the economic loss to society would be enormous. This massive detention would result in many asymptomatic individuals being denied employment and the opportunity to support their dependents for an indefinite period.

Not only would the forced isolation of all infected persons have enormous costs, it would also produce limited results. Because the AIDS antibody test cannot identify persons who have recently contracted the virus,[8] any system of universal screening is likely to miss a substantial number of infected persons. As a consequence, the forced isolation of those believed to be seropositive would give the rest of the population a false sense of security. Some people would be tempted to engage in risky behavior, believing incorrectly that all infected individuals had been placed under quarantine.

PERSONS WITH AIDS

Placing only those who had been diagnosed with full-blown AIDS in isolation would avoid many of the problems associated with a quarantine of all seropositive individuals. Identifying persons with AIDS would be a relatively simple task because AIDS is a reportable disease, and attending physicians and hospitals are required to submit the names of patients diagnosed with this ailment to the United States Public Health Service (Curran, Clark and Gostin, 1987). In addition, the costs associated with this type of quarantine would be substantially less because significantly fewer individuals would be involved. However, this approach would be totally ineffective because it would not isolate the great majority of infected persons, those who appear healthy yet can transmit the virus. Under these circumstances, the courts might rule that because such a quarantine is underinclusive in scope and does not protect public health, it would amount to confinement based merely on illness, and thus would violate the Constitution.[9]

INFECTED PERSONS WHO CONTINUE TO ENGAGE IN RISKY BEHAVIOR

Several states have enacted statutes that authorize the forced isolation of those infected persons who continue to engage in high-risk behavior. Unlike traditional public health measures that gave officials broad discretion to isolate persons, these modern statutes often provide subjects with a considerable amount of due process protection (Gostin, 1989). In addition, the forced isolation of these few recalcitrant individuals does not pose many of the problems that would plague a broader quarantine. Nonetheless, opponents still raise a number of objections.

For one thing, predicting future behavior is difficult. Because a person has engaged in high-risk behavior in the recent past does not necessarily mean that he or she will continue to do so in the future. Individuals who are seropositive are believed to remain infectious for the rest of their lives. Therefore, a quarantine based on past behavior could conceivably last for an indefinite period.

Second, widespread use of this approach could discourage members of high-risk groups from cooperating with public health officials. The strategy for controlling the AIDS epidemic has been to encourage persons who may be at risk to seek voluntary testing and counseling. If a positive test result could later be the basis for being placed in quarantine, there would be little incentive to learn one's HIV status.

Third, enforcement of this type of quarantine could entail massive intrusion by both public health officials and courts into the most private aspect of our lives, i.e., the bedroom. In order to learn whether high-risk activities were occurring, it would be necessary for officials to delve into such questions as which sexual acts were being performed by infected persons[10] and whether condoms were being used.

Finally, any quarantine based on behavior is likely to be selective in nature. As previously noted, there are approximately 1.4 million persons infected with HIV in the United States. Because public health officials have no way of monitoring the conduct of so many people, only in rare cases will they learn about risky behavior on the part of infected individuals. As a consequence, this type of quarantine could easily become a tool for the selective harassment of unpopular or outspoken members of high-risk groups who were infected with the AIDS virus.

Despite these concerns, it might be argued that such behavior-based statutes are advisable to placate the public and prevent passage of more draconian measures. "Horror stories" have already appeared in which law enforcement personnel and public health authorities have argued that, despite intense public concern, they are powerless to take action against infected individuals who continue to engage in high-risk activities (*New York Times*, 12/26/85). These situations will test the ability of public officials to fashion policy based on medical evidence and rational policy concerns, rather than caving in to public demands to get tough on AIDS. The publicity surrounding the behavior of persons who continue to engage in high-risk sexual activities can serve an important educational objective, reinforcing the message that everyone has an obligation to avoid the types of behavior that can put one at risk of contracting HIV (i.e., unsafe sex and needlesharing).

HOMOSEXUAL/BISEXUAL MALES

Sixty-eight percent of adult/adolescent persons with AIDS in the United States are homosexual or bisexual males (Centers for Disease Control, 1989:9). Epidemiological studies have reported that almost one-half the gay men in certain neighborhoods of San Francisco are infected with HIV (Winkelstein, Samuel, Padian et al, 1987). However, because of the long incubation period for AIDS, it is clear that many of these individuals were infected several years ago. Recent evidence strongly suggests that gay men have changed their sexual behavior and that the rate of new infection has been declining among this group (McKusick, Wiley, Coates et al., 1985; Winkelstein, Samuel, Padian et al., 1987:687).

As the AIDS epidemic has developed, the gay community has taken the lead in encouraging its members to avoid unsafe sex. As a consequence, any quarantine directed at homosexuals would isolate many uninfected persons as well as many individuals who do not currently engage in high-risk behavior. Even if a quarantine of gay males were desirable (which it is not), it would not be feasible. How would gay males be identified? What level of proof would be required to determine sexual preference? Would decisions with respect to isolation be based on rumors? The potential for denial of civil liberties, harassment, and persecution inherent in such a policy would be enormous.

Despite the draconian nature of this type of quarantine, it would have little practical effect. The gay community is a fairly self-contained entity. To date, only 5 percent of the adult/adolescent AIDS cases reported in the United States have involved heterosexual transmission (Centers for Disease Control, 1989:9). Five times as many females have been infected through sexual contact with IVDUs, as opposed to contact with bisexual males (Friedland and Klein, 1987:1129). Any quarantine directed at gay men would probably miss many bisexual individuals. Because these deeply closeted males often lead straight lives (i.e., are married or have girlfriends), they would not be identified as gay and thus not be subject to isolation.

INTRAVENOUS DRUG USERS

The National Institute on Drug Abuse (NIDA) estimates that there are 1.28 million IV drug users in the United States and that 70 percent are black or Hispanic (Stengel, 1987:13). Because they often share needles and syringes, many of these IVDUs have become infected with HIV. Twenty-seven percent of persons with AIDS have intravenous drug use as a risk factor (Centers for Disease Control, 1989:9). Among minorities, almost one-half of AIDS cases have been linked to IVDU, in contrast to just 14 percent among whites (Centers for Disease Control, 1989:9).

IVDUs (most of whom are heterosexual) are a threat to both the persons with whom they share needles and to their sex partners. Sixty-one percent of the AIDS cases involving heterosexual transmission among persons born in the United States involve individuals who report sexual contact with an IVDU (Haverkos and Edelman, 1988: 1925). Because intravenous drug abuse occurs most often in poor, inner-city neighborhoods, black females are 11 to 13 times more likely than whites to be infected (Friedland and Klein, 1987:1128). In addition, the overwhelming majority of pediatric AIDS cases are linked to mothers who are either intravenous drug users or the sex partners of IVDUs (Moss, 1987:389).

It might seem that the forced isolation of IVDUs would be wise public policy. However, more careful consideration reveals that this course of action would not be advisable. For one thing, the hardships associated with a quarantine directed at IVDUs would be felt most heavily in the black and Hispanic communities. Such a move would be perceived by many as a racially motivated attempt to fight the epidemic by detaining hundreds of thousands of blacks and Hispanics.

Other problems would make this plan unworkable. In addition to the enormous financial costs that would be incurred, there is the question of who would be considered eligible for quarantine under this approach. Would society attempt to isolate only current users, or anybody who had a history of IVDU since 1978, when the AIDS virus first appeared in the United States? Quarantining only current users would miss many former users who have become infected through needlesharing. Attempting to identify all persons who have injected drugs since the late 1970s would be an impossible task.[11] Furthermore, neither approach would be effective, because many seropositive sex partners of these persons would remain at large in the community.

There is a final consideration. HIV is not transmitted through intravenous drugs, but through the sharing of contaminated needles and syringes. Therefore, those at risk are not IVDUs per se, but IVDUs who have shared needles or syringes. It would not be possible to identify such individuals without widescale mandatory HIV screening and all the problems that widespread testing would entail.[12] Clearly, it would seem preferable to allow IVDUs to purchase sterile needles. Preliminary data suggest that the rate of HIV infection among IVDUs is substantially lower in those states that permit over-the-counter sale of hypodermic needles (Raymond, 1988:2620). In addition, studies conducted in cities where sterile needles have been made available to IVDUs indicate that the rate of new infection among this group tends to decline after these programs are introduced (Raymond, 1988). Such an approach is far less costly and would not entail the massive deprivation of liberty that is inherent in a policy of quarantine.

FEMALE PROSTITUTES

Many street prostitutes are IVDUs. As a consequence, a substantial number have become infected with the AIDS virus. In fact, almost all prostitutes who have become infected report a history of intravenous drug use (Cohen, Alexander and Wofsy, 1988:20). In general, the proportion of infected prostitutes in a given community is related to the prevalence of HIV infection found among IVDUs in that locale (Cohen, Alexander and Wofsy, 1988). Because the average female prostitute sees approximately 1,500 male customers per year (Bergman, 1988:782–783), concern has been expressed that sex workers are a potential source of HIV infection. If that were the case, the forced isolation of these individuals might be considered as one option for preventing the transmission of the virus. However, a closer examination of the facts reveals that such a course of action would be ill advised.

There are over 100,000 arrests for prostitution each year in the United States. The AIDS virus has been present in the U.S. since at least 1978. Indeed, there are a handful of heterosexual males who claim to have become infected through contact with female prostitutes. However, not a single case to date has been definitely traced to a specific prostitute (Cohen, Alexander and Wofsy, 1988:18). If sexual contact with female prostitutes were an important source of HIV transmission, there should have been hundreds (if not thousands) of cases reported by now in which this activity was a risk factor (Bergman, 1988:783).

Although AIDS is predominantly a sexually transmitted disease (STD) in the United States, there is little evidence that female prostitutes are infecting their male customers (Cohen, Alexander and Wofsy, 1988). Several reasons explain this apparent anomaly. First of all, HIV is highly unlikely to be transmitted as a result of a single heterosexual encounter involving vaginal intercourse (Hearst and Hullen, 1988). Second, many prostitutes have been educated about safer sex and are using condoms to prevent infection (Rosenberg and Weiner, 1988:422). Third, the AIDS virus appears to be transmitted with less efficiency from females to males than in the opposite direction (Friedland and Klein, 1987:1129). Finally, studies have indicated that oral sex (which presents little risk of viral transmission—Lyman, Winkelstein et al., 1986:1703) is the most common sexual activity requested of prostitutes and that anal sex (which presents a high risk—Winkelstein, Lyman, Padian et al., 1987:324) is not commonly performed (Rosenberg and Weiner, 1988:42).

Historically, prostitutes have often been blamed for the spread of sexually transmitted diseases (STDs). During the First World War, 30,000 female prostitutes were placed in quarantine to protect military personnel from becoming infected with venereal disease (Brandt, 1986: 233). Soldiers were told that "a German bullet is cleaner than a whore" (Brandt, 1988:368). Nonetheless, the rate of STDs rose dramatically during the war (Brandt, 1986: 233). Another quarantine directed at female prostitutes would be equally ineffective in controlling the spread of HIV infection. Public officials should resist the temptation to take punitive action against these individuals as a means of appearing tough in the battle against AIDS. Intensive educational programs that teach prostitutes how to reduce the risk of transmission are more likely to be effective as a means of protecting the community.

SUMMARY

All the forms of quarantine that have been examined would involve heavy social costs, and none would contribute significantly to curbing the AIDS epidemic. Even the forced isolation of seropositive individuals who continue to engage in high-risk behavior is not likely to have a meaningful impact on the spread of the virus. Almost all cases of HIV transmission through sexual contact are unintentional. With 1.4 million infected persons in the United States, this epidemic is not going to be curbed by selecting a handful of bizarre and atypical cases for quarantine. Instead, the solution lies in providing more resources for educational programs that seek to reduce the incidence of high-risk behavior, greater support of medical research, and solving the problems associated with intravenous drug use.

REFERENCES

Bergman, Beth. (1988). AIDS, prostitution, and the use of historical stereotypes to legislate sexuality. *The John Marshall Law Review.* Vol. 21, pp. 777–830.

Blendon, Robert J. and Karen Donelan. (1988). Discrimination against people with AIDS: The public's perspective. *The New England Journal of Medicine.* Vol. 319, No. 15, pp. 1022–1026.

Brandt, Allan M. (1988). AIDS in historical perspective: Four lessons from the history of sexually transmitted diseases. *American Journal of Public Health.* Vol. 78, No. 4, pp. 367–371.

Brandt, Allan M. (1986). AIDS: From social history to social policy. *Law, Medicine & Health Care.* Vol. 14, Nos. 5–6, pp. 231–242.

Centers for Disease Control. (1989). *HIV/AIDS Surveillance.* U.S. Department of Health and Human Services, August.

Centers for Disease Control. (1987). Human immunodeficiency virus infection in the United States: A review of current knowledge. *Morbidity and Mortality Weekly Report.* Vol. 36, No. S-6 (December 18).

Cohen, Judith, Priscilla Alexander, and Constance Wofsy. (1988). Prostitution and AIDS: Public policy issues. *AIDS & Public Policy Journal.* Vol. 3, No. 2, pp. 16–22.

Curran, William J., Mary E. Clark, and Larry Gostin. (1987). AIDS: Legal and policy implications of the application of traditional disease control measures. *Law, Medicine & Health Care.* Vol. 15, Nos. 1–2, pp. 27–35.

Friedland, Gerald H., Brian R. Saltzman, Martha F. Rogers et al. (1986). Lack of transmission of HTLV-III/LAV infection to household contacts of patients with AIDS or AIDS-related complex with oral candidiasis. *The New England Journal of Medicine.* Vol. 314, No. 6, pp. 344–349.

Friedland, Gerald H. and Robert S. Klein. (1987). Transmission of the human immunodeficiency virus. *The New England Journal of Medicine.* Vol. 317, No. 18, pp. 1125–1135.

Gostin, Larry O. (1989). Public health strategies for confronting AIDS: Legislative and regulatory policy in the United States. *Journal of the American Medical Association (JAMA).* Vol. 261, No. 11, pp. 1621–1630.

Gostin, Larry and William J. Curran. (1986). The limits of compulsion in controlling AIDS. *Hastings Center Report.* Vol. 16, No. 6, pp. 24–29.

Haverkos, Harry W. and Robert Edelman. (1988). The epidemiology of acquired immunodeficiency syndrome among heterosexuals. *JAMA.* Vol. 260, No. 13, pp. 1922–1929.

Hearst, Norman and Stephen B. Hulley. (1988). Preventing the heterosexual spread of AIDS: Are we giving our patients the best advice? *JAMA.* Vol. 259, No. 16, pp. 2428–2432.

Hellinger, Fred J. (1988). Forecasting the personal medical care costs of AIDS from 1988 through 1991. *Public Health Reports.* Vol. 103, No. 3, pp. 309–319.

Institute of Medicine. (1986). *Confronting AIDS: Directions for public health, health care, and research.* National Academy Press.

Lyman, David, Warren Winkelstein, et al. (1986). Minimal risk of transmission of AIDS-associated retrovirus infection by oral-genital contact. *JAMA.* Vol. 255, No. 13, p. 1703.

McKusick, Leon, James A. Wiley, Thomas J. Coates, et al. (1985). Reported changes in the sexual behavior of men at risk for AIDS, San Francisco, 1982–84—The AIDS behavioral research project. *Public Health Reports.* Vol. 100, No. 6, pp. 622–629.

Moss, A. R. (1987). AIDS and intravenous drug use: The real heterosexual epidemic. *British Medical Journal.* Vol. 294, pp. 389–390.

New York Times. (1985). Prostitute seized in Chicago is said to have spread AIDS. P. A21, col. 6 (Dec. 26).

Parmet, Wendy E. (1985). AIDS and quarantine: The revival of an archaic doctrine. *Hofstra Law Review.* Vol. 14, pp. 53–90.

Petricciani, John C. and Jay S. Epstein. (1988). The effects of the AIDS epidemic on the safety of the nation's blood supply. *Public Health Reports.* Vol. 103, No. 3, pp. 236–241.

Raymond, Chris Anne. (1988). U.S. cities struggle to implement needle exchanges despite apparent success in European cities. *JAMA.* Vol. 260, No. 18, pp. 2620–2621.

Rosenberg, Michael J. and Jodie M. Weiner. (1988). Prostitutes and AIDS: A health department priority? *American Journal of Public Health.* Vol. 78, No. 4, pp. 418–423.

Stengel, Richard. (1987). The changing face of AIDS: More and more victims are black or Hispanic. *Time.* August 17 (pp. 12–14).

Winkelstein, Warren, David Lyman, Nancy Padian, et al. (1987). Sexual practices and the risk of infection by the human immunodeficiency virus: The San Francisco men's health study. *JAMA.* Vol. 257, No. 3, pp. 321–325.

Winkelstein, Warren, Michael Samuel, Nancy S. Padian, et al. (1987). The San Francisco men's health study: III. Reduction in human immunodeficiency virus transmission among homosexual/bisexual men, 1982–1986. *American Journal of Public Health.* Vol. 76, No. 9, pp. 685–689.

NOTES

[1] The Human Immunodeficiency Virus (HIV) is the cause of AIDS. Asymptomatic carriers are often referred to as "seropositives."

[2] There is a technical distinction between the terms "quarantine" and "isolation." Strictly speaking, the former refers to the isolation of healthy individuals who have been exposed to a communicable disease whereas the latter refers to the isolation of infected persons who have the capacity to infect others. However, this article will use these terms interchangeably to refer to the forced isolation of persons who are presumed to be infectious because public health statutes and common parlance often do not make any distinction (Gostin and Curran, 1986).

[3] However, almost all these cases predate the modern concern by the courts with the protection of individual rights, see Parmet (1985).

[4] Approximately 90 percent of the AIDS cases in the United States have occurred among persons in two risk groups: gay/bisexual males and intravenous drug users (Centers for Disease Control, 1989).

[5] Conceivably, persons placed under quarantine could be ordered to remain in their own homes. However, this policy would require that the premises be constantly monitored to insure compliance and to prevent others who might engage in high-risk behavior from entering. It would do little to prevent the sexual transmission of the disease to a partner who resided in the household.

[6] The drug AZT has been shown to prolong the lives of persons with AIDS as well as to delay the onset of symptoms in some asymptomatic individuals.

[7] The lifetime costs of medical treatment for a person with AIDS are approximately $60,000; see Hellinger (1988).

[8] It generally takes between 6 and 12 weeks from the time of exposure for the body to produce antibodies to HIV; see Petricciani and Epstein (1988).

⁹ The mere fact that an individual is ill, or physically unattractive or socially eccentric, does not justify commitment; see *O'Connor v. Donaldson* 422 U.S. 563 (1975).

¹⁰ Not all sex acts risk transmission of the AIDS virus, only those that involve the transfer of certain body fluids between partners (i.e., blood or semen).

¹¹ Even if all such persons could be identified, this group would include many individuals who do not currently engage in any type of high-risk behavior.

¹² For a discussion of the problems inherent in a system of mandatory screening, see Institute of Medicine (1986: 120–122).

SECTION SIX

Intravenous Drug Use and AIDS

Increasingly, new AIDS cases in the United States arise from intravenous drug abuse. We find these basic facts:

1. Most heterosexually acquired cases are the female sex partners of IVDUs.
2. Most pediatric cases are newborn infants of females who are IVDUs or the sexual partners of IVDUs.
3. Drug use is responsible for the disproportionate impact of the epidemic on Blacks and Hispanics.

Health officials believe that intravenous drug use could transmit the virus into the general population. It is crucial, then, to control the spread of HIV within this group.

As a result, in some cities outreach programs have been developed to help IVDUs reduce high-risk behavior. Some programs encourage drug users not to share needles, others provide information about how to sterilize drug injection equipment. In some communities, outreach workers have even provided users with bleach so that users could clean their "works."

The proposal that has generated the most heated controversy is the suggestion to provide IVDUs with sterile needles. While proponents see this strategy as a means of reducing the incidence of needle sharing (and thus, slowing the spread of the virus), critics contend that this policy shows that society is willing to tolerate drug use. Further, critics assert that IVDUs will share needles anyway, even when sterile needles are available.

The readings in Section VI tackle the dilemma of how to prevent AIDS transmission among intravenous drug users. The first selection, "Target Groups for Preventing AIDS Among Intravenous Drug Users" by Des Jarlais and Friedman examines the characteristics of the various subgroups of IVDUs. They believe that the same HIV prevention strategy will not be effective with each subgroup. And—contrary to popular notion—the authors present evidence that IVDUs can change their behavior. Both self-report data and the existence of a black market in sterile needles in New York City are cited to support the view that IVDUs will take measures to protect themselves from AIDS.

The second selection, "Can Public Policies Limit the Spread of HIV among IV Drug Users?" by Conviser and Rutledge examines various ways to control the transmission of the AIDS virus among this group. The authors make the point that the goals of promoting public health and curtailing drug use are not mutually exclusive. Further, that programs teaching addicts how to clean their needles tend to increase the demand by users for drug treatment.

The third selection is the recommendation of the Report of the Presidential Commission on the Human Immunodeficiency Virus Epidemic regarding drug use. The Commission recommends that "treatment on demand" be in the forefront of the national effort to fight HIV infection associated with IVDU. There are between 1.2 and 1.3 million intravenous drug users in the United States; only 148,000 are enrolled in treatment at any given time. In some cases, addicts must wait up to six months on a waiting list in order to receive treatment.

The final selection, "U.S. Cities Struggle to Implement Needle Exchanges Despite Apparent Success in European Cities" by Chris Anne Raymond examines the experiences of two American cities (New York and Portland, Oregon) that have decided to adopt experimental needle-exchange programs. The author discusses the mechanics of how these pilot programs operate and what we hope to learn. Preliminary evidence from European cities suggests that needle-exchange programs do not lead to an increase in drug usage.

13

Target Groups for Preventing AIDS Among Intravenous Drug Users

Don C. Des Jarlais and Samuel R. Friedman

EPIDEMIOLOGY

HIV is transmitted among IV drug users primarily through the sharing of the equipment ("works") used for injecting drugs (Cohen, Marmor, Des Jarlais, Spira, Friedman, & Yancovitz, 1985; Friedland, Harris, Small, Shine, Moll, Reiss, Darrow, & Klein, 1985; Weiss, Ginzburg, Goedert, Biggar, Mohica, et al., 1985). The virus can also be transmitted through heterosexual activity (Luzi, Ensoli, Turbessi, Scarpatti, & Aiuti, 1985; Redfield, Markham, Salahuddin, Wright, Sarngadharan, et al., 1985). IV drug users are the primary source of heterosexual transmission of AIDS in the United States: 60% (163/273) of the heterosexual transmission cases reported to the Centers for Disease Control (CDC) through April 18, 1986 involved an IV drug user as the likely source of the virus (A. Hardy, personal communication, 1986).

The virus can also be transmitted to children perinatally (Lapointe, Michaud, Pekovic, Chausseau, & DuPuy, 1986). IV drug use in a parent is the major risk for AIDS among children in the United States, accounting for slightly over half (150 of 278) of pediatric AIDS cases (reported through April 18, 1986; A. Hardy, personal communication, 1986).

The New York City metropolitan area has by far the greatest concentration of IV drug users who have developed AIDS. There have been 1,869 cases of AIDS

Reprinted from *Journal of Applied Social Psychology*, 1987, 17, 3, pp. 251–268. Copyright © 1987 by V.H. Winston & Sons, Inc., all rights reserved.

Requests for reprints should be sent to Dr. Don C. Des Jarlais, State of New York, Division of Substance Abuse Services, 55 W. 125th Street, New York, NY 10027.

in IV drug users from New York and 490 from New Jersey reported to the U.S. CDC through April 18, 1986. There were an additional 781 cases from a total of 37 different states, and 147 cases from Europe through December 31, 1985 reported to the European Coordinating Center (A. Hardy, CDC, personal communication, 1986; IV drug users who also have male homosexuality as a risk factor—1,568 in the U.S. and 35 in Europe—are not included in these totals).

While the actual cases of AIDS among IV drug users have so far been concentrated in the New York area, studies of HIV seroprevalence (indicating infection by the virus) shows a great potential for cases throughout the U.S. and Western Europe. Research in Edinburgh (Robertson, Bucknall, Welsby, Roberts, Inglis, Peutherer, & Brettle, 1986) and Italy (Angarano, Pastore, & Monno, 1985) show seroprevalence rates of greater than 50%, while studies from Zurich (Schupbach, Haller, Vogt, Luthy, Joller, Oelz, Popovic, Sarngadharan, & Gallo, 1985) and the Federal Republic of Germany (W. Hoeckmann, personal communication, 1986) show rates between 20% and 40%. Studies in San Francisco and Chicago show approximately 10% seroprevalence in those cities (Spira, Des Jarlais, Bokos, Onichi, Kiprov, & Kalyanaraman, 1985), while studies from Washington, D.C. and New Orleans show 7% and 2%, respectively (Ginzburg, personal communication, 1986).

Studies using historically collected blood indicate that the virus can spread relatively rapidly among IV drug users in a community. We examined serum samples from IV drug users collected from 1969 through 1984 for New York City. Testing of these samples showed no presence of HIV antibody in samples from 1969 through 1976. The first seropositive sample was collected in late 1978. There was then a rapid rise, from approximately 20% seropositive in samples collected in late 1978 and 1979 to 40% seropositive in samples collected in 1980, and 50% in samples collected in the following years (Novick, Kreek, Des Jarlais, Spira, Khuri, Ragunath, Kalyarnaraman, Gelb, & Miescher, 1986).

Similar rapid spread of HIV among IV drug users appears to have occurred in Edinburgh. Seroprevalence rates in the Robertson et al. study (1986) went from essentially zero to 50% in less than two years. In contrast, seroprevalence rates in San Francisco appear to have held at around 10% through 1985 (R. Chaisson, personal communication, 1986). This epidemiologic research shows both an opportunity and a great need for immediate efforts to prevent the virus from saturating IV drug-use groups in many different communities.

THE IV DRUG-USE SUBCULTURE

Successful prevention efforts will need to be based on an understanding of the social psychology and physiology of IV drug use. The scientific literature on these topics is immense, so we will confine our review here to those aspects we believe are most closely related to preventing AIDS.

There is a common misconception that IV drug users have no social organization. A multi-billion dollar industry, however, does not persevere without some forms of social organization. IV drug use has been traditionally described as a "subculture" within sociological and anthropological research (e.g., Agar, 1973; Combs, Fry, & Lewis, 1976; DuToit, 1977; Johnson, 1980; Weppner, 1977). While the concept of "subculture" does not have an overly precise definition, it is used to denote a distinct group with its own set of values, roles, and status allocation that exists within a larger society (Johnson, 1973, 1980). From the perspective of its members, participating in the subculture is a meaningful activity (rather than a psychopathology), an "escape from reality," or an "illness" (Preble & Casey, 1969).

Although there is considerable regional and ethnic variation, IV drug use clearly constitutes a deviant subculture within the U.S. (Agar, 1973). Possession and sale of drugs are violations of the law, as are many of the activities undertaken to obtain money for purchasing the drugs. In addition to legal differences between IV drug users and members of conventional society, there is an empathy barrier. Most members of conventional society, even those who use illicit drugs, have great difficulty imagining themselves injecting drugs or doing what IV drug users are believed to do to obtain money for drugs. Most members of conventional society find it easier to empathize with victims of drug-related crimes than with IV drug users. Thus, IV drug users are not just considered different, but are often objects of fear, mistrust, hostility, scorn, and, to a limited extent, pity. This psychological and social distance between the IV drug-use subculture and conventional society contributes to a climate of generalized mistrust between the two groups.

There is a precarious balance between trust and mistrust among IV drug users themselves. They need a degree of interpersonal trust so that they can conduct the business of acquiring drugs, equipment, and locations for injecting and for social validation of the worth of "getting high." But they also have a widespread mistrust of other IV drug users. Among the many reasons for this mistrust are competition for scarce goods (drugs and the money to buy them), use of informants by law-enforcement agencies, carryover of the "hustling" (use of deception and/or limited violence to obtain money) of "straights" (non-drug users) to the hustling of other drug users, and the use of violence to settle disputes.

Another very important limitation of trust among IV drug users is their varying commitment to the values of the subculture. As with any subculture, new members are not expected to be fully socialized into the group. It is also quite difficult to be a "successful" IV drug user in terms of obtaining money and drugs, avoiding the law, maintaining some positive relationships with non-users (particularly family and sexual partners), and not becoming "strung out" from excessive drug use. Because of these great difficulties, many IV drug users will at least temporarily attempt to stop injecting drugs, either on their own or by entering a treatment program. Persons who enter treatment are usually seen as having failed at being IV drug users, and (at least temporarily) lose the respect and trust of those who continue injecting drugs. Persons who succeed in treatment also come to denigrate current IV drug users so that the mistrust becomes mutual.

IV drug users rely on oral communication. There are few written documents and few print channels of communication. They rely on the spoken word for two main reasons: Since much of what they do is illegal, written documents would be incriminating; and many of them have difficulties in reading and writing. Part of the oral nature of the subculture is a specialized argot. While some terms have been incorporated into the slang of conventional society (e.g., "O.D." for overdose), the argot generally tends to inhibit communication between members of the subculture and conventional society.

It should be noted that, prior to AIDS, death was already a frequent occurrence within the IV drug-use subculture. Estimates of the annual death rate among IV drug users not in treatment range from 3.5% to 8% (Des Jarlais, 1984). Although AIDS clearly poses a threat of a protracted, painful, and often socially isolated death (compared to the rapid, painless death associated with an overdose), there is some tendency to generalize the fatalistic acceptance of death within the subculture to AIDS. AIDS, however, represents a more frequent and qualitatively different way of dying. It serves as much greater motivation for behavior change than any previous health threat associated with IV drug use.

The sharing of works is deeply embedded in the IV drug use subculture. Such sharing serves both social bonding and economic functions. Sharing among "running partners" (persons who cooperate to obtain drugs and the money needed to purchase them) can symbolize their cooperative effort. The legally restricted supply of sterile needles and syringes for injection also encourages multiple users for the same works. (See Des Jarlais, Friedman, & Strug, 1986, for a more complete discussion of the roles of needlesharing within the pre-AIDS IV drug-use subculture.) Reducing some types of needlesharing (e.g., the purely pragmatic use of rented works in a shooting gallery) will be easier than reducing the sharing among running partners or sexual partners, where a close social bond is involved.

The most difficult situation in which to prevent the use of possible contaminated works occurs when an IV drug user is experiencing withdrawal symptoms (Des Jarlais, Friedman, & Strug, 1986). While narcotic withdrawal is not life threatening, it includes anxiety and severe physical discomfort. Injection of a narcotic will provide almost instantaneous relief. Thus, when an IV drug user is undergoing withdrawal and has the drug to inject, he or she will be severely tempted to use whatever works are readily available.

In general, the characteristics of IV drug use as a deviant subculture will require specifically designed prevention programs. The differences and hostility between the subculture and conventional society make cooperative efforts between public health authorities and IV drug users difficult. Language and literacy problems reduce the potential effectiveness of written communications. The generalized mistrust within the subculture makes collective self-organization to promote the health of the group as a whole difficult (Friedman & Des Jarlais, in press; Friedman, Des Jarlais, Sotheran, Garber, Cohen, & Smith, 1987). That there are many aspects of the IV drug-use subculture that make AIDS prevention difficult should not, however, be used as a rationale to justify not making prevention efforts.

CURRENT FINDINGS ON BEHAVIOR CHANGE AMONG IV DRUG USERS

In addition to skepticism based on the social and physiological reasons that makes AIDS prevention difficult, there are common stereotypes that IV drug users are concerned only about drugs and/or are basically "self-destructive" and not likely to respond to prevention efforts. These stereotypes create a great inertia against AIDS-prevention efforts. The extent to which these beliefs were true prior to AIDS is a matter of considerable disagreement, but they certainly should not be generalized to the AIDS epidemic.

AIDS has created a new and qualitatively different fear of death among IV drug users. This type of death is protracted, usually painful, and often preceded by social isolation. Dying from AIDS has none of the elements of escapism that can be seen in an overdose death.

A number of recent studies indicate that the majority of IV drug users can be expected to change their behavior in order to avoid exposure to the AIDS virus.

In the fall of 1984, we collected data from a sample of New York City IV drug users in treatment, regarding their knowledge of AIDS and responses to the epidemic (Friedman et al., 1987). These subjects had not received any special education/prevention programming at the time of data collection. Essentially all of the subjects knew of AIDS, and over 90% knew that it could be transmitted through the sharing of needles for injecting drugs. Fifty-nine percent reported that they had changed their behavior in order to reduce the likelihood of being exposed to the virus. The major changes in behavior consisted of greater use of sterile needles, greater cleaning of previously used needles, and reduction in the sharing of needles.

Selwyn and colleagues (Selwyn, Cox, Feiner, Lipschutz, & Cohen, 1985; P. Selwyn, personal communication, 1986) more recently conducted a study of AIDS knowledge and behavior change among patients in a methadone maintenance program and in a detention center detoxification program. The findings were similar: 97% were aware that sharing needles could transmit AIDS, and over 60% reported that they had changed their drug/needle use in order to reduce the risk of developing AIDS.

Evidence of behavior change among IV drug users in response to AIDS is not confined to self-reports of IV drug users in treatment. Evidence for the increase in use of sterile needles in New York City has also come from interviews with persons selling needles in the "copping areas" (areas where drugs can be purchased) and from the emergence of a market in "counterfeit" sterile needles in which a used needle is washed out and placed in the original package, which is then resealed

(Des Jarlais, Friedman, & Hopkins, 1985). "Free" sterile needles, in the form of 2-for-1 sales and free needles with purchases of $25 and $50 bags of heroin, are now being used as a marketing tactic in New York City (Des Jarlais & Hopkins, 1985).

Only preliminary data are available from studies of AIDS-related behavior change outside of New York City. These studies also support the idea that IV drug users will change their behavior because of AIDS. In New Jersey, where there have been 538 cases of AIDS among heterosexual IV drug users and 81 cases among homosexual male IV drug users (through May 1, 1986), the threat of the disease has become one of the major reasons for entering treatment. Approximately half of the IV drug users entering treatment since the last half of 1985 reported that AIDS was one of their reasons for entering treatment (J. French, personal communication, 1986).

There have been only 18 cases of AIDS among IV drug users in San Francisco (through April 1986, with gay males who inject drugs excluded), and the seroprevalence is estimated to be approximately 10% (R. Chaisson, personal communication, 1986). Yet even here, ethnographic research with IV drug users not in treatment shows that the majority knows of the disease and realizes that it can be transmitted through sharing works. A "substantial minority" has already reduced their sharing of works in order to avoid exposure to the virus (Biernacki & Feldman, 1986).

The current research on behavior change among IV drug users thus consistently supports the idea that many of them will modify their behavior in order to avoid exposure to the AIDS virus. These changes have occurred prior to formal AIDS-prevention programs aimed at IV drug users and suggest that more extensive prevention efforts would produce greater risk reduction.

PREVENTION TARGET GROUPS

While IV drug users can generally be considered to form a single subculture with some geographic and ethnic variations, we want to emphasize the need for targeting different subgroups within the subculture. As noted above, individual IV drug users have varying commitment to the subculture at different points in time, and AIDS-prevention efforts will be more effective if they utilize these different levels of commitment.

IV Drug Users in Treatment

IV drug users in treatment programs are among those with the least commitment to the subculture, though they must still be considered at risk for exposure to HIV. Many will drop out of treatment prior to successful completion, and many in ambulatory treatment will continue to inject drugs despite being in treatment. The injection of cocaine is a particular problem for persons in ambulatory treatment, since at present there is no effective chemotherapy that blocks the effects of cocaine. IV drug users in treatment are also more easily reached with information about AIDS than those not in treatment.

A critical part of AIDS prevention among IV drug users in treatment is prior education efforts for the staff of the treatment programs. All staff in contact with persons at increased risk need to be able to provide accurate basic information about AIDS. This includes the viral causation of AIDS, the long latency period, early symptoms, the fact that clinical AIDS is only the most severe manifestation of HIV infection, and the specifics of the modes of transmission of the virus. They should know that casual contact does not transmit the virus and that the traditional means of cleaning needles and syringes (rinsing with nonsterile water) does not kill the virus. Finally, they should know the "safe-sex" guidelines relevant to prevention of homosexual and heterosexual transmission.

Staff should never be sources of misinformation. They need to maintain credibility with persons at increased risk and may permanently lose credibility if they appear to be spreading misinformation. In the rapidly changing AIDS field, with the frequent news stories that do not provide full explanations of various "new findings," this can be difficult. Staff need to have a sense of what they do *not* know about AIDS, as well as what they do know. The treatment program as a whole will need a resource/referral source through which difficult questions can be answered.

Staff need more than just knowledge; they should be able to communicate the information accurately, without embarrassment, and without either sensationalizing or denying the seriousness of AIDS. This means having "worked through" their own emotional reactions to the epidemic, including fears that they themselves might contract the illness through casual contact or from their own previous IV drug use, and the emotional reactions that AIDS evokes even in persons not at risk for viral exposure.

Admitting that clients or patients in treatment are at risk for IV drug use is difficult for many treatment program staff, since it may seem to undermine the basic treatment message that drug-abuse problems can be overcome. This does not, however, justify the absence of AIDS education/prevention activities. Too many drug-abuse treatment clients either drop out of treatment or inject drugs at some level while in treatment to ignore the opportunity of providing needed information while they are in treatment. For residential programs, the most opportune time for such prevention/education efforts may be at intake, where the knowledge can serve to reinforce motivation not to inject drugs. For ambulatory treatment programs, where clients and patients must be considered at risk for injecting drugs while in treatment, prevention/education at intake and periodically throughout treatment would both be appropriate.

To be most effective, prevention efforts for persons at increased risk will involve more than sharing information. The modes of transmission of the virus involve private behaviors, and the disease is quite capable of arousing strong emotions. In this situation, education about AIDS may easily merge with counseling on transmission-related behavior. Even drug-abuse treatment staff who are competent to provide counseling on drug injection may not be competent to provide counseling on sexual and in utero transmission of HIV. They should, however, be able to recognize when a client or patient needs counseling in these areas and be able to make an appropriate referral.

While it is necessary to provide AIDS education/prevention to persons in drug-abuse treatment, controlling the epidemic will require prevention efforts aimed at those who are not in treatment. Relatively few illicit drug injectors are in treatment at any point in time, and once the virus becomes established in a geographic area, many IV drug users will be exposed before they come into treatment. Thus, it will be necessary to mount effective IV drug use/AIDS-prevention efforts outside of treatment settings.

Persons at Risk for Initiation into IV Drug Use

The ideal point for prevention of AIDS among IV drug users would be to prevent initiation into IV drug use. This would not only prevent needlesharing transmission of HIV, it would also prevent the many other health and social problems associated with IV drug use. Educational programs about the dangers of AIDS and IV drug use have been developed in New York City for use in junior and senior high school. While we support the development of these programs, we also feel that they are not likely to be greatly effective. First, drug-prevention programs based on fear arousal have not been successful in the past (Schaps, DiBartolo, Paley, & Churgin, 1978), particularly if the fear is associated with a low-probability event. Second, many persons who eventually become IV drug users drop out of school well before they make decisions about injecting drugs.

Prevention programs targeted at reducing initiation into IV drug use may have to operate outside of school settings. They include discussions of experiences with noninjected drugs as part of the behavioral processes that lead to drug injection. Such programs may need to focus on teaching skills needed to resist social pressures to begin injecting drugs (similar to the cigarette smoking prevention programs that focus on teaching the social skills to resist initiation into cigarette smoking; e.g., Botvin & Eng, 1980; Botvin, Eng., & Williams, 1980). Such programs undoubtedly would be more expensive than the in-school programs. They would also pose some difficult policy/strategic questions: Should they focus only on drug injection (the AIDS danger) or should they be broader and include any use of such drugs as cocaine and heroin, or broader still and focus on any illicit drug use? Preventing noninjected drug abuse is a valid public health goal in itself, but may dilute efforts to reduce the AIDS-specific problem in initiation into drug injection.

Current IV Drug Users Who Wish to Enter Treatment

Fear of AIDS, among other reasons, will undoubtedly lead significant numbers of IV drug users to seek treatment for their drug use. For the U.S. as a whole, however, the availability of treatment was significantly less than the demand prior to the AIDS epidemic. Expanding the treatment system could significantly reduce transmission of HIV among IV drug users. Users who had not been exposed would greatly reduce their chances of being exposed, and users who had already been exposed would greatly reduce their chances of exposing others. The economics of treating AIDS (currently estimated to be between $100,000 and $150,000 per case; Hardy, 1986) versus providing drug-abuse treatment (approximately $3,000 per patient year) also argues for expansion of the treatment network.

Unfortunately, there are real factors other than finances that currently limit the availability of drug-abuse treatment. Drug-abuse treatment has general approval within American society, but is particularly subject to the "NIMBY" (not in my backyard) phenomenon. In addition, methadone maintenance treatment, which tends to be the most acceptable treatment modality to large numbers of IV drug users, also tends to have the least degree of in-my-neighborhood acceptance. Any public association of IV drug use with AIDS is likely to increase the difficulties in finding acceptable locations for new drug-abuse treatment programs. Finally, if there is to be significant reduction of HIV transmission through increased treatment, the program expansion will have to be on a large scale. Based on our New York experience, we would estimate that there are approximately four IV drug users not in treatment for every one currently in treatment. Thus, to control HIV transmission among IV drug users through additional treatment would require a massive expansion of the treatment system.

IV Drug Users Who Do Not Wish to Enter Treatment

Many current IV drug users wish to reduce their chances of exposure to HIV, but will not enter treatment or refrain from all drug injection. (As noted above, there are also IV drug users in treatment who will continue some level of drug injection. Much of this section also applies to them.) As will be reviewed below, even though many IV drug users will not eliminate their drug injection, they will nevertheless reduce sharing of works and/or increase their use of sterile works as a way of reducing their risk of developing AIDS.

Whether legal restrictions on the sale of sterile hypodermic needles should be reduced in order to reduce transmission of HIV among IV drug users has been the subject of much public discussion in New York, New Jersey, and other states. There are only 11 states in the country that require prescriptions for the purchase of hypodermics (National Association of Boards of Pharmacy, 1983). Increasing the legal availability of hypodermic needles has received some support among public health officials, but has generally been opposed by law-enforcement officials, who predict that it would lead to greater IV drug use.

The actual effects of increasing the legal availability of sterile needles are unknown. Almost no data have been collected about the relationship between the legal availability of sterile needles and levels of IV drug use prior to the AIDS epidemic; and we have serious doubts that such earlier data can be generalized to the epidemic situation. The actual effects of an increased legal availability on reducing HIV transmission and levels of IV drug use may depend greatly on the specific methods of changing the legal availability and the simultaneous presence of other AIDS-prevention efforts.

A second method of attempting to reduce HIV transmission among IV drug users who are not ready to enter treatment would be education about not sharing needles and on how to properly "clean" needles in order to kill HIV. Printed materials containing this information (after emphasizing that stopping drug injection is the only certain method of avoiding HIV exposure) are being used in several states. Some of these materials have been criticized as "encouraging IV drug use." Again, only empirical study will show the extent to which such educational materials and training either reduce HIV transmission or affect levels of IV drug use.

Heterosexual Partners and Children of IV Drug Users

Space limitations do not permit a full discussion of the complex questions related to preventing AIDS among the heterosexual partners and children of IV drug users, but we will outline some of the relevant issues. As discussed in the earlier section on epidemiology, IV drug users are the primary source of HIV transmission to heterosexual partners and children in the U.S.

Both the heterosexual partners and children are relatively large groups. A study of sexual relationships of male IV drug users in New York City found that almost 80% of them had their primary sexual relationship with women who did not inject drugs themselves. The size of the female heterosexual partner population was estimated to be at least half the size of the IV drug-use population (Des Jarlais, Chamberland, Yancovite, Weinberg, & Friedman, 1984). IV drug users also have considerable numbers of children. A recently completed New York study of the children of methadone maintenance patients found an average of almost two children per patient, and a quarter of the patients indicated that they expected to have additional children (Deren, 1985). The incidence of surveillance-definition AIDS in both heterosexual partners and children has been low compared to the numbers of partners and children at risk—which suggests that these modes of transmission may be less likely to lead to AIDS than drug injection—but the incidence follows the same exponential increase as the cases in IV drug users (Des Jarlais et al., in preparation).

Preventing AIDS among the sexual partners and children of IV drug users will clearly be a necessary part of overall public health control of the epidemic. The behavior changes needed to prevent heterosexual and in utero transmission are at least as complex and difficult as those associated with drug-injection transmission. Disruption of ongoing sexual relationships and foregoing having children would involve considerable psychological costs and would require more intensive prevention resources than are needed for dissemination of information. Until more is known about the probabilities of heterosexual and in utero transmission, it is difficult to provide any guidelines for the trade-offs of risk reduction and psychological costs. The same "safe sex" guidelines used for homosexual transmission (avoidance of bodily fluid transfer and anal intercourse, use of condoms), and, for women who are HIV-antibody positive, postponing voluntary pregnancies until more is known about transmission to children, would seem to be minimal recommendations for prevention in the heterosexual partners and children groups.

The prevention of in utero transmission is one clear case where HIV-antibody testing may be of specific use. Women who are contemplating pregnancy should be provided with the opportunity for voluntary testing, with strict protection of the confidentiality of the results.

ETHNIC AND RACIAL DIFFERENCES

At several places in this article, we have noted that ethnic differences among IV drug users will have to be considered in prevention efforts. These ethnic differences are intellectually separate from, but confounded with, social class factors. In general, the delivery of prevention services to minority groups has been inadequate in the U.S., and the problems are likely to be at least as great for AIDS, if not greater. The subject of ethnicity and AIDS is sufficiently complex to justify a separate article (which is in preparation), so we will make only a few comments here.

Compared to their percentage of the total population, blacks and Hispanics are overrepresented among AIDS cases in the U.S. as a whole. This is particularly true for the IV drug-related cases, of which 80% have occurred among blacks and Hispanics (A. Hardy, personal communication, 1986).

There is a great lack of information on how best to incorporate ethnicity and racial considerations into AIDS prevention efforts for IV drug users and their sexual partners. Printed materials about AIDS and IV drug use have been translated into Spanish, and black and Hispanic ex-addicts have worked as health educators for IV drug users. Information is needed on what else should be done. Much of the needed knowledge may be specific to local geographic areas. Questions for "needs assessment" research include:

1. the extent to which AIDS is perceived to be a disease of gay white males and/or of IV drug users and/or of heterosexuals;

2. attitudes toward the various "safe sex" practices;
3. the social integration of IV drug users within the ethnic group and the larger community, including how attitudes toward IV drug users combine sympathy, fear, and denial of a problem; and
4. the integration of the ethnic minority into the larger community, which may involve increased discrimination against the group as a potential outcome of a perceived association between the group and AIDS.

SEX DIFFERENCES

Sex differences in planning AIDS/IV drug use-prevention programs are also sufficiently complex to deserve a full analysis, so we will make only limited comments here. To some extent, gender considerations interact with ethnic considerations, since sex roles vary across ethnic groups. There are some factors that are similar across ethnic groups. In many ethnic groups, a woman who injects drugs is more highly stigmatized than a man who injects drugs, including the assumption that a woman who injects drugs is also a prostitute. Conflict between drug use and child-rearing responsibilities may be more intense for women in many ethnic groups. Many women who inject drugs are dependent on a male sexual partner as a source of drugs, and they share drug-injection equipment primarily with that man. Since the woman is likely to have less power in the relationship, taking precautions against HIV transmission—both via shared drug equipment and heterosexual activity—may be particularly difficult if the man objects.

How best to incorporate ethnic/racial and sex differences in AIDS-prevention programs is an area where additional research is urgently needed. Given the rapidity with which HIV can spread among IV drug users, using seroconversion rates as the outcome measures in evaluating prevention efforts that incorporate ethnic and sex differences may be too costly in time and money. It will often be more appropriate to use focus groups and self-reported behavior changes to evaluate potential effectiveness.

DISCUSSION

Research has not yet demonstrated what are the most effective means of preventing AIDS among IV drug users, but there are several tentative generalizations that seem to hold. First, the mass media seem to be able to convey the basic information that AIDS is deadly and that it can be spread through the sharing of equipment for injecting drugs. (Pamphlets and posters can supplement the mass media for this message.) This basic information will produce a significant amount of behavior change among IV drug users, but probably not enough to do more than slow the spread of the virus within the group and prevent exposure in a small minority of IV drug users.

Secondly, prevention and education campaigns need to include very specific information. Some of the behavior changes that IV drug users report undertaking to avoid AIDS may not be effective. For example, methods of cleaning needles such as rinsing with water or using a wire to remove clotted blood are not sufficient to kill HIV. If IV drug users are to sterilize their equipment, they will have to be taught the specific information needed to do so.

A third generalization about prevention/education programs for IV drug users is that they should incorporate face-to-face communication. The use of ex-addicts as health educators is currently under way in New Jersey, New York, Maryland and the Netherlands. The use of current or ex-addicts should make it easier to communicate the specific details noted above to permit the recipient of the information to ask clarifying questions, and to avoid the literacy and argot problems found among many IV drug users. Face-to-face communication would also permit the health educator to modulate the emotional tone of the message in accordance with the response of the recipient. The seriousness of AIDS needs to be stressed, but not to the point where so much anxiety is aroused that denial becomes the dominant response.

A final aspect of preventing AIDS among IV drug users concerns the perceived conflict between preventing AIDS and "encouraging drug use." Some form of this conflict will probably occur among almost all groups active in preventing AIDS among IV drug users, from public health officials to drug-abuse treatment staff to ex-addict health educators.

SUMMARY

In the absence of any effective treatment or vaccine, control of the AIDS epidemic must be through prevention efforts. Since IV drug users constitute the second largest risk group in the United States and are the primary source of transmission to heterosexual partners and children, overall control of the epidemic will require control within the IV drug-use group.

Because of the social organization of IV drug users in the U.S., there are greater constraints on prevention efforts with this group than with others. Present research, however, shows that IV drug users in New York City and elsewhere do modify their behavior in response to the threat of AIDS. Even so, efforts at prevention that have begun within the IV drug-use subculture need to be reinforced by programs undertaken by public health and drug-abuse treatment and prevention personnel.

Persons at risk for HIV exposure through IV drug use do not constitute a homogeneous group. Different prevention activities need to be targeted for these different groups. Special prevention efforts also need to be devised for persons who have not yet started IV drug use, heterosexual partners (who do not themselves inject drugs), and potential parents who may have been exposed to HIV.

Public health efforts aimed at preventing AIDS among IV drug users may be limited by perceptions that some AIDS-prevention efforts may actually "encourage" illicit drug use. Such perceptions may be held both among the general public and among some members of the drug-abuse treatment/prevention community. At present, relevant data on the accuracy of these perceptions are almost nonexistent. AIDS has created a qualitatively different risk of death associated with IV drug use, and previous beliefs about what does and does not encourage IV drug use cannot safely be generalized to the AIDS situation. The dilemma about preventing adverse health consequences of drug use versus "encouraging" drug use can be applied to any treatment of adverse health consequences of drug use (e.g., using naloxone to treat acute overdoses). AIDS, however, magnifies the scale of the dilemma on several dimensions—it is specific to IV drug use rather than to all forms of drug use; some successful prevention can probably be achieved without any overall reduction in drug injection (i.e., reducing the use of contaminated needles); the adverse consequences may occur after successful elimination of IV drug use, thus undermining the hope needed in drug-abuse treatment programs; and the fatal consequences are not limited to the drug user, but may also include sexual partners and children.

Specific approaches to these prevention policy questions will vary according to the different target groups for preventing AIDS among IV drug users, the extent to which HIV has spread among the local IV drug users, the feelings of individual prevention workers, the philosophy of the sponsoring organization, and the local political climate. The problem is certainly large enough to permit a wide variety of approaches, and there are not yet sufficient data to identify the single "best" prevention approach. Individuals working to prevent AIDS among IV drug users, their sexual partners and their children need to believe in the validity of what they are personally doing, but will also need to be able to keep an open attitude to forthcoming data showing relative effectiveness of the different approaches. In the meantime, the AIDS problem is of sufficient urgency that we should be trying and assessing a very wide variety of prevention programs.

REFERENCES

Agar, M. H. (1973). *Ripping and running: A formal ethnography of urban heroin addicts*. New York: Seminar Press.

Angarano, G., Pastore, G., Monno, L. (1985). Rapid spread of HTLV-III infection among drug addicts in Italy. *Lancet*, 8467(II), 1302.

Biernacki, P., & Fieldman, H. (1986, April). *Ethnographic observations of IV drug use practices that put users at risk for AIDS*. Presented at the XVth International Institute on the Prevention and Treatment of Drug Dependence, Amsterdam/Noordwijkerhout, the Netherlands.

Botvin, G. J., & Eng, A. (1980). A comprehensive school-based smoking prevention program. *Journal of School Health*, 50, 209–213.

Botvin, G. J., Eng, A., & Williams, C. L. (1980). Preventing the onset of smoking through life skills training. *Preventive Medicine, 9*, 135–143.

Cohen, H., Marmor, M., Des Jarlais, D., Spira, T., Friedman, S., & Yancovitz, S. (1985, April). *Behavior risk factors for HTLV-III/LAV seropositivity among intravenous drug users.* Presented at the International Conference on the Acquired Immune Deficiency Syndrome (AIDS). Atlanta, GA.

Combs, R. H., Fry, L. J., & Lewis, P. G. (Eds.). (1976). *Socialization in drug abuse.* Cambridge, MA: Schenkman.

Deren, S. (1985). *A description of methadone maintenance patients and their children.* New York: New York State Division of Substance Abuse Services.

Des Jarlais, D. C. (1984). Research design, drug use and deaths: Cross study comparisons. In G. Serban (Ed.), *Social and medical aspects of drug abuse* (pp. 229–236). New York: SP Scientific.

Des Jarlais, D. C., & Friedman, S. R. (in press). AIDS and therapeutic communities: Policy implications.

Des Jarlais, D. C., Friedman, S. R., & Hopkins, W. (1985). Risk reduction for the acquired immunodeficiency syndrome among intravenous drug users. *Annals of Internal Medicine, 103*, 755–759.

Des Jarlais, D. C., Friedman, S. R., Spira, T. J., Zolla-Pazner, S., Marmor, M., Holzman, R., Mildvan, D., Yancovitz, S., Mathur-Wagh, U., Garber, J., El-Sadr, W., Cohen, H., Smith, D., & Kalyanaraman, V. S. (1986). A stage model of HTLV-III infection in intravenous drug users. In L. J. Harris (Ed.), *Problems of Drug Dependence 1985: Proceedings of the 47th Annual Meeting, The Committee on Problems of Drug Dependence, Inc.* Rockville, MD: National Institute on Drug Abuse, NIDA Research Monograph 67.

Des Jarlais, D. C., Friedman, S. R., & Strug, D. (1986). AIDS among intravenous drug users: A sociocultural perspective. In D. Feldman & T. Johnson (Eds.), *The social dimensions of AIDS: Methods and theory* (pp. 111–126). New York: Praeger.

Des Jarlais, D. C., & Hopkins, W. (1985). Free needles for intravenous drug users at risk for AIDS: Current developments in New York City. *New England Journal of Medicine, 313*, 23.

Des Jarlais, D. C., Chamberland, M. E., Yancovitz, S. R., Weinberg, P., & Friedman, S. R. (1984). Heterosexual partners: A large risk group for AIDS. *Lancet, 8415*(II), 1346–1347.

DuToit, B. M. (Ed.). (1977). *Drugs, rituals and altered states of consciousness.* Rotterdam: A. A. Balkema.

Friedland, G. H., Harris, C., Small, C. B., Shine, D., Moll, B., Reiss, R., Darrow, W., & Klein, R. (1986). Intravenous drug users and the acquired immunodeficiency syndrome (AIDS): Demographic, drug use and needle sharing patterns. *Archives of Internal Medicine, 145*, 837–840.

Friedman, S. R., & Des Jarlais, D. C. (in press). Knowledge of AIDS, behavioral change, and organization among intravenous drug users. Stichting Drug Symposium.

Friedman, S. R., Des Jarlais, D. C., & Sotheran, J. L. (1986). AIDS health education for intravenous drug users. *Health Education Quarterly, 13*, 383–393.

Friedman, S. R., Des Jarlais, D. C., Sotheran, J. L., Garber, J., Cohen, H., & Smith, D. (1987). AIDS and self-organization among intravenous drug users. *International Journal of the Addictions, 22*, 201–220.

Goldstein, P., Hunt, D. E., Des Jarlais, D. C., & Deren, S. (in press). Health consequences of drug use.

Hardy, A. M., et al. (1986). The economic impact of the first 10,000 cases of acquired immunodeficiency syndrome in the United States. *Journal of the American Medical Association, 255,* 209–211.

Johnson, B. D. (1973). *Marijuana users and drug subcultures.* New York: Wiley.

Johnson, B. D. (1980). Toward a theory of drug subcultures. In D. Letieri (Ed.), *Theories on drug abuse.* Rockville, MD: National Institute on Drug Abuse, NIDA Research Monograph 38.

Lapointe, N., Michaud, J., Pekovic, D., Chausseau, J. P., & DuPuy, J. M. (1986). Transplacental transmission of HTLV-III virus. *New England Journal of Medicine, 312,* 1325–1326.

Luzi, G., Ensoli, B., Turbessi, G., Scarpati, G., et al. (1985). Transmission of HTLV-III infection by heterosexual contact. *Lancet,* 8462(II), 1018.

Marmor, M., Des Jarlais, D. C., Friedman, S. R., et al. (1985). The epidemic of acquired immunodeficiency syndrome (AIDS) and suggestions for its control in drug abusers. *Journal of Substance Abuse Treatment, 1,* 237–247.

National Association of Boards of Pharmacy. (1983). *Survey of state pharmaceutical laws, 1983–1984.* Chicago: Author.

Novick, D., Kreek, M. J., Des Jarlais, D. C., Spira, T. J., Khuri, E. T., Ragunath, J., Kalyarnaraman, V. S., Gelb, A. M., & Miescher, A. (1986). Abstract of clinical research findings: Therapeutic and ethical aspects. In L. J. Harris (Ed.), *Problems of Drug Dependence 1985: Proceedings of the 47th Annual Meeting, The Committee on Problems of Drug Dependence, Inc.* Rockville, MD: National Institute on Drug Abuse, NIDA Research Monograph 67.

Preble, E., & Casey, J. H. (1969). Taking care of business: The heroin user's life on the street. *International Journal of the Addictions, 4,* 1–24.

Redfield, R. R., Markham, P. D., Salahuddin, S. Z., Wright, D. C., Sarngardharan, M. G., & Gallo, R. C. (1985). Heterosexually acquired HTLV-III/LAV disease (AIDS-related complex and AIDS): Epidemiologic evidence for female-to-male transmission. *Journal of the American Medical Association, 254,* 2094–2096.

Robertson, J. R., Bucknall, A. B. V., Welsby, P. D., Roberts, J. J. K., Inglis, J. M., Peutherer, J. F., & Brettle, R. P. (1986). Epidemic of AIDS-related virus (HTLV-III/LAV) infection among intravenous drug users. *British Medical Journal, 292,* 527–529.

Schaps, E., Dibartolo, R., Palley, C., & Churgin, S. (1978). *Primary prevention research: A review of 127 program evaluations.* Walnut Creek, CA: Pyramid Project, Pacific Institute for Research and Evaluation.

Schupbach, J., Haller, O., Vogt, M., Luthy, R., Joller, H., Oelz, O., Popovic, M., Sarngadharan, M. G., & Gallo, R. C. (1985). Antibodies for HTLV-III in Swiss patients with AIDS and pre-AIDS and in groups at risk for AIDS. *New England Journal of Medicine, 312,* 265–270.

Selwyn, P. A., Cox, C. P., Feiner, C., Lipschutz, C., & Cohen, R. (1985, November 18). *Knowledge about AIDS and high-risk behavior among intravenous drug abusers in New York City.* Presented at annual meeting of the American Public Health Association, Washington, D.C.

Spira, T. J., Des Jarlais, D. C., Bokos, D., Onichi, R., Kiprov, R., & Kalyanaraman, V. S. (1985, April). *HTLV-III/LAV antibodies in intravenous drug users—Comparisons of high and low risk areas for AIDS.* Presented at the International Conference on the Acquired Immune Deficiency Syndrome (AIDS), Atlanta, GA.

Weiss, S. H., Ginzburg, H. M., Goedert, J. J., Biggar, R. J., Mohica, B. A., & Blattner, W. A. (1985, April). *Risk for HTLV-III exposure and AIDS among parenteral drug abusers in New Jersey*. Presented at the International Conference on the Acquired Immune Deficiency Syndrome (AIDS), Atlanta, GA.

Weppner, R. S. (Ed.). (1977). *Street ethnography*. Beverly Hills, CA: Sage.

14

Can Public Policies Limit the Spread of HIV Among IV Drug Users?

Richard Conviser and John H. Rutledge

Within the last year it has become clear that the virus responsible for the AIDS epidemic (HIV) has been spreading most rapidly among intravenous drug users (IVDUs). The spread of HIV occurred earlier among New Jersey IVDUs than it did in other parts of the United States or the world. By the end of 1983, over 40% of New Jersey's reported AIDS cases had been among heterosexual IVDUs, and as of July 1987, the percentage of New Jersey's 2,229 AIDS cases directly attributable to drug use alone was 45%. Another 6% of New Jersey's cases were among homosexual IV drug users, bringing to more than half the proportion of New Jersey's cases in which drug use was a risk factor. Add to this the cases resulting from either sexual transmission by IVDUs or perinatal transmission by IVDUs or their sex partners, and drug use becomes a factor in about 60% of New Jersey's AIDS cases. That this epidemic has not even begun to run its course is suggested by data on seropositivity among New Jersey's estimated 40,000 IVDUs. Among those presenting themselves for drug treatment in parts of northern New Jersey in 1984, seropositivity rates exceeded 50%.[1] Thus, thousands more of New Jersey's IVDUs are likely to develop AIDS in the next decade, along with many of their sex partners and children. Heroic measures are required if the further spread of HIV from IV drug use is to be prevented. Caring for those already infected will burden both the state's health care facilities and those who have to pay for the care. Given the increasing amounts of public support that will be required, the epidemic will touch,

Reprinted from Journal of Drug Issues, Vol. 19, Number 1, (Winter 1989), pp. 113–128. Copyright © 1989 by the *Journal of Drug Issues*. Reprinted with permission.

167

CAN PUBLIC POLICIES LIMIT THE SPREAD OF HIV AMONG IV DRUG USERS?

indirectly, upon everyone in the state. The growth of New Jersey's AIDS epidemic is shown in Chart 1.

In comparison, figures for the United States as a whole show that heterosexual IVDUs accounted for only 17% of the country's adult AIDS cases (as of April 20, 1987) and that homosexual IVDUs added 8% to the percentage of cases possibly attributable to drug use. Seropositivity rates among IVDUs tested in several regions of the United States in 1986–87 varied widely, from 61% in Harlem and Brooklyn, New York to 29% in Baltimore, 5% in Denver, 2% in San Antonio, 1.5% in southern California, and 0% in Tampa, Florida (Lange et al., 1987). In New York City, by mid-1987, IVDUs accounted for 36% of the more than 10,000 cases of AIDS (Sullivan, 1987). Of newly diagnosed AIDS cases in New York City, 47% were among IVDUs. Outside of the northeast, however, few cases of AIDS had shown up among IVDUs by early 1987. In San Francisco, as of the beginning of 1987, the number of IVDUs among reported AIDS cases was miniscule relative to the number of homosexual males with AIDS—thirty-three IVDUs vs. 2,680 gay men. But alternate test site results in San Francisco produced estimates that 10–15% of drug abusers there were seropositive (compared to 40–45% of homosexual men).[2] This

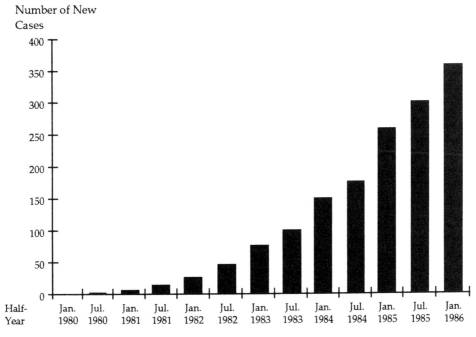

CHART 1
New Cases of AIDS among IVDUs and Others in New Jersey

suggests that the second wave of the AIDS epidemic in San Francisco will be among IVDUs, a fact that public health officials there recognize.[3]

In Europe the picture is very much the same. Among the twenty-seven western European countries currently reporting to the World Health Organization Collaborating Centre on AIDS, the proportion of AIDS cases directly attributable to IV drug use among heterosexuals increased from 12% to 15% in the last quarter of 1986. (Homosexual IVDUs added 3% to this total.) Heterosexual IVDUs accounted for a majority of AIDS cases in only two countries—57% in Italy and 53% in Spain. The next highest percentage—15%—was in Austria. But the proportion of reported AIDS cases among heterosexual IVDUs in western European countries had reached its current level from only 1% at the end of 1984 and 7% at the end of 1985 (WHO Collaborating Centre on AIDS, 1987). Seropositivity rates among IVDUs in European cities varied widely, from 5% in Glasgow, Scotland and 6% in south London (Webb et al., 1987) to over 50% in Edinburgh, Scotland and nearly 80% in Milan, Italy.[4] Rates of HIV infection in many western European cities had risen—Glasgow's 5% in late 1986, for example, was up from only 1% in early 1986, and south London's 6% in May 1987 was up from 0.7% in May 1986. These considerations suggest that the second wave of the HIV epidemic—among IVDUs, their sex partners, and their children—is swelling in Europe as well.

The first wave of HIV infection in the United States, among homosexual males, has slowed considerably as a result of concerted action from within the homosexual community to end high-risk sexual practices. In San Francisco, seroconversion rates among gay men in one sample were in double digits in the early 1980s (Russell, 1987). But figures from 1987 show that the seroconversion rate there has fallen to under 1% annually. Incidence rates for other sexually transmitted diseases in the San Francisco gay community, such as rectal gonorrhea, have also dropped off markedly (Silverman, 1987).[5] These changes bespeak substantial behavior changes toward safer sexual practices among gay men, and the San Francisco results are mirrored in survey results from other large American cities as well (Fox, 1987). However, the community resources that have contributed to behavior changes among gay men—political and voluntary organizations, a gay press, high levels of literacy, visible role models—are largely absent from the drug-using population.

In addition to an absence of community resources, the IVDUs population shares two characteristics that tend to thwart any attempt to produce behavior change among them. The first is that they are addicts. This requires that they devote their energies primarily toward assuring a continuing supply of drugs. The second is that their use of intravenous drugs is a criminal act. Probably, by virtue of their shared activity, IV drug users would form a subculture in any case (Friedman et al., 1986). But in making this activity illegal, the state makes the subculture a deviant one, driving drug users underground and limiting the access health care workers have to them.

169

CAN PUBLIC POLICIES LIMIT THE SPREAD OF HIV AMONG IV DRUG USERS?

The criminalization of drug use produces distrust among users, partly by creating a scarcity of drugs (contributing to their distrust of each other) and partly by putting users at odds with the law (contributing to their distrust of others as possible informers). It also results (along with illiteracy) in the preponderance of oral rather than written communications among IVDUs. There may be relatively small groups of people with whom drug users form strong friendships. The sharing of works (needles and syringes) that is instrumental in spreading the HIV infection is an important symbol of social bonding among these friends. This bonding makes needlesharing behavior difficult to change (Friedman et al., 1986:383). All of these factors—the spread of HIV among IVDUs through needlesharing and its potential spread among their sex partners, the underground character of the IVDUs subculture, and the subcultural importance of needlesharing—add up to present a major challenge to policymakers and public health officials who would stop the spread of the epidemic.

POLICY OPTIONS

It has become clear to key officials in many places that effective control of the HIV epidemic will hinge upon their bringing about changes in the behavior of IVDUs. Dr. Stephen Joseph, Health Commissioner of New York City, has said of the United States that "There will be no slowing of the transmission of the AIDS virus, or of preventing seepage of the virus into the general population, without a meaningful war on drugs . . . The future of the AIDS epidemic in New York and elsewhere in the nation lies in the AIDS–intravenous drug use connection" (Sullivan, 1987).

The ways public officials have chosen to deal with this issue have varied considerably from one country to another. A key factor in their responses has been whether they give more importance to containing the HIV epidemic or to curtailing drug use. Those who place a higher priority on containing the epidemic may, for this purpose, be inclined to overlook the illegality of intravenous drug use; these officials are willing to provide means for addicts to stop sharing needles whether or not they give up using drugs. Those who are committed primarily to eradicating drug use, on the other hand, often favor more punitive measures against addicts. These officials require that addicts give up their addictions as the price for public health protection.[6] In many places, the response to the epidemic has fallen somewhere between these polar extremes. This may represent an ambivalence on the part of officials concerning which goal is the more important, or it may represent a compromise between public health workers who favor the former position and policymakers who favor the latter.

While there are always good reasons that can be offered for a polity's public health response to the AIDS crisis, it is evident that not all responses are equally effective. A comparison of the course of the epidemic in Edinburgh with that in Glasgow suggests that highly punitive treatment of IVDUs may worsen the HIV epidemic. In both Scottish cities, over-the-counter sales of needles and syringes are legal, at the discretion of individual pharmacists. However, police in the Lothian Region of Scotland, which includes Edinburgh, have been far stricter in their treatment of addicts than those in the Strathclyde Region, which includes Glasgow. In Edinburgh, police arrested addicts for carrying needles, going so far as to sit in unmarked cars in front of the pharmacies that sold needles in order to pick up addicts. This drove many addicts into shooting galleries where they could share needles—as many as fifty addicts to a needle. Between 1983 and 1984, the seropositivity rate among addicts in Edinburgh grew from 3% to an estimated 50%. In contrast, in Glasgow, where addicts carrying needles have been left alone by the police, seroprevalence has remained relatively low (5% in late 1986), as addicts have been able to confine their sharing of works primarily to smaller local groups.[7]

There are three basic non-punitive strategies that public officials can follow in an effort to curtail the spread of HIV through shared needle use. The first is to reduce the *demand* for needles by bringing addicts into drug detoxification treatment. This option is intended to get addicts to give up injecting drugs, either by becoming drug-free or by participating in substitution therapy. The latter involves the oral administration of methadone, a drug that blocks heroin craving. Few policy makers object to drug-free programs, while support for substitution therapy varies, both among states within the United States and from one country to another. In the United Kingdom, for example, there has traditionally been little substitution therapy.

The political support that is often voiced for increasing drug treatment program slots does not always translate into appropriations to create such slots. Consequently, drug treatment programs in many parts of the United States are oversubscribed and often have long waiting lists as well.[8] Moreover, few addicts are ready to give up drugs, and many are unable or unwilling to afford the payments typically required for entry into drug detoxification programs. In New Jersey, initial intake fees range from $50 to $175. However, even addicts who do participate in such programs sometimes shoot drugs, and most return to using drugs once they have attempted an initial course of detoxification. For this reason, New Jersey has contracted with many of the state's drug treatment programs to provide AIDS education to program participants. Of the state's eighty-nine programs, twenty-eight (including fourteen detoxification programs) have staff who educate incoming clients about AIDS transmission, symptoms, and prevention. These twenty-eight programs contain a majority of the state's drug treatment slots. Thus, most of the IVDUs who return to using drugs are at least informed about how to avoid exposure to HIV. AIDS education is also offered to continuing clients by designated staff members at these twenty-eight programs.

A second strategy to halt the sharing of needles is to ensure a plentiful *supply* of sterile needles for those who do shoot drugs. This can be facilitated by legalizing over-the-counter sales of needles and syringes, although the cost of works

171

CAN PUBLIC POLICIES LIMIT THE SPREAD OF HIV AMONG IV DRUG USERS?

may still deter some from purchasing them. Needle exchange programs, requiring that used works be returned when new ones are given out, remove this obstacle. Some policy makers object to legal needle sales and exchange programs on the grounds that they appear to condone drug use. Such objections are commonly registered in the United States.[9] However, many other countries have moved in recent years to increase the supply of needles as a way of fighting the HIV epidemic.

Perhaps the most liberal needle distribution policies are to be found in the Netherlands, where addicts' entitlement to health services is regarded as more fundamental than any stigmatization that might attach to them because of their behavior. Various government-sponsored programs in the Netherlands are oriented toward preventing needlesharing among addicts: legal needle sales, needle exchange programs, drug-supply and drug-substitution therapies, mobile methadone treatment vans, and information campaigns conducted with the participation of junkie unions.[10] In the needle exchange program, the number of needles exchanged has grown from 25,000 in 1984 to a projected 600,000 in 1987 (Buning, 1987).

In the United Kingdom, where national health plans entitle all citizens to basic health care, the responses have been largely pragmatic ones. England, Wales, and Scotland are instituting experimental needle-exchange programs and promoting the legal availability of needles; Australia has begun a needle-exchange program in New South Wales and plans to have such programs in all states soon (Wodak et al., 1987); and New Zealand will soon legalize the sale of needles and syringes.[11] Free access to needles and substitution therapies have been available in Italy for several years (Dal Conte et al., 1987), and France legalized the sale of needles in mid-1987 on a one-year trial basis.

Supporters of needle exchanges point out that no increase in drug use has been evident in places where they have been instituted (Des Jarlais, 1987). Preliminary findings from Amsterdam suggest that exchange program participants reduce their needlesharing more than non-participants (Buning, 1987). However, given the social bonding described above, simply increasing addicts' access to works still provides no guarantee that the works will not be shared. Dal Conte et al. (1987) pointedly note that a free needle policy alone will not prevent the spread of HIV among IVDUs. Preliminary results from an Amsterdam study support this view: among prostitute IVDUs studied in 1983–84, seropositivity was 23%; in this same group in 1985–86, seropositivity had risen to 39% (van den Hoek et al., 1987).

To our knowledge, no needle exchange program had been instituted anywhere in the United States prior to 1988. In the spring of 1986, the New Jersey Department of Health cosponsored a conference on "AIDS in the Drug Abuse Community and Heterosexual Transmission" at which several speakers from the Netherlands described needle exchange programs there. The conference inspired some discussion within the Departments of Health of New Jersey and New York

City about instituting such programs on a very limited basis to assess their effects. Even while such programs were under discussion, they received national attention in the news media. This attention may have been premature, since it elicited political reactions before proponents of the programs could fully work out rationales and protocols for them. Many elected officials anticipated that constituent response to the programs would be overwhelmingly negative, and they let it be known that the programs would receive little legislative support. Additionally, within the New Jersey Department of Health, preliminary evaluations indicated that other techniques for reducing the spread of HIV among IVDUs would be more cost-effective. A needle-exchange program was finally instituted on an experimental basis in New York City in 1988.

A third strategy, meant to affect neither the supply of needles nor the demand for them, is to provide IVDUs with information about how to prevent the spread of HIV by sterilizing needles and syringes between uses. These can be sterilized effectively with a variety of substances, including bleach, alcohol, and hydrogen peroxide. Given the constraints mentioned above that make it difficult for addicts to give up drugs and needlesharing, this third strategy had promise to be the most effective of all. However, some people who work with addicts object to providing information on sterilizing works on the ground that they believe it is inconsistent with their central message to give up drugs altogether. This objection is commonly raised by staff members at New Jersey's drug-free treatment programs, in which opposition to the use of any drugs at all sometimes reaches a religious fervor. Consequently, the needle sterilization portion of the AIDS education curriculum tends to be de-emphasized at the drug-free programs. In methadone maintenance programs, on the other hand, one addictive drug (methadone) is already being substituted for another (heroin). Staff members at these programs tend to be more supportive of needle sterilization messages as a pragmatic way of protecting the health of IVDUs.

Providing addicts with information about safer needlesharing practices does not ensure that they will act on that information. Indeed, a key challenge facing those who would change addicts' behavior is motivating them to act on information about how to protect their health and that of others. We will take needle sterilization campaigns as our jumping-off point for a broader discussion of this issue.

INNOVATIVE HEALTH EDUCATION TECHNIQUES TO MOTIVATE IVDU BEHAVIOR CHANGE

It was noted above that there is little trust in the IVDUs subculture and that oral messages are more common there than written ones. These factors limit the credibility that IVDUs place on mass media messages intended to bring about behavior change. Moreover, the mass media would be an inappropriate place to locate messages about sterilizing works for intravenous drug use. Effective campaigns to

173

CAN PUBLIC POLICIES LIMIT THE SPREAD OF HIV AMONG IV DRUG USERS?

teach addicts how to sterilize their works should involve face-to-face contact with people they are able to trust. In New Jersey, such campaigns have been conducted since 1984 by ex-addict street workers, who work in the areas they had frequented as addicts and for the private drug treatment programs in which they have been enrolled. This makes them familiar to many of those they seek to reach. The street workers, affiliated with the twenty-eight drug treatment programs alluded to above, urge addicts to stop sharing works. They also provide IVDUs with specific oral and written information about how to sterilize works if they do share them. Referral for treatment is available from the "Health Educator" street workers if it is requested. Many of those entering treatment reportedly do so after having contact with a Health Educator.

The intake fees charged by New Jersey's drug treatment programs were imposed in 1981 as a result of cutbacks in federal funding. Department of Health personnel believed that the imposition of these fees most seriously limited access to drug treatment among inner city males—the very group at highest risk for HIV infection in the state. Consequently, a voucher program was instituted late in 1986 and—because of high demand—repeated early in 1987 to bring this group into treatment. Coded vouchers were distributed by Health Educators that entitled their bearers to get priority in entering drug detoxification programs and to have the intake fees for their treatment provided by the state. A study has confirmed the success of the voucher program in bringing the targeted population into treatment. Approximately 40% of those presenting vouchers had never before been in a detoxification program, and another 40% had not been in such a program since the fees had first been imposed (Jackson and Rotkiewicz, 1987). All IVDUs presenting vouchers for treatment were required to take an hour-long AIDS education course from an "AIDS Coordinator" at the treatment center.

Cities offering street worker outreach programs similar to New Jersey's include New York, Baltimore, and San Francisco. San Francisco's Community Health Outreach Workers (CHOWs), who are ethnically matched to the populations of the neighborhoods in which they work, distribute small bottles of full-strength bleach whose labels give instructions for cleaning works. San Francisco's program was begun midway between two studies of drug use patterns among the city's addicts. These studies record an increase in the percentage of addicts reporting that they had sterilized their needles with bleach from 3% in 1986 to 68% in 1987, and an increase in the percentage cleaning works in all possibly safe ways from 37% to 76% (Watters, 1987). Program personnel have concluded that "IV drug users are concerned about AIDS and do change their behavior when offered reasonable strategies to protect themselves in a non-judgmental setting. Essential to this behavior change is the ongoing interaction with CHOWs, who support and monitor clients in their communities" (Feldman and Biernacki, 1987). A New York observer has argued, even more strongly, that instruction in AIDS-safe injection practices seems to increase demand for treatment (Des Jarlais, 1987). Once again, this suggests that the alternatives of promoting public health and curtailing drug use need not be mutually exclusive.

The cultural sensitivity that has been shown in street outreach programs is a critical factor in bringing about change in addicts' risk-reducing behavior. Considerations from learning theory suggest why this is so. Behavior change requires not only that people have appropriate cognitive information, but also that they form appropriate attitudes toward that information.[12] The limited initial success of anti-smoking campaigns should make this point evident. Attitudes provide the link between information and behavior: as advertising techniques amply demonstrate, the desired behavior must be made to seem attractive to those in whom it is desired. Thus, prevention efforts should focus on helping people desire to change. Risk-reducing messages that come from people with whom addicts can identify, and those that receive peer support (Phair, 1987), make behavior change more likely. A study by Friedman (cited by Des Jarlais, 1987), suggests that addicts' adoption of risk-reduction practices correlates highly with that of their acquaintances.

However, peer support is often difficult to come by among addicts. The clearest evidence of social organization among IVDUs comparable to voluntary gay organizations comes from the Netherlands, where there are about thirty-five junkie unions.[10] Some of these were formed six years ago in reaction to a proposal for forced detoxification of IVDUs (Friedman et al., 1987). In addition to IVDUs, they involve ex-addicts, relatives, and friends. Five years ago these unions were instrumental in establishing the Netherlands' first needle-exchange programs and in passing out leaflets about the risks of hepatitis B infection. When the government recognized the AIDS epidemic in 1984 and 1985, it acknowledged the unions as having an important potential for AIDS prevention. They became involved in public forums and in prevention activities like preparing a booklet for distribution to addicts. While few IVDUs participate in the unions, many are reached by their messages. The existence of junkie unions points to the possibility of bringing about change in the IVDUs subculture by creating milieux supportive of self-protection, stopping behavior that puts others at risk, and legitimating and building AIDS organizations (Friedman et al., 1987). However, attempts to form such unions in the United States (such as ADAPT in New York City) have met with very limited success.

In New Jersey, especially when its Health Educator program began in 1984, it was difficult to get addicts outside the northeastern part of the state to pay attentionto the Health Educators' risk reduction message. Few addicts in other areas were personally acquainted with anyone who had AIDS, and that made it easier for them to remain ignorant of their risk or to deny it. A similar pattern was reported initially in gay populations and probably typifies other areas where the HIV epidemic among IVDUs is in its early stages. A 1987 study in south London, for example, showed that only 25% of the addicts questioned had known about the

175

CAN PUBLIC POLICIES LIMIT THE SPREAD OF HIV AMONG IV DRUG USERS?

risk of HIV transmission through needlesharing for more than a year (Webb et al., 1987). But as a result of increased evidence of AIDS among addicts and a generally higher level of societal awareness of the epidemic, New Jersey's IVDUs have become more receptive to information about risk reduction.[13] Over half of all addicts coming into treatment centers for detoxification cite a fear of AIDS as a primary reason for their wanting to give up drugs. In addition to addressing IVDUs, the AIDS Coordinators at these treatment centers also provide AIDS education courses for program staff and for community groups and agencies.

While New Jersey's Health Educators and AIDS Coordinators work for private drug treatment programs, the funding for these positions comes from the state Department of Health. This reveals a unique feature of New Jersey's AIDS program: it represents a deliberate decision by a government agency to combine the two approaches—containing the HIV epidemic and curtailing drug use—described earlier in this article. Typically, drug treatment programs focus on controlling the use of drugs in their own treatment populations. But in New Jersey these programs also exert public health leadership in the drug community as a whole through the health educators and counselors. The shift in the orientation of drug programs toward public health is attributable to the way state agencies are organized. In New Jersey, the Division of Narcotic and Drug Abuse Control is located in the Department of Health; in most other states, it is not. In addition, because of the character of its affected population, New Jersey's AIDS program was located in its Division of Narcotics until it became a separate division in 1988. This organizational structure promoted public health concerns for IVDUs. An additional state-funded program, that became operational in mid-1987, sends two mobile health vans into urban areas that have high concentrations of addicts. In these areas, many people do not have access to primary care physicians. Each van is staffed by a physician and a social worker and provides medical examinations and information, educational materials, and appropriate referrals.

HOW MUCH BEHAVIOR CHANGE IS THERE AMONG IVDUs?

The evidence that educational efforts decrease needlesharing among IVDUs offers some grounds for optimism about the possibility of slowing the spread of the HIV epidemic. But a closer examination of that evidence and other factors suggests that the optimism must be tempered severely. First, several studies show that decreases in needlesharing are smallest among the youngest addicts (Dal Conte et al., 1987; Des Jarlais, 1987; Webb et al., 1987). This group is the least likely to have had previous exposure to the virus and thus is at the greatest risk of contracting it for the first time through needlesharing. This risk is, of course, highest where seroprevalence among IVDUs is highest. It is not easy to tell a "running buddy" that one does not wish to share a needle with him because he may be carrying the AIDS virus (Des Jarlais, 1987). Second, many of those who decrease their needlesharing do not abandon it altogether. This is partly because addicts undergoing withdrawal tend not to be very fussy about where their next fix is coming from, even if there is a risk of exposure to the virus. Third, those IVDUs who have had the most personal contact with the disease—i.e., those in the areas where the incidence of AIDS is highest—are the most likely to recognize the risks of needlesharing and act on that knowledge. But it is in the places where seroprevalence, and hence direct acquaintance with people with AIDS, is low that a cessation of needle sharing can do the most good to limit the epidemic's spread.

Studies on sexual practices among gay and bisexual men in areas with a relatively low incidence of AIDS sound a similar cautionary note in this regard. A failure to use condoms in these places is far more common than in places where the epidemic is farther along, largely because the men can rationalize this failure on the ground that there have been few cases of AIDS locally (Valdiserri et al., 1987). The long latency period of the virus can be forgotten at people's convenience. None of these cautionary notes is a reason to abandon efforts to educate IVDUs about the risks of needlesharing. But all of them should serve to remind us of how difficult it can be to change behavior. If the epidemic is to be controlled, far more massive programs need to be mounted to bring addicts into treatment and to try to prevent intravenous drug use in the first place.

Thus far, our discussion has been limited to the second wave of the HIV epidemic, among IVDUs. But we would be remiss if we did not also draw attention to its looming third wave, among the sexual partners of IVDUs and their children. While the numbers of heterosexual partners and infants with AIDS are not yet large, in areas of high drug use it is among them that the epidemic is growing the most quickly. In New Jersey, since 77% of IVDUs with AIDS are black or Hispanic, it is racial and cultural minorities that will be most seriously affected. Through the first half of 1987, 80% of the state's reported pediatric AIDS cases and 85% of the cases of AIDS through heterosexual contact have been among blacks or Hispanics.

At present, bringing about the behavior change required to halt the epidemic on this front seems even more difficult to accomplish than ending needlesharing. In a San Francisco study, the proportion of IVDUs reporting that they used condoms more than half the time in intercourse increased from 4% in 1986 to 14% in 1987 (Watters, 1987). Thus, even in this group that had contact with street outreach workers, the vast majority of intercourse reportedly involved a risk of transmitting HIV. IVDUs typically find it difficult to talk openly with street workers about contraceptive practices, and many male IVDUs are resistant to using condoms.[14] It is also difficult for women to broach the subject of condom use with their (possibly) IVDUs sexual partners, and their attempts to do so sometimes meet with a violent response.[15]

Behavior change in this area has to overcome numerous obstacles, including a general reticence in our culture to discuss intimate sexual behavior, social class and ethnic barriers to such discussions, and sexism. Worth and Rodriguez (1987) report that Hispanic women typically defer to their male partners to make decisions relating to sexual practices. "Puerto Rican women interviewed in drug treatment programs [on New York's Lower East Side] professed the wish to have their partners use condoms, but felt unable to ask them to do so for fear of being rejected or superseding their defined role" (Worth and Rodriguez, 1987:6). Empowering women to reduce their risks of being exposed to HIV by their spouse or partner IVDUs is, thus, not likely to be accomplished readily; this area has yet to get the attention it requires. Worth and Rodriguez (1987:7) propose that successful AIDS prevention and education campaigns within the Hispanic community must originate there and "be delivered by the existing Hispanic leadership and communication network." In New Jersey, there are plans to contract out funds for AIDS prevention messages targeted at women to existing groups in black, Hispanic, and Haitian communities. Some of these groups have already been involved in providing AIDS education and other public health messages, such as pregnancy prevention.

It may be that the HIV epidemic will ultimately reduce the marginalization of the drug subculture in many societies, though not before the epidemic has taken a substantial toll in lives. Given the threat of heterosexual transmission of HIV from IVDUs, some policymakers are beginning to recognize that there might be a social responsibility to provide for the health of IVDUs—because it has implications for the health of others, most of whom have not engaged in any illegal behavior. But no measures to halt the HIV epidemic among IVDUs are likely to succeed unless they involve the addicts themselves in changing their behavior. The greater sympathy and understanding this will require on the part of public health officials and policymakers could provide an opening to make a serious effort to understand and eradicate the social conditions that give rise to drug addiction in the first place. In that way a tragedy could be turned into an opportunity.

NOTES

1 The rates of seropositivity of New Jersey's IVDUs varied inversely with the distance of test sites from New York City, the major source of heroin in the region, from over 50% to a low of under 2% at Camden in Southern New Jersey. All data for the preceding discussion were supplied by the Office of Research and Evaluation, Division of Alcohol, Narcotic and Drug Abuse Control, New Jersey Department of Health.

2 John Newmeyer, Ph.D., Haight-Ashbury Free Medical Clinic, personal communication.

3 David Wordegar, Commissioner, San Francisco Department of Public Health, personal communication.

4 Scottish data from Drs. David Goldberg and John Emslie, Communicable Disease (Scotland) Unit, Ruchill Hospital, Glasgow, personal communication. Italian data from Anna Lucchini, Universita degli Studi-Instituto Malattie Infettive, Turino, International Working Group on AIDS and IV Drug Use, III International Conference on AIDS.

5 Note that seroconversion rates cannot remain in double digits for long before a population has converted entirely.

6 Of course, as will be explored below, addicts who continue to use drugs are not the only ones denied public health protection by this option.

7 Dr. David Goldberg, personal communication. The earlier onset of the epidemic in Edinburgh may be a consequence of its maritime location. However, the difference in growth rates seems principally attributable to police practices. More recently, Lothian Region police have eased up in their arrests of addicts carrying works. In the local drug-using groups in Glasgow, seropositivity rates at the end of 1986 ranged from 0% to about 20%.

8 New York City responded to its "emergency" in mid-1987 by increasing its methadone treatment program slots by 10%.

9 Governor Michael Dukakis of Massachusetts "said he was . . . opposed to the distribution of sterile needles to intravenous drug abusers. 'We should be getting them off drugs,' he said." *New York Times,* June 30, 1987, p. B4.

10 Wouter De Jong, International Working Group on AIDS and IV Drug Use, III International Conference on AIDS, Washington, D.C.

11 British Isles information from Robert Covell, International Working Group on AIDS and IV Drug Use, III International Conference on AIDS. Australian information from Wodak et al. (1987). New Zealand information from Richard J. Meech, Chairman, AIDS Advisory Committee, personal communication. The New Zealand policy shift follows a study that suggested needle sharing was continuing among those shooting drugs 10–50 times in three months because of the limited availability of needles.

12 The discussion in this paragraph draws on materials supplied by Dr. Bernard Branson, Medical Director, Health Education Resources Organization (HERO), Baltimore, MD. HERO has innovated in providing attitudinally sensitive materials to promote the use of condoms.

13 Joyce Jackson (personal communication) reports that the news of Rock Hudson's death from AIDS greatly increased addicts' interest in risk-reduction messages. The authors would like to acknowledge the contributions of Joyce Jackson to both the development of New Jersey's health educator program and the description of it in this article. We would also like to acknowledge the help of Eileen Palsho Nieves, Bob Baxter, and E. Steven Saunders in preparing the article.

14 Joyce Jackson and Bob Baxter, New Jersey Department of Health, personal communication.

15 L. Allen Grooms, Jr., Washington Area Council on Alcohol and Drug Abuse, personal communication.

REFERENCES

Buning, Ernst C. (1987). Prevention Policy on AIDS among Drug Addicts in Amsterdam. Poster session at III International Conference on AIDS, Washington, D.C., June 1–5.

Dal Conte, Ivano, A. Lucchini, S. Colombo, D. Guiliani, E. Nigra, and R. Diecidue. (1987). HIV Infection in Drug Addicts: An Epidemiologal Study in Turin, North Italy. Poster session at III International Conference on AIDS, Washington, D.C.

Des Jarlais, Don. (1987). Current Issues in Drug Abuse and AIDS. Roundtable Discussion, III International Conference on AIDS, Washington, D.C.

Feldman, Harvey W. and Patrick Biernacki. (1987). AIDS Community Outreach for Intravenous Drug Users. Poster session at III International Conference on AIDS, Washington, D.C.

Fox, Robin, D. Ostrow, R. Valdisseri, M. Van Raden, B. Visscher and B. F. Polk. (1987). Changes in Sexual Activities Among Participants in the Multicenter AIDS Cohort Study. III International Conference on AIDS, Washington, D.C.

Friedman, Samuel R., Don C. Des Jarlais and Jo L. Sotheran. (1986). "AIDS Health Education for Intravenous Drug Users." *Health Education Quarterly,* 13, 4 (Winter): 383–393.

Friedman, Samuel R., W. De Jong, D. C. Des Jarlais, C. D. Kaplan and D. S. Goldsmith. (1987). Drug Users' Organizations and AIDS Prevention: Differences in Structure and Strategy. Poster session at III International Conference on AIDS, Washington, D.C.

179

CAN PUBLIC POLICIES LIMIT THE SPREAD OF HIV AMONG IV DRUG USERS?

Jackson, Joyce and L. Rotkiewicz. (1987). A Coupon Program: AIDS Education and Treatment. III International Conference on AIDS, Washington, D.C.

Lange, W. Robert, B. J. Primm, F. S. Tennant, J. T. Payne, C. M. Luney and J. H. Jaffee. (1987). The Geographic Distribution of Human Immunodeficiency Virus (HIV) Antibodies in Parenteral Drug Abusers (PDAs). Poster session at III International Conference on AIDS, Washington, D.C.

Phair, John. (1987). The Role of Health Care Providers in Preventing AIDS and AIDS Hysteria. Workshop at AMA Conference on AIDS and Public Policy: A Community Response, Chicago, April 20–22.

Russell, Cristine. (1987). Map of AIDS' Deadly March Evolves from Hepatitis Study. *Washington Post*, February 1, 1987, pp. A1, A14.

Silverman, Mervyn. (1987). The AIDS Epidemic. AMA Conference on AIDS and Public Policy: A Community Response, Chicago.

Sullivan, Ronald. (1987). Citing "State of Emergency," New York Starts Drug-Clinic Program to Fight AIDS. *New York Times*, June 12, 1987, p. B4.

Valdiserri, Ronald O., D. Lyter, C. Callahan, L. Kingsley, and C. Rinaldo. (1987). Condom Use in a Cohort of Gay and Bisexual Men. III International Conference on AIDS, Washington, D.C.

van den Hoek, Johanna A. R., R. A. Coutinho, A. W. Zadelhoff, H. J. A. Van Haas, N. Trecht and J. Goudsmit. (1987). Prevalence, Incidence and Risk Factors of HIV-infection among Drug Addicts in Amsterdam. Poster session at III International Conference on AIDS, Washington, D.C.

Watters, John. (1987). Preventing Human Immunodeficiency Contagion Among Intravenous Drug Users: The Impact of Street-Based Education on Risk-Behavior. III International Conference on AIDS, Washington, D.C.

Webb, G., H. Burgess, S. Sutherland, J. Strang and T. J. McManus. (1987). Prevalence of HIV among the Infectable Drug Using Population in South London and Factors Influencing Its Spread. Poster session at III International Conference on AIDS, Washington, D.C.

WHO Collaborating Centre on AIDS. (1987). AIDS Surveillance in Europe, Report no. 12, Situation by 31st December 1986.

Wodak, Alex D., K. Dolan, A. Imrie, J. Gold, B. M. Whyte and D. A. Cooper. (1987). HIV Antibodies in Needles and Syringes Used by Intravenous Drug Users. Poster session at III International Conference on AIDS, Washington, D.C.

Worth, Dooley and R. Rodriguez. (1987). Latina Women and AIDS. SIECUS Report Research Note, January–February: 5–7.

15

Drug Abuse and the HIV Epidemic

The Presidential Commission on the Human Immunodeficiency Virus Epidemic

O ur nation's ability to control the course of the HIV epidemic depends greatly on our ability to control the problem of intravenous drug abuse. Intravenous and other drug abuse is a substantial carrier for infection, a major port of entry for the virus into the larger population. Although intravenous drug abusers constitute only 25 percent of AIDS cases in the United States, 70 percent of all heterosexually transmitted cases in native-born citizens comes from contact with this group. In addition, 70 percent of perinatally transmitted AIDS cases are the children of those who abuse intravenous drugs or whose sexual partners abuse intravenous drugs. And the situation is rapidly worsening as the number of infected drug abusers grows daily.

Among the more tragic manifestations of this epidemic are the infected infants of intravenous drug abusers. Most of these children die in their first few years of life. Many never leave the hospital. Their time on this earth begins with a few months of drug withdrawal in an isolation unit and ends after a series of painful illnesses. Because few have visitors in the hospital, the nurses, physicians, social workers, and volunteers who staff our pediatric acute care units become father, mother, and friend to these children. By 1991 there are expected to be 10,000 to 20,000 cases of AIDS among infants and children.

But they represent only the beginning of the tragedy if this nation does not move to address its entire drug abuse problem. The Commission recognizes that

---

"Drug Abuse and the HIV Epidemic" is Section I of Chapter 8: Societal Issues of the *Report of the Presidential Commission on the HIV Epidemic*, submitted June 24, 1988.

alcohol and drug abuse in all their manifestations represent a threat since the use of alcohol or any drug which impairs judgment may lead to the sexual transmission of HIV. The United States continues to have the highest rate of illicit drug use among young people of any country in the industrialized world. Our drug problem pervades all elements of society. A recent study has demonstrated that drug abuse is a problem for both suburbs and inner cities, for all races and at all income levels. Without a coordinated and sustained response, America as a whole faces a bleak future.

In addition to the devastation that drug abuse represents for the individual, the family and the community, the purely financial cost of drug abuse—in terms of providing health care, reduced productivity, law enforcement, plus theft and destruction of property—is estimated at $60 billion annually. This remarkable figure does not include the staggering costs of providing health care for drug abusers with HIV infection.

A number of efforts to curb drug abuse have been initiated. The First Lady's highly visible "Just Say 'No' " campaign, for example, has successfully drawn our nation's attention to the devastation of drug abuse and called on America's youth to reject drugs. Such efforts need to be strengthened and increased. In addition, more needs to be done in providing treatment for those already addicted.

But curbing drug abuse will require major commitments from many sources. It will require, first, that individual drug abusers take personal responsibility for their own well-being. Treatment systems, to be effective, require the commitment of individual drug abusers to the treatment regimen. It will also require a major commitment from federal, state, and local governments, as well as parents, educators, and community leaders to work together to initiate new prevention and education programs and to build community support for eliminating drug abuse and drug trafficking.

The Commission's recommendations are designed to develop a comprehensive, ten-year strategy to deal with the nation's intravenous and other drug abuse problems. This will be accomplished by increasing treatment capacity, increasing research into treatment modes, strengthening primary prevention and early intervention programs, and conducting aggressive outreach programs in HIV-related education and prevention. The Commission recommends a system which can accommodate a treatment-on-demand response for intravenous drug abusers.

Provision of Treatment Services

The Commission believes it is imperative to curb drug abuse, especially intravenous drug abuse, by means of treatment in order to slow the HIV epidemic. Because a clear federal, state, and local government policy is needed, the Commission recommends a national policy of providing "treatment on demand" for intravenous drug abusers.

This policy would need to be a long-term commitment, and the funding should come from a 50 percent federal and 50 percent state-and-local matching program. The spending should be accompanied by the institution of a national campaign to promote community acceptance of treatment programs.

Given the fact that temporarily alleviating the health effects of symptomatic HIV infection can cost as much as $100,000 per person and that imprisonment costs an average of $14,500 per person per year, and even without considering the previously cited astronomical costs of drug abuse to the nation, the investment necessary to provide for intravenous drug abuse "treatment on demand" is sound public policy. Current treatment modes for intravenous drug abusers, including methadone maintenance and drug-free residential communities, reduce illicit drug use, improve employment among addicts, reduce crime rates, and improve social functioning.

Obstacles to Progress

The Commission has identified the following obstacles to progress in providing drug treatment services nationwide:

- The National Institute on Drug Abuse (NIDA) estimates that 6.5 million people are now using drugs in a manner which significantly impairs their health and ability to function. Of these, 1.2 to 1.3 million are intravenous drug abusers. At any given time there are probably not more than 250,000 drug abusers in treatment, of whom 148,000 are intravenous drug abusers. The lack of treatment capacity has produced long waiting lists for treatment, in some cases up to six months, in three out of four cities in the United States. During this waiting period many intravenous drug abusers continue to use drugs intravenously several times each day, increasing their risk of contracting and spreading HIV, and in many cases diminishing their resolve to enter treatment.
- Treatment capacity in most parts of the country can be increased by approximately 20 percent with the addition of treatment funds. But further expansion could exceed the capacity of the nation's existing infrastructure and may require an increase in "brick and mortar" funds and a concerted effort to recruit and train more personnel.
- A substantial commitment of funds by federal, state, and local governments, plus private care providers, is needed to expand expeditiously the quantity and improve the quality of the treatment system. Further, collaboration among all these sources is needed to design innovative plans for reducing barriers to expansion. This expansion should incorporate treatment models which have been demonstrated to be cost-effective. As an interim emergency measure, it may be necessary to establish minimal

service or "holding" clinics, but as soon as possible patients must be admitted to programs with full services, including psychological counseling and medical care.

- Rates of effectiveness of treatment are directly related to retention in treatment. Attention must be paid to improving the quality of treatment to retain clients until they are rehabilitated.
- The presence of HIV infection in the drug-abusing population has generated a decline in the overall health of this population, with dramatic increases in deaths from bacterial pneumonia, tuberculosis, endocarditis, nephritis, and a variety of other infections.
- Establishment of community-based treatment programs has been hampered by the "not-in-my-neighborhood" syndrome.
- Many community services which could give much needed support to clients in drug treatment programs are not well coordinated.
- The treatment field needs more trained staff and in-service training. HIV infection has increased the already heavy burdens on those in this field. In addition to their regular duties, they now face the need to educate their clients on HIV-related issues, risk reduction activities, and, in many cases, the psychosocial needs of dying clients.
- The special needs of women of childbearing age have become more pronounced, emphasizing the need for programs for addicted women, addicted pregnant women, and their children.

RECOMMENDATIONS

In response to these obstacles, the Commission recommends the following improvements in providing drug abuse treatment, with emphasis in every instance on appropriate HIV-related education and prevention:

8–1   In the near term, the National Institute on Drug Abuse, in conjunction with state agencies, local drug abuse officials, and representatives of drug treatment providers, should develop a plan for increasing the capacity of the drug treatment system so that the goal of treatment-on-demand can be met. The plan should designate an implementing office with the staff and technical capacity to guide implementation of the plan. The plan should provide for matching funding on a 50 percent federal and 50 percent state-and-local basis. It should have elements for a phased, targeted increase in programs insuring the quality of care and mechanisms to evaluate progress and make appropriate adjustments.

8–2   The Alcohol, Drug Abuse, and Mental Health Block Grant program should continue to be the mechanism for disbursing treatment funds. However, provisions must be made for expediting disbursements and targeting the money to those areas with the largest numbers of intravenous drug abusers. If using the block grant mechanism would cause undue delays in accomplishing this, consideration should be given to such methods as state and citywide contracts that could later be folded into the block grants.

8–3   The Alcohol, Drug Abuse, and Mental Health Block Grant funds should be directed to activities that stimulate and help patients to enter the treatment system. These activities should include, but not be limited to: aggressive outreach services to drug abusers; telephone hotlines that provide treatment information and initial access to treatment programs; centralized assessment, referral, or intake units; linkages between drug abuse programs and community service agencies, criminal justice and correctional systems, employers, schools, churches, clinics for treatment of sexually transmitted diseases, prenatal clinics, mental health professionals, marriage, family, and sexual counselors and therapists, hospice care, HIV crisis networks and coalitions; and mechanisms for identifying, developing, and cataloguing treatment resources within the community.

8–4   Federal constraints on funds for constructing, expanding, and renovating facilities for intravenous drug treatment should be made more flexible in response to increased treatment needs. In addition, a wide range of federal and local financing arrangements for community-based treatment programs should be considered.

8–5   Since an estimated 1.2 million intravenous drug abusers are concentrated in 24 cities in the United States, treatment should be quickly expanded in those cities by having state, city, local, and community officials identify facilities which could be used for treatment centers. These should include hospitals, clinics, and other health-related sites. Approximately 2,500 new facilities may need to be developed this way.

8–6   As an interim step until new treatment facilities can be developed, state drug abuse agencies should consider contracting with allied health professionals and social workers or organizations to serve as case managers for drug abuse clients. Case managers, who need not be affiliated with traditional drug abuse facilities, could procure medical, educational, job training and social services, and other necessary services, from existing community resources. They could assess client needs, develop individualized treatment plans, procure services, and monitor service delivery. The federal government should provide demonstration funds for projects that use the case management approach to bring external community resources into treatment plans.

8–7   The National Institute on Drug Abuse should develop model demonstration programs that are community-based. These should focus on ethnic and minority populations that have been disproportionately affected by the HIV epidemic, and on the treatment needs of teenaged intravenous drug abusers. In addition, grants should be made to communities which are designing and implementing treatment programs that integrate community services and have the support of community leaders.

8–8 More emphasis needs to be placed on matching treatment with the specific needs of clients. Drug addiction is a disease of the whole person involving multiple areas of function. To be effective, any treatment approach must ultimately address many dimensions of the client. Those who fund and administer treatment programs should become more flexible, focusing not only on drug abuse behaviors, but also on other dimensions of the client's life (e.g., educational and vocational deficiencies and family problems) that may contribute to drug abuse. Services should not be limited to those that can be provided within a program's own facilities or by its own staff. There should be more extensive use of services available in local communities which can help to rehabilitate the drug abuser. This will require a focus on continuity of care, whether services are provided in one facility or in a number of community facilities. Community care facilities which receive public funds should be required to coordinate services with drug treatment programs and should be monitored by appropriate authorities.

8–9 Treatment programs should try different strategies to encourage patients to participate. These should include: extended hours of operation, operation during unusual hours, mobile treatment units, 24-hour satellite clinics in medical facilities, and storefronts in communities. Results of these efforts should be carefully evaluated.

8–10 Effective drug treatment, especially in this HIV epidemic, includes dealing not only with the health care needs of patients but also of their families. Treatment should include on-site primary services or referrals to community health centers, mental health centers, and other accessible community-based resources.

8–11 Comprehensive programs should be made available for women who are intravenous drug abusers and are of childbearing age, pregnant, or mothers. These programs should provide treatment as well as prenatal and postnatal care, day care facilities, family planning, HIV testing, counseling, and child welfare services. It is essential that these services be provided during extended hours.

8–12 Drug treatment programs must aggressively provide HIV prevention and risk reduction education to clients and their sexual partners. Information must be provided on the dangers of needle and paraphernalia sharing, the immunosuppressive effect of drugs (including nonintravenous drugs and alcohol), sexual transmission, and risks to the unborn. Voluntary HIV testing should be strongly encouraged for clients, their sexual partners, children of intravenous drug-abusing mothers, and children of sexual partners of intravenous drug abusers. Any such testing must be accompanied by a counseling program. Collaborative efforts should be established to routinely refer released prisoners to drug treatment programs near their homes, for HIV services as well as drug intervention, if such prisoners are known to have a history of drug use.

8-13 Political and community leadership should be exerted to reduce barriers to the establishment of community treatment facilities in appropriate locations. In communities where there are high rates of drug abuse and a proven need for drug abuse rehabilitation programs, but continued resistance to their establishment, health commissioners should review the possibility of invoking emergency health measures to overcome this inertia and resistance.

8-14 Quality assurance in drug abuse treatment programs needs to be reexamined. Quality of care needs to be better defined by the drug abuse treatment field and standards for programs and practitioners need to be established or refined. States should reexamine their licensing procedures for drug abuse treatment programs. The federal government should support studies of treatment outcome and the development of scientifically based quality assurance mechanisms.

8-15 A significant increase in trained personnel will be needed to implement new programs. Approximately 59,000 persons will be needed to join the ranks of drug abuse workers. New staff training programs should be developed at universities, community colleges, vocational and technical schools, and through internships in existing drug programs and the training of ex-addicts. Curricula dealing with education, prevention, and treatment of substance abuse and HIV should be developed throughout the educational systems for physicians, nurses, and social service workers. Federal leadership is needed to foster and identify model curricula for training programs as well as establishing the fields of drug abuse prevention, treatment, and research as viable and rewarding professions.

8-16 Staff development and training for drug abuse treatment providers must include education and skill development related to HIV, such as education in the modes of HIV transmission and prevention.

8-17 State judicial and correctional systems should consider assigning individuals to drug treatment programs as a sentence or in connection with sentencing. For persons convicted of drug-related offenses or those convicted on non-drug-related offenses but found to be drug abusers, the convicted person should be placed in a drug treatment program in those instances where probation authorities recommend alternatives to imprisonment. To assure program compliance, the convicted person should serve a prison sentence for violating the terms of the drug treatment program. Those who are incarcerated should be referred upon release to drug treatment facilities near their homes.

16
U.S. Cities Struggle to Implement Needle Exchanges Despite Apparent Success in European Cities

Chris Anne Raymond

Philosophical arguments are seldom settled by numbers. In the case of drug abusers and acquired immunodeficiency syndrome (AIDS), many public health experts say the numbers support their view that, in the absence of effective means to eliminate intravenous (IV) substance abuse, the next best thing is to help addicts inject more safely. Opponents say that distributing free needles and syringes will encourage drug use and send the wrong message at a time when the nation appears increasingly concerned about the impact of illicit substance abuse.

After numerous false starts, two cities in this country—New York and Portland, Ore.—are poised to put the issue to the test. But given the politically charged environment, it is far from certain that the results of those tests will change minds.

They may save lives, though. As many as 4.5 million men and women are "in the direct line of fire"—as IV drug users or their sexual partners—for human immunodeficiency virus (HIV) infection, says an unpublished 1988 report of the New York County Lawyers Association, using figures compiled by the National Institute on Drug Abuse and other surveys.

NEEDLES AND INFECTION

The association has come out in favor of lifting the legal ban of over-the-counter sales of hypodermic needles. An analysis prepared by the group's Committee on

Reprinted from *Journal of the American Medical Association*, Vol. 260, No. 18, November 11, 1988, pp. 2620–2621. Copyright 1988, American Medical Association.

Law Reform of 17 states with large, urban, minority populations—the group most associated with IV drug use—shows that the average rate of infection with HIV was 31% in states that ban sale of needles, compared with 5% in states that do not have such laws. While no causal relationship can be drawn, the group argues that needle laws have been a major stumbling block in initiatives to lessen the spread of AIDS in the drug-using community.

In New York City, a two-month-long stumble was finally righted at the end of August, when, after a mandatory 45-day waiting period for public comment, and some additional persuasion of narcotics prosecutors, authorization of a needle-exchange pilot project became official (*JAMA* 1988; 259:1289–1290).

The program will take place at four health care facilities in the city. None is or will become a drug-treatment center, according to Stephen C. Joseph, MD, the city's public health commissioner. Two of the sites will give addicts clean needles in exchange for used ones; two sites will serve as controls.

The study will follow about 400 drug addicts. Half will receive needles and counseling and the other half will get information about AIDS risk behaviors, be issued condoms, and will be encouraged to undergo treatment for substance abuse.

"PERMISSION" CARDS

Participants will carry an identification card allowing them to possess needles. The cards have a number, which can be matched by police with a master log of numbers and photographs maintained by the program directors.

Joseph says that the pilot project, using surveys, self-reports, and serologic analysis of returned equipment, will assess several issues: Do people come into the program and stay? Do they go on into treatment? And do they modify their drug use, equipment sharing, and sexual behavior? He adds that it will take from six to nine months to determine the answers to these questions, but admits that as the program is set up "we won't have statistical data on this go-round. This is a feasibility study. We will not be able to answer the public health questions in terms of really staving the spread of the AIDS virus, or the adverse effects [increase in drug using population]."

Meanwhile, a Portland social service agency, OutsideIn, with funding from the American Foundation for AIDS Research, has set up a broader, more sophisticated needle-exchange program that awaits only a liability insurance policy to get under way. OutsideIn, one of the oldest free clinics in the United States, provides medical and prenatal care and has a drop-in center offering mental health and employment counseling to homeless teenagers.

Portland has a much lower estimated HIV seroprevalence rate in its IV drug-using population than does New York City—about 7% vs 50% or more. Health experts there say that there are 7000 to 10,000 IV drug users in the city, which is considered a primary point of entry into the country of potent Mexican heroin.

Although HIV seropositivity rates are still low, an ongoing epidemic of acute hepatitis B infection focused among drug users suggests that their injecting practices favor the spread of infectious diseases, including AIDS. Experience in New York and in Europe indicates that once the HIV virus is present among IV drug users, it spreads quickly.

According to the agency's executive director, Kathy Oliver, MUS (Master of Urban Studies), the Portland project owes its existence to two factors: "OutsideIn had access to a difficult-to-reach, very vulnerable population" and little local opposition to the experiment. "Politically, it was no big deal. Oregonians tend to be somewhat independent . . . the law enforcement people said this isn't a legal issue and we see no reason to take a public stand," Oliver said. Oregon does not ban sale of drug paraphernalia.

POSING TWO QUESTIONS

The Portland project will assess two questions: Does the program reduce the spread of HIV? And does it encourage IV drug use in people not previously practicing such behavior? Four cohorts will be followed up. Two will be used to assess the question of HIV spread, two to address the question of encouraging new drug use.

The first group will consist of 125 participants in the Portland needle-exchange program, who will answer questions concerning drug use and sexual behavior and who will be tested for hepatitis B exposure. Results of the latter test will serve as a marker for new IV drug use and as an avenue for counseling. Part of the blood sample, with all identifying information removed, will be tested for HIV antibodies.

A second cohort will be recruited from 12 cities where needle-exchange programs do not exist, and, to the extent possible, it will be matched to the first cohort in terms of age, race, and length and patterns of drug use. The cities will include those involved in AIDS education efforts funded by the National Institute on Drug Abuse Community Outreach Demonstration Projects.

The third group, of 125 persons in Portland with history of noninjecting drug use, will receive counseling, answer questions about their behavior, and give a blood sample like those in the first cohort.

The fourth group will include persons from New York City who are considered at high risk for beginning to inject drugs; they are part of a Centers for Disease Control (Atlanta) study of drug sniffers. Like the noninjecting Portland group, they will receive AIDS-prevention education. They will not have legal access to injecting equipment.

Even in Portland, some persons have objected to the program, raising questions about its efficacy and ethics. One of the most outspoken critics of such programs, special narcotics prosecutor Sterling Johnson, Jr., of New York City, has been quoted in the *New York Times* as saying he opposes the programs with "every breath I take" for sending the wrong message and that he doubts that any drug injector is capable of deciding to use clean equipment while experiencing intense physical craving.

Responding to Johnson's view that needle exchanges will encourage new drug use, Joseph says that "there aren't any data to back it up." Johnson could not be reached for comment despite repeated phone calls.

The data that are available from needle exchange programs under way in Europe do not support the critics. At the Fourth International AIDS Conference held in Stockholm this year, investigators from the Netherlands, Sweden, England, Austria, and Scotland presented data on their early experience with needle- and syringe-exchange programs.

Several consistent trends emerged from these studies. The programs tend to attract persons who have not had any previous contact with drug treatment programs. "[Drug abusers] are drawn to clean needle programs and then into treatment programs . . . so actually, the rates of IV drug use go down," says David Corkery, a spokesperson for the American Foundation for AIDS Research in New York City. There is no indication in these studies of an increase in the IV drug-using population in cities with exchange programs.

Where HIV testing has been done, the seroprevalence rate shows a marked decline after introduction of the exchange program. Furthermore, self-reported rates of needlesharing and sexual intercourse without condoms, to the extent that they are reliable, show a downward trend.

Observers of the U.S. IV drug-using population point to some indirect evidence to suggest that abusers can and do change their risk behavior. Sellers of illegal needles in New York City report an increase in sales, with at least one fourth of them specifically citing AIDS concern as the reason; some even have been observed using AIDS as a sales pitch.

The street price of clean needles has gone up, and some dealers repackage used needles as new to increase their value. All this suggests growing concern among drug users about the risk of needlesharing (*Ann Intern Med* 1985; 103:755–759).

Despite the apparent success of the European programs, even supporters acknowledge that there are hurdles that may be difficult to overcome in transplanting the model to the United States. Many European countries have traditionally taken a more pragmatic, less repressive stance toward drug users and this may contribute to their success in bringing in participants. Few other countries have the "shooting galleries" common in cities like New York, where dozens of addicts pass one needle among themselves shortly after a drug purchase.

In addition, there is more to sharing of needles than mere supply: it also is a cultural ritual in the drug community. Merely increasing needle supplies will not necessarily stop the practice of sharing, note observers of the IV drug use subculture.

Finally, the latency period between HIV infection and AIDS symptoms increases the difficulty of linking specific risk behaviors to health consequences in the minds of drug users.

Despite these caveats, supporters of the programs, including many government health officials and a panel of the National Academy of Sciences' Institute of Medicine, say that anything that helps reduce risk is worth trying. "We can't answer it [the question of efficacy] with complete authority without trying it here," Oliver notes. The New York County Lawyers Association puts it more bluntly: "AIDS is far more lethal than intravenous drug use."

SECTION SEVEN

AIDS
and Corrections

$\mathbf{M}$ost inmates with AIDS have histories of IV drug abuse (as opposed to homosexuality or bisexuality). In fact, of the institutional cases (3,136 as of 1988; Hammett, 1989:9)* over half have occurred in the mid-Atlantic region of the United States (Hammett, 1989:12), an area where the seroprevalence rate among IVDUs is quite high. Although inmates who have been incarcerated continuously since the beginning of the epidemic are not often acquiring the disease in prison, nonetheless we remain concerned that correctional institutions could become breeding grounds for the spread of the virus.

What will work to safeguard prisoners? The first article in this section, "Issues and Controversies with Respect to the Management of AIDS in Corrections" by Mark Blumberg examines what correctional administrators have been forced to confront:

1. Is the virus being transmitted in prison?
2. Should HIV screening be mandatory?
3. Should seropositive inmates be segregated?
4. Who should have access to files about the HIV antibody status of inmates?
5. Should institutions distribute condoms?

The second article in this section, "AIDS and Prisoners' Rights Law: Deciphering the Administrative Guideposts" by Allen F. Anderson looks at the legal issues

---

*Hammett, Theodore M. (1989). *1988 Update: AIDS in Correctional Facilities.* Washington, D.C.: National Institute of Justice, June.

surrounding the quality of inmate care, the confidentiality of institutional medical records, the constitutionality of segregating infected inmates, and institutional liability for transmission of the virus. The author shows how established case law can be applied and in most instances how courts have shown considerable deference to correctional administrators in the formulation of policy in this area.

The final article in this section is an excerpt from the National Institute of Justice monograph "AIDS in Probation and Parole" authored by Dana Eser Hunt. The chapter is entitled "Confidentiality, Legal and Labor Relations Issues" and focuses on the impact of AIDS on the work of community corrections personnel. For example, what responsibility do probation and parole officers have to notify third parties who may be placed at risk due to the high-risk behavior of their paroled clients? Could the agency be held civilly liable if a sex partner of a probationer or parolee became infected with HIV? This article will be useful to community corrections administrators who must formulate policy for dealing with AIDS.

17

Issues and Controversies with Respect to the Management of AIDS in Corrections

Mark Blumberg

INTRODUCTION

In the United States, AIDS cases have predominated among gay or bisexual males and intravenous (IV) drug users. Because correctional institutions contain a large number of inmates who have a history of IV drug use, and because homosexual behavior is a reality in jails and prisons, many have feared that these facilities would contribute to the spread of this disease. To assess the actual spread of the virus, in each of the last 3 years the National Institute of Justice (NIJ), in conjunction with the American Correctional Association (ACA), has surveyed all 50 state prison systems, the Federal Bureau of Prisons (FBOP) and more than 30 large county/city jail systems to determine the number of inmates who have been diagnosed with full-blown AIDS (Hammett, 1986; 1987; and 1988). The findings from these annual surveys indicate that the number of AIDS cases is increasing in the nation's correctional facilities, but at a slower pace than in the general population. As of October 1, 1987, a cumulative total of 1,964 confirmed cases had been reported. This represents an increase of 59 percent over the previous year's cumulative total of 1,232 inmates diagnosed with full-blown AIDS, comparable with a rate of increase of 61 percent for the population as a whole (Hammett, 1988:23).

This is a slightly revised version of an article that appeared in the Spring-Summer (1989) edition of the *Prison Journal*.

The author would like to express his gratitude to Kenneth Haas, Allen Sapp, and Scott Christianson for providing helpful comments and ideas.

Even though the number of persons with AIDS in prisons and jails has not reached the levels initially feared, the long incubation period associated with this disease has created apprehension that the worst is yet to come. As a consequence, correctional administrators have been forced to confront a variety of new and complex issues as they struggle to develop policies that will prevent transmission of AIDS within the institutional setting. Many of these are issues that the outside society has also faced: mandatory testing, whether to segregate infected inmates, who should have access to the results of positive HIV tests, the appropriate content of educational programs designed to slow the spread of AIDS (i.e., whether to teach abstinence or "safer sex"), and the question of condom distribution. At the heart of the debate is this question: Should prisons and jails adhere to the practices of the larger society, or is the institutional environment sufficiently unique that deviations from these policies are acceptable?

This chapter examines some of the key issues that AIDS poses for policymakers and administrators in the field of corrections. After a brief discussion of the relevant medical and social aspects of the HIV epidemic, the scope of the problem in correctional facilities is explored. The relationship between AIDS in prisons and jails and IV drug use is examined. In addition, various studies that have attempted to determine whether the virus is being transmitted within the institution are highlighted. This is followed by an examination of the pros and cons of various policy options that are designed to prevent the transmission of this disease within the correctional system. The controversies that have been raging in the field of corrections over such practices as mass screening, the segregation of infected inmates, confidentiality requirements, condom distribution and the release of prisoners with AIDS are reviewed.[1]

THE NATURE OF THE HIV EPIDEMIC

Scope

Previously, it was noted that between 1 and 1.5 million Americans have become infected with HIV, the viral agent that causes AIDS (CDC, 12/18/87:804). The great majority of these seropositives[2] appear healthy but are able to infect others. Because the incubation period is so lengthy (mean = seven years), it is not known what proportion of seropositive persons will eventually develop full-blown AIDS. A recent study suggests the percentage may be as high as 99 percent (Lui, Darrow and Rutherford, 1988:1334). At this time, the available data indicate that more than 40 percent will progress to this stage within 10 years and that a similar proportion will develop symptoms of HIV infection that are expected eventually to result in full-blown AIDS (Institute of Medicine, 1988: 35–36).

Mode of Transmission

HIV is transmitted only through certain forms of sexual contact, through inoculation with infected blood, or from an infected mother to a newborn infant (Friedland and Klein, 1987). There is overwhelming evidence that casual contact with infected persons does not transmit AIDS. Studies of individuals who resided in the same household as AIDS patients and who shared plates, cooking utensils, toilets and other objects over an extended period of time have concluded that not a single individual has become infected by such close contact (Friedland et al., 1986).

In the United States, approximately 90 percent of AIDS cases have been reported among two risk groups: homosexual/bisexual males and IV drug users (Centers for Disease Control, 1/23/89:1). Despite exaggerated claims to the contrary (Masters and Johnson with Kolodny, 1988), there is little evidence to suggest that the disease is breaking out of the high-risk groups into the general population. Only four percent of the cases have been linked to heterosexual transmission (Centers for Disease Control, 1/23/89:1), and the great majority of these have occurred among the female sex partners of IV drug users (Friedland and Klein, 1987:1129).

Treatment

At present, there is no cure for AIDS and no vaccine to protect against the virus. In fact, most public health experts do not believe that a general vaccine to prevent AIDS will be available until the mid-1990s, at the earliest (Weisburd, 1987:329). Physicians are able to treat some of the opportunistic infections that plague AIDS patients. However, the only drug approved to treat AIDS itself is azidothymidine (AZT). This drug has been shown to prolong the lives of persons with AIDS as well as to delay the onset of symptoms in some individuals infected with HIV. The costs of AZT and other medical treatment for AIDS patients are very high. A recent study estimated that the lifetime medical costs (including AZT) for each person with AIDS will rise to approximately $61,800 by 1991 (Hellinger, 1988:309).

Social Stigma

Because AIDS is a horrible disease and because it is associated in the public mind with practices that are viewed as immoral by many people (i.e., homosexuality and drug addiction), a great social stigma has attached to it. Infected persons have often been treated as outcasts and subjected to discrimination. Many cases have been reported in which persons with AIDS or individuals merely carrying HIV have been unable to buy insurance, denied housing, terminated from employment, forced to leave school or subjected to other forms of harassment.

THE RELATIONSHIP BETWEEN AIDS
IN CORRECTIONS AND IV DRUG USE

Outside the institution, male homosexual behavior is the most common risk factor associated with AIDS. Approximately 70 percent of all reported case have occurred among members of this risk group (Centers for Disease Control, 1/23/89:1). Among inmates, however, IV drug use is the key risk factor for developing AIDS. Almost all cases have occurred in prisoners with a history of IV drug use. With the exception of California, IV drug users constitute the majority of inmates with AIDS in all states (Greenspan, 1988:7). In addition, the largest concentration of confirmed cases has been reported in those states (New York and New Jersey) where the rate of seroprevalence[3] among addicts tends to be high. Epidemiological data indicate that between 50 and 60 percent of IV drug users in New York City and northern New Jersey are seropositive, as compared with a rate of less than 5 percent in most other sections of the nation (CDC, 12/18/87:2). Because "shooting galleries"[4] are typically found in the northeast, a substantial proportion of addicts in this region have become infected with HIV.

IV drug use also accounts for the disproportionate number of minority persons affected by this disease. The National Institute on Drug Abuse (NIDA) estimates that 70 percent of the nation's 1.28 million IV drug addicts are black or Hispanic (Stengel, 8/17/87:13). Forty-two percent of AIDS patients are members of these groups (CDC, 3/89:11), approximately double their representation in the general population. One-third of the AIDS cases among minorities are attributed to IV drug use, compared with just five percent among whites (Stengel, 8/17/87:13). Among men with AIDS whose risk factor is not homosexual behavior, the ratio of blacks to whites is 12.0 to 1; for Hispanics, 9.3 to 1 (CDC, 12/18/87:10).

Minorities constitute an even greater proportion of those diagnosed with AIDS in the correctional setting. One reason is the greater prevalence of IV drug use in poor, disadvantaged neighborhoods. Another is that prison and jail populations contain a disproportionate number of minorities as well as IV drug users. Whatever the reasons, the fact remains that this epidemic has placed a tragic burden on some of the most powerless individuals in our society.

TRANSMISSION OF HIV WITHIN INSTITUTIONS

Most epidemiological studies have concluded that the rate of seroprevalence within the general inmate population is low—less than 3 percent (Hammett, 1988:29).[5] Nonetheless, many correctional administrators remain concerned that seropositive inmates will transmit HIV to others within the institution either through homosexual activity, or by sharing contaminated needles or tattoo equipment. Although no cases have been documented in which an inmate seroconverted[6] during incarceration, "logic and common sense both suggest that even in the best managed correctional institutions, there may be at least some transmission of the AIDS virus occurring among inmates" (Hammett, 1987:15). On the other hand, there is little doubt that incarcerated IV drug users face far less risk of becoming infected with HIV than do those addicts who remain on the street.

Several states have attempted to determine through HIV testing whether the virus is being transmitted within the institution. These studies indicate that very few prisoners who have been continuously incarcerated since the beginning of the epidemic are infected. Maryland authorities observed that only two of 137 such inmates were seropositive (Vaid, 1987:238). Similar findings have been reported in New York and Florida (Hammett, 1988:31). However, because the upper limit of the incubation period for AIDS has not been established, it is uncertain whether these inmates actually seroconverted during incarceration.

Mass HIV screening of all inmates *both* upon entry and at release has been instituted in four states (Alabama, Idaho, New Hampshire and West Virginia— Greenspan, 1988:6). These data should eventually provide some indication of how frequently the AIDS virus is being transmitted within the prison. However, because Alabama is the only state among these systems with a substantial number of AIDS cases, it is questionable whether these findings will be generalizable to those systems that contain the largest number of inmates with AIDS (New York, New Jersey, and Florida).

MASS SCREENING

In the U.S., public health authorities have attempted to control the spread of HIV through education, voluntary testing and by counseling persons at high risk. With the exception of immigrants and military personnel, most testing has been conducted on a voluntary basis. From the beginning of the epidemic, correctional administrators have debated whether this approach is appropriate in prisons and jails. Before discussing the controversy regarding mandatory testing, it is necessary to touch upon the available medical technology for diagnosing HIV.

The current blood test is not able to predict which seropositive individuals are likely to develop full-blown AIDS, nor at what point symptoms may appear. The test cannot detect the AIDS virus, merely the presence of antibodies to HIV. Because the human immune system will generally not develop antibodies until 6 to 12 weeks[7] after exposure (Petricciani and Epstein, 1988:236), persons tested during this period will be seronegative[8] despite the fact that they are able to infect others. These results are commonly referred to as "false negatives." They pose a real concern for any program of mass screening.

Mandatory mass screening involves testing all inmates or all incoming inmates for HIV infection. A more limited version involves testing only members of high-risk groups (homosexuals, IV drug users, or prostitutes). Proponents argue that mass screening is the best way to identify seropositive inmates. Such a policy provides correctional administrators with an opportunity to target education and prevention programs. In addition, infected individuals can be placed under special supervision to ensure that they do not transmit the virus to others. Supporters of this policy argue that institutions must take action to identify infected inmates and to prevent the spread of this virus, or face civil liability. Finally, it has been suggested that mass screening could provide a more accurate projection of how many cases of full-blown AIDS will eventually develop. This will enable correctional officials to plan more effectively and to seek an appropriate level of funding to meet future needs.

Critics of mass screening do not accept these rationale. They assert that education and prevention programs must be directed toward *all* inmates, and that all prisoners should be encouraged to refrain from high-risk behavior, not just those identified as seropositive. Furthermore, opponents of mass screening decry the practice of segregating infected individuals from the inmate population. Because any system of mass screening would produce some false negatives, it is not possible even to identify all infectious inmates. The problems that this raises with respect to any segregation policy are discussed in the next section.

Opponents of mass screening are also skeptical about the civil liability concern. They note that institutions already have rules that prohibit those types of conduct which can transmit HIV (i.e., sexual contact and IV drug use). As a consequence, inmates who engage in these practices do so at their own risk. Most correctional lawyers argue that the institution would not be held liable unless an inmate became infected through a sexual assault (Hammett, 1987:35).

The claim that correctional institutions must be able to project accurately the number of future AIDS cases is not disputed. However, critics of mass screening note that anonymous testing procedures can satisfactorily achieve this goal. In fact, the Centers for Disease Control (CDC) are now utilizing this procedure to determine the prevalence of HIV in ten geographically diverse institutions across the nation (*Corrections Digest*, 6/1/88:1). Blood samples will be coded in such a manner as to ensure that prison officials do not learn the names of infected inmates.

Opponents of mass screening also fear that it will create a class of outcasts within the institution, with seropositive inmates subjected to harassment, discrimination and perhaps even violence within the prison, and to difficulties in obtaining employment and housing upon release. Finally, they argue that such a policy is not a wise expenditure of resources.

There is also the question of how prisoners will respond to the knowledge that they are seropositive. Because institutions contain a substantial number of individuals with sociopathic personalities, it can be argued that inmates who learn they are carrying a deadly virus might be more likely to engage in predatory behavior.

In recent years, the pressure to conduct widespread testing of inmates has come from politicians, not state correctional officials (Greenspan, 1988:8). In some cases, state legislators have proposed statutes that require mandatory testing over the objections of correctional and public health officials. Both the National Association of State Corrections Administrators (Vaid, 1986:3) and the National Commission on Correctional Health Care (*Criminal Justice Newsletter*, 5/2/88:3) have gone on record as opposing this policy. However, the recent finding that the drug AZT delays the onset of symptoms in certain HIV-infected individuals may greatly change the nature of this debate. The case for testing is much stronger now that medical science has something to offer many of those who test positive. Whether such testing should be done on a voluntary or a mandatory basis is an issue that will probably continue to be hotly debated by policymakers.

It will be interesting to see whether lawmakers continue to press for mandatory HIV testing in correctional institutions now that AZT has been demonstrated to be beneficial for many asymptomatic carriers of HIV. As noted earlier, this drug is extremely expensive; the average cost of treating one patient can be several thousand dollars per year. With the universe of individuals who can benefit from this medication now greatly expanded, politicians may become less interested in identifying infected inmates. In fact, the pressure to conduct testing may come increasingly from inmates whose past behavior has put them at risk of developing AIDS. Whether institutions will be required to provide testing on demand and AZT to those seropositive inmates who could benefit from this drug is something that the courts are likely to be asked to decide.

SEGREGATION

In addition to the controversy over testing, correctional administrators must also decide whether to separate infected prisoners from the inmate population. Segregation can be undertaken for medical reasons,[9] to protect an infected individual from violence, or as a general policy to prevent the transmission of HIV within the institution. It is the latter rationale which raises controversy and is thus the focus of our attention.

Proponents of segregation assert that this is necessary to prevent the transmission of HIV within the institution. Advocates make the following arguments:

1. Previous research indicates that homosexual activity is a fact of life in prison. Nacci and Kane (1983:35) report that 30 percent of male inmates have had a homosexual experience as an adult in prison. Data from another institution (Wooden and Parker, 1982:50–51) indicated that 65 percent of the male prisoners have had sex with another male during their current period of incarceration.[10]
2. Other sexually transmitted diseases (e.g., rectal gonorrhea) are sometimes transmitted in the correctional setting.
3. Tattooing, although prohibited in most institutions, is a common practice;[11] illicit drug use probably takes place as well.

4. Studies conducted within various institutions conclude that a small proportion of inmates are sexually assaulted during incarceration (see Bowker, 1980:2–3).

Civil libertarians are opposed to the practice of segregation except for valid medical reasons or in cases involving protective custody. They argue that because HIV is not spread through casual contact, separate facilities are unnecessary. In fact, the CDC opposes special housing for AIDS patients except when medically necessary. Critics contend that institutional segregation undermines the basic public health message that AIDS is not transmitted except through intimate contact.

Opponents of this practice also express concern because infected inmates are often placed in substandard living quarters and denied an opportunity to participate in certain work assignments or rehabilitation and recreation programs, or to be eligible for work-release. Furthermore, because these prisoners are excluded from many institutional programs, they may also lose the opportunity to earn "good time" credit toward early release.

The problem of false negative HIV test results has already been noted. Vaid (1987) has suggested that a policy of mandatory testing and segregation could actually be counterproductive for this reason. Because individuals who remained in the general prison population would be perceived as HIV-free, inmates might be encouraged to continue engaging in high-risk behavior. Furthermore, such a policy could conceivably place seropositive inmates in greater jeopardy as well. Believing that they have little to lose, these individuals might continue to engage in risky activities. However, it is possible that repeated exposure to the virus may increase the likelihood that a seropositive individual will eventually develop full-blown AIDS (Gostin, 1986:11).

Segregation raises other problems as well. Critics note that it can become very expensive. In those jurisdictions that have a large number of infected inmates, this policy may require the development of what is in fact a second corrections system. Officials may be required to duplicate many existing institutional programs. As the number of cases continues to grow over the next few years, this could become an administrative nightmare.

Clearly, correctional administrators have a legal as well as an ethical responsibility to pursue policies that minimize the transmission of HIV within the institution. However, it is questionable whether a blanket policy of segregation is the best way to accomplish this objective. As an alternative, prison and jail administrators could reduce the incidence of high-risk behavior through such steps as increased supervision, hiring more correctional officers, intensive educational programs, and harsh penalties for sexual assault (Vaid, 1987:238). In addition, the classification process can be used to identify both inmates who are likely to engage in predatory behavior and those who are likely to be victimized. Bowker (1980:11) notes that the latter are "more likely to be middle class, young, inexperienced, convicted of minor property offenses, and slight of build." This is important information for correctional officials who wish to place potentially vulnerable prisoners under special supervision.

CONFIDENTIALITY

Policymakers must also decide who should have access to information about HIV antibody status. Clearly, the attending physician must have these results if the inmate is to be provided with proper medical attention. The case for disclosure to other personnel within the institution is far less compelling. Although correctional officers have sometimes asserted that they have a right to know who is seropositive, relatively few systems routinely disclose this fact to line officers (Hammett, 1988:97). In fact, state law in some jurisdictions prohibits the disclosure of HIV test results without the written authorization of the infected party.

Correctional officers base their case for disclosure on the rationale that this knowledge is necessary if they are to be able to take appropriate precautionary measures when interacting with seropositive inmates. The latter, on the other hand, are genuinely concerned that they will be subjected to threats, ridicule, or even attack if their condition becomes known. Policymakers are thus confronted with the task of balancing these competing concerns. In those jurisdictions that do not prohibit disclosure, does the officer's right to know outweigh the inmate's right to privacy? Are line officers put at increased risk when they are forced to operate without this medical information?

Examination of the circumstances under which HIV is and is not transmitted suggests that the inmate's right to privacy should take precedence over the employee's right to know. For one thing, this virus is not transmitted through casual contact. The basic modes of transmission are now clearly understood. If correctional officers become infected as a result of their employment, it is quite probable that they have engaged in activities with inmates that would be cause for dismissal even if AIDS were not a concern. Second, educational programs have been designed to teach staff to take proper infection control measures with all inmates (e.g., wearing latex gloves when contact with blood or other body fluids is anticipated). Providing institutional personnel with a master list of seropositive prisoners could create a false sense of security for persons working in the facility. Correctional officers may fail to take adequate precautions when appropriate in dealing with unlisted inmates. Because the available technology for detecting HIV antibodies in newly infected persons in unreliable, this would not be a wise course of action.

Whatever policy is followed with respect to notification of line officers, institutions must ensure that the antibody status of infected inmates does not become known within the general prison population. Administrators should clearly enunciate policies that prohibit medical personnel and others from making disclosures to unauthorized individuals. Care must also be exercised in the handling of master lists that contain the names of seropositive inmates. These should be stored in locations that are not accessible to inmates. However, despite the best efforts of correctional administrators, the identity of some infected individuals is still likely to become known. On occasion, inmates will disclose their HIV status to others. In other instances, the fact that an inmate has been denied the opportunity to participate in a particular activity or release program will tip off the institution's rumor mill. Finally, in cases where an individual has progressed to ARC (AIDS-related complex) or full-blown AIDS, the physical manifestations of the disease may become obvious to other inmates. Therefore, educational programs, as part of their mission, must articulate the message that infected prisoners pose no danger to other individuals within the facility as long as high-risk behaviors are avoided.

DISTRIBUTION OF CONDOMS

Another important decision that correctional administrators must confront is condom distribution.[12] Because condoms can reduce the risk of HIV infection, many educational campaigns outside the prison have emphasized the use of condoms as a means of avoiding exposure to the virus. Such campaigns have often been controversial, with critics charging that they encourage people to engage in casual sexual activity. The debate over "safer sex" vs. abstinence is even more intense in the area of corrections. Although most correctional systems allow inmates to be provided with safer sex information (generally through outside speakers), only New York City, Mississippi, and Vermont actually make condoms available for use by inmates within the institution[13] (Hammett, 1988:92).

Advocates of condom distribution assert that homosexual behavior is a fact of life in many institutions and that officials should give inmates access to these devices as a means of protecting them from disease. They point to desperate attempts by inmates who "are fashioning makeshift condoms out of trash can liners, bread wrappers and other plastic bags" in an attempt to protect their health (*Criminal Justice Newsletter*, 7/1/88:5).

Critics of condom distribution note that sexual activity is prohibited within institutions and that many states have statutes that criminalize homosexual behavior. They argue that this step would imply tacit approval of such conduct by correctional administrators. There is also concern how the public might react, and fear that inmates might use condoms to make weapons or hide contraband (Hammett, 1988:92). Finally, there is the question of whether condoms actually offer significant protection against HIV infection during anal intercourse (CDC, 3/11/88:136).

Those jurisdictions that have chosen to distribute condoms report few problems. New York City has not experienced any cases in which inmates used condoms to make weapons or conceal contraband (Hammett, 1988:92). Inmates receive condoms from medical personnel, who must dispense AIDS information and counseling about safer sex along with prophylactic devices (*Criminal Justice Newsletter*, 7/1/88:6). The same policy is followed by Vermont officials.

RELEASE OF PERSONS WITH AIDS

Denial of Parole

How should persons with AIDS be treated with respect to parole? Some argue that infected inmates should be denied release on parole (Vaid, 1987:250) because they present a serious danger to the health of others, and the state has an obligation to protect its citizens from infection. However, others assert that to deny parole solely on medical grounds would constitute punishment based on illness, and would therefore violate the Constitution (*Robinson v. California*, 1962).[14] Because HIV is not transmitted through casual contact, persons in the community could protect themselves by not engaging in the types of high-risk behavior that spread this disease. Following this line of reasoning, it would only be appropriate to deny release to a convicted sex offender who was infected with the virus. Other parolees would pose no greater risk to the public than the one million other seropositives already in the population.

Early Release

Some have made the opposite claim, that inmates with AIDS who present no danger to the community should be eligible for early release from prison. Recently, the New York State Division of Parole announced that 50 seriously ill prisoners had been released as soon as they became eligible for parole (Sullivan, 3/7/87:1). Under the New York policy, release is not automatic; inmates must demonstrate evidence of good conduct and must not present a danger to the community. The state argues that this policy demonstrates compassion toward those who are terminally ill.

Although most jurisdictions with a large number of institutional AIDS cases have not followed the lead of New York, there are several reasons why correctional administrators may wish to consider this approach. For one thing, the cost of treatment for prisoners with AIDS is high, and inmates are not eligible for Medicaid reimbursement or social security disability. As a consequence, correctional systems that must care for many individuals with AIDS will face enormous budgetary pressures. Second, there is the issue of whether prisons and jails can provide satisfactory medical care. Gido and Gaunay (1987) have concluded that inmates with AIDS in New York survive, on the average, less than half as long as such patients on the outside (p. 28). This raises the question of whether institutions are able to provide the kinds of treatment that these patients require. Third, there is a humanitarian consideration: Should gravely ill individuals who pose no risk to the community be forced to spend their final days in prison, isolated from family and friends?

Claims of humanitarian treatment may cut both ways, however. Most inmates suffering from AIDS are not only ill, they are also from the most disadvantaged segments of our society. Few of these individuals come from families with economic resources. Because of their physical condition, they are unable to obtain employment or qualify for health insurance. Some are likely to have trouble finding suitable housing if released and may end up on the street. Under these circumstances, there is reason to believe that early release is not always in the best interests of inmates suffering from full-blown AIDS. Although some correctional systems may be tempted to release these individuals en masse in order to be relieved of the substantial medical expense that treatment for AIDS entails, this temptation should be resisted. Such a policy would be short-sighted. In addition to the hardships that some of these inmates would be forced to endure, the actual savings would be minimal. For the most part, releasees will still be treated at state expense, whether through Medicaid or in public hospitals. Any policy of early release that is truly based on humanitarian concerns must take into consideration the individual circumstances of each particular case.

Conditions of Parole

The HIV epidemic poses other parole-related issues as well. Specifically, may a parolee who continues to engage in high-risk behavior be subject to revocation for this reason? On the one hand, it can be asserted that the purpose of parole is to prevent the commission of additional crimes and that revocation under these circumstances is therefore inappropriate. However, others argue that the purpose of parole is to protect the community, regardless of the nature of the threat. This debate is complicated by the fact that twelve states have enacted statutes that make it a crime to knowingly expose another person to HIV (Weisenhaus, 8/1/88:1). Is it therefore appropriate to revoke parole for this behavior only in those jurisdictions?

Disclosure

Finally, there is the question of disclosure. What obligation does a parole officer have to notify a spouse or sex partner that a releasee is infected with HIV? This is similar to the dilemma that currently confronts physicians. Does the well-being of others outweigh the need to protect patient confidentiality? Clearly, there is no simple answer. In some states, there are statutes that prevent disclosure of HIV test results to third parties without consent. Parole officials in these jurisdictions can protect the health of persons who may be at risk by counseling inmates that they have an ethical obligation to notify all potential sex or needle partners of their HIV status.

CONCLUSION

It is apparent that the AIDS epidemic has generated a great deal of discussion and controversy regarding the proper management of this disease within the nation's prisons and jails. Some correctional systems have responded to this challenge by instituting mass screening for HIV and segregating inmates infected with the virus. Although these measures are viewed by most public health officials as inappropriate for dealing with AIDS, others say that the unique circumstances of the institution justify this response.

Correctional officers have sometimes expressed concern that they will become infected with HIV as a result of various risks that they face on the job. It has been suggested that staff could become infected as a result of bites, by being spat upon, by having feces thrown at them by inmates, or in the course of breaking up fights between prisoners. However, an examination of the dynamics under which HIV is transmitted indicates that all these modes of transmission are highly unlikely. Three consecutive surveys of correctional institutions by the National Institute of Justice (NIJ) indicate not a single case of occupational transmission in the United States (Hammett, 1988:15). With thousands of seropositive inmates in correctional facilities, a compelling case can be made that if occupational transmission were a serious risk in prisons and jails, it would have manifested itself by now.

HIV is a very difficult virus to transmit. Laboratory tests reveal that HIV is not commonly found in the saliva of infected persons (Ho, Byington, Schooley et al., 1985), and that when present, it is found in such minute quantities as to make transmission by biting or spitting extremely improbable. The virus cannot pass through intact skin. Assaults against staff that involve the throwing of bodily waste pose even less danger, because HIV is not present in feces (Hammett, 1988:15). Although it is theoretically possible for a corrections officer to become infected as a result of a cut received in the course of terminating a fight (if one of the participants is seropositive), the fact that this has never occurred suggests that the threat is more theoretical than real. Staff members who consistently follow prescribed CDC (11/15/85) infection control procedures (i.e., ensuring that open wounds are bandaged, wearing gloves when contact with blood or other body fluids is anticipated, etc.) face far less risk from AIDS than from stab wounds or other traditional risks associated with their job.

Not only is the fear of occupational transmission unwarranted, there is also little evidence to suggest that this virus is being sexually transmitted between inmates within the institution. Almost all prisoners diagnosed with AIDS have a history of intravenous drug use prior to entering the institution. In addition, seroprevalence studies indicate that few, if any, inmates who have been continuously confined since the beginning of the AIDS epidemic are infected. As previously noted, the rate of AIDS cases is rising at a slightly lower rate in prisons and jails than in the general population. Taken together, this evidence suggests strongly that our correctional institutions have not become breeding grounds for this disease as was initially feared. In fact, for those inmates who have a history of intravenous drug use, the institution probably provides a more secure environment than they would encounter on the street.

NOTES

[1] Readers who are interested in learning what practices are actually being followed by most correctional facilities with respect to HIV testing, segregation, and confidentiality requirements are advised to consult Hammett (1988).

[2] The term "seropositive" refers to individuals whose blood test indicates that they have been exposed to the human immunodeficiency virus (HIV), regardless of whether they manifest symptoms of illness.

[3] The term "seroprevalence" refers to the proportion of individuals in a specific group who are seropositive.

[4] "Shooting galleries" are locations where drug users gather to rent needles and syringes. It is not uncommon for the same equipment to be shared by numerous addicts in a short period of time.

[5] The rate of seroprevalence is somewhat higher in those jurisdictions (e.g., New York) that have a substantial number of intravenous drug users within their correctional population (*Criminal Justice Newsletter*, 4/15/88).

[6] The term "seroconvert" refers to a positive HIV blood status by an individual who formerly was not infected.

[7] Some persons do not develop antibodies until several months after exposure to the virus.

[8] The term "seronegative" refers to those individuals whose HIV blood test indicates that they have not been exposed to the virus.

[9] Because AIDS patients have an impaired immune system, they sometimes must be isolated to protect them from infectious conditions that do not threaten healthy persons.

[10] These statistics may overstate the risk of HIV transmission within prisons and jails. Wooden and Parker (1982:54) note that the overwhelming majority of inmates in their sample (80 percent) report not having been the passive partner in anal sex. Studies that have examined the sexual practices of gay men observe that this type of behavior poses the greatest risk of viral transmission (Winkelstein, Lyman, Padian, et al., 1987).

[11] Although there are no documented cases of HIV transmission as a result of sharing tattoo needles (Vaid, 1987:230), there is concern that this common practice among inmates may be quite risky.

[12] A policy that would generate far more controversy is the distribution of clean needles to inmates. Not only would this create a security problem, it would be a tacit admission that authorities are unable to stop the smuggling of illicit drugs into the institution. Not surprisingly, this step has not been considered by any correctional facility.

[13] The state of Washington dispenses condoms, but only for conjugal visits. In addition, some jurisdictions provide inmates with condoms upon release (Hammett, 1988:92).

[14] The U.S. Supreme Court noted that even one day in jail for the "crime" of having a common cold would constitute cruel and unusual punishment (*Robinson v. California*, 370 U.S. 660).

REFERENCES

Bowker, Lee H. (1980). *Prison victimization.* Elsevier, New York.

Centers for Disease Control. (1989). *HIV/AIDS Surveillance.* U.S. Public Health Service (March).

———. (1989). *AIDS weekly surveillance report.* U.S. Public Health Service (Jan. 23).

———. (1988). Condoms for prevention of sexually transmitted disease. *Morbidity and Mortality Weekly Report.* Vol. 37, No. 9 (March 11).

———. (1987). Human immunodeficiency virus infection in the United States. *Morbidity and Mortality Weekly Report.* Vol. 36, No. 49 (Dec. 18).

———. (1985). Recommendations for preventing transmission of infection with human T-lymphotropic virus type III/lymphadenopathy-associated virus in the workplace. *Morbidity and Mortality Weekly Report.* Vol. 34, pp. 681–86 (November 15).

Corrections Digest. (1988). CDC funding study to measure the spread of AIDS in U.S. prison population. (June 1).

Criminal Justice Newsletter. (1988). Of inmates from New York City, 15% show exposure to AIDS virus. (April 15).

———. (1988). Correctional health group urges no mass screening for AIDS. (May 2).

———. (1988). Condoms for inmates at issue in Philadelphia, San Francisco. (July 1).

Friedland et al. (1986). Lack of transmission of HTLV-III/LAV infection to household contacts of patients with AIDS or AIDS-related complex with oral candidiasis. *The New England Journal of Medicine.* Vol. 314 (Feb. 6).

Friedland, Gerald H. and Robert S. Klein. (1987). Transmission of the human immunodeficiency virus. *The New England Journal of Medicine.* Vol. 317 (Oct. 29).

Gido, Rosemary and William Gaunay. (1987). *Acquired immune deficiency syndrome: A demographic profile of New York State inmate mortalities, 1981–1986.* N.Y. State Commission of Correction (Sept.).

Gostin, Larry. (1986). AIDS policies raise civil liberties concerns. *National Prison Project Journal* (Winter), pp. 10–11.

Greenspan, Judy. (1988). NPP gathers statistics on AIDS in prison. *National Prison Project Journal* (Summer), pp. 5–8.

Hammett, Theodore M. (1986). *AIDS in correctional facilities: Issues and options.* National Institute of Justice, Washington, D.C. (April).

———. (1987). *AIDS in correctional facilities: Issues and options,* 2nd edition. National Institute of Justice, Washington, D.C. (May).

———. (1988). *AIDS in correctional facilities: Issues and options,* 3rd edition. National Institute of Justice, Washington, D.C. (April).

———. (1988b). *Precautionary measures and protective equipment: Developing a reasonable response.* National Institute of Justice, Washington, D.C. (Jan.).

Hellinger, Fred J. (1988). Forecasting the personal medical care costs of AIDS from 1988 through 1991. *Public Health Reports.* Vol. 103 (May–June):3.

Ho, David D., Roy E. Byington, Robert T. Schooley, et al. (1985). Infrequency of isolation of HTLV-III virus from saliva in AIDS. *The New England Journal of Medicine.* Vol. 313, No. 25 (December 19), p. 1606.

Institute of Medicine. (1988). *Confronting AIDS: Update 1988.* Washington, D.C.: National Academy Press.

Lui, Kung-Jong, William W. Darrow and George W. Rutherford, III. (1988). A model-based estimate of the mean incubation period for AIDS in homosexual men. *Science.* Vol. 240 (June 3).

Masters, William and Virginia Johnson with Robert Kolodny. (1988). *Crisis: Heterosexual behavior in the age of AIDS.* Grove Press.

Morgan, W. Meade and James W. Curran. (1986). Acquired immunodeficiency syndrome: Current and future trends, *Public Health Reports.* Vol. 101, No. 5 (Sept.–Oct.).

Nacci, Peter L. and Thomas R. Kane. (1983). The incidence of sex and sexual aggression in federal prisons, *Federal Probation.* Vol. 47, No. 4 (Dec.), pp. 31–36.

Petricciani, John C. and Jay S. Epstein. (1988). The effects of the AIDS epidemic on the safety of the nation's blood supply. *Public Health Reports.* Vol. 103, No. 3 (May–June).

Rosellini, Lynn and Erica E. Goode. (1987). AIDS: When fear takes charge. *U.S. News and World Report.* (Oct. 12), pp. 62–70.

Stengel, Richard. (1987). The changing face of AIDS: More and more victims are black or Hispanic. *Time.* (Aug. 17), pp. 12–14.

Sullivan, Ronald. (1987). New York State paroles 50 men sick with AIDS. *New York Times.* (March 7), section I, p. 1.

Vaid, Urvashi. (1986). Balanced response needed to AIDS in prison. *National Prison Project Journal.* No. 7 (Spring), pp. 1–5.

———. (1987). "Prisons." In Burris Dalton and the Yale AIDS Law Project (eds.), *AIDS and the law: A guide for the public.* Yale University Press, pp. 235–250.

Weisburd, Stefi. (1987). AIDS vaccine: The problems of human testing. *Science News.* Vol. 131, No. 21 (May 23).

Weisenhaus, Doreen. (1988). The shaping of AIDS law. *The National Law Journal.* Vol. 10, No. 47 (Aug. 1).

Winkelstein, Warren, Jr., David M. Lyman, Nancy Padian, et al. (1987). Sexual practices and risk of infection by the human immunodeficiency virus: The San Francisco men's health study. *Journal of the American Medical Association.* Vol. 257, No. 3 (Jan. 16).

Wooden, Wayne S. and Jay Parker. (1982). *Men behind bars: Sexual exploitation in prison.* Plenum Press, New York.

18

AIDS and Prisoners' Rights Law: Deciphering the Administrative Guideposts

Allen F. Anderson

SCOPE AND PURPOSE

It is often said that a society's ills are mirrored in its prisons. This notion, though somewhat hackneyed, is nonetheless true concerning acquired immune deficiency syndrome (AIDS), with the exception that the mirror should be a magnifying glass. Prisons are, indeed, a confluence of high risk populations and practices[1] that form a particularly volatile, closed environment for the spread of the disease.

Unfortunately, the full impact of the human immunodeficiency virus (HIV) has yet to be felt by the American prison system. Medical researchers, though making significant progress in understanding the disease, are far from finding a cure. Diagnosed cases in the population at large are increasing geometrically: the number doubles approximately every fifteen months (Sullivan and Field, 1988:147). Yet, even these figures are an underestimation of the true reach of the disease when one considers the so-called "iceberg effect" (Daniels, 1987:85): that is, taking into consideration asymptomatic carriers and those with persistent generalized lymphadenopathy (PGL) and other non-specific symptomology.[2] With American prisons in a period of burgeoning growth that is expected to continue beyond the turn of the century, it seems logical that greater and greater numbers of those carrying the virus will be incarcerated, thus leading to a greater potential for exposure by other inmates. As Margolis (1988:59) has warned, the "increasing incidence of AIDS among IV drug abusers and among minority communities, who

Reprinted with permission from *The Prison Journal*, Vol. LXVIX, No. 1 (Spring-Summer 1989), 14–26.

are overrepresented in the population of correctional institutions, should lead to serious concern and continual monitoring and surveillance."

To complicate the picture, a new type of carrier-inmate is emerging as prosecutors use the criminal law in response to certain acts of HIV-positive offenders. Increasingly, such individuals are being prosecuted for the reckless/intentional exposure or spread of the disease to victims or unsuspecting partners under the traditional crimes of homicide, assault, attempted homicide or assault, and reckless endangerment, as well as new AIDS-specific public health crimes (see generally Sullivan and Field 1988).[3] Attempts have even been made to prosecute attacks by AIDS carriers as an assault with a deadly weapon.[4] This means that carriers are being sent into the penal system, not because of some act tangential to their disease, but for the very reason that they have acted with a disregard for others concerning it. This disregard, in many cases, could be expected to continue during incarceration.

The AIDS epidemic has undoubtedly made an already complicated environment even more challenging for prison administrators as they attempt to develop and implement policies that will prevent the spread of the disease among the inmate population, provide for the adequate care of afflicted inmates, and protect staff. As might be expected, prisoners are taking issue with these policies in the courts.[5] The issues being raised, however, are not unique to the virus. As noted by Messitte (1989:202), "the AIDS crisis, for the most part, does not present new legal issues." As long as policy and practice are honed and polished with prior case law in mind from the more generic areas of prisoners' rights law (i.e., medical care, conditions of confinement, etc.), then prison officials are on relatively solid legal ground. Coughlin (1988:66) concludes that "judges are interested in assuring quality care, access to programming, other normally available inmate privileges and grievance mechanisms and assurance that confidentiality is maintained. Administrators who honor these interests stand a good chance of winning litigation."

The purpose of the present article is to review and analyze the main categories of prison case law related to the AIDS problem, and identify judicial concerns which, if met, will simplify official responses to challenges caused by the presence of the disease. However, before these specific areas of litigation are covered, a foundation for administrative action must be laid, that is, the constitutional criteria for the limitation of those rights retained by an individual after incarceration.

THE CONSTITUTIONAL TOUCHSTONE

Today, in contrast to the philosophy of the old "hands-off* doctrine,"[6] "convicted prisoners do not forfeit all constitutional protection by reason of their conviction

---

*Under the "hands-off doctrine," courts did not interfere with the exercise of discretion by correctional administrators operating jails and prisons. This doctrine was observed until the late 1960s.—Ed.

and confinement in prison" (*Bell v. Wolfish* at 545). When official policy or practice contravenes "a fundamental constitutional guarantee, federal courts will discharge their duty to protect" that guarantee (*Procunier v. Martinez* at 405–406). However, the unique goals and demanding circumstances of the prison environment necessitate that the enforceable rights that are retained by inmates be limited in scope. A prisoner's "(l)awful incarceration brings about the necessary withdrawal or limitation of many privileges and rights, a retraction justified by the considerations underlying our penal system" (*Price v. Johnston* at 285). The withdrawal or limitation of constitutional rights must be done with a spirit of "mutual accommodation" in which rights are balanced against the legitimate needs and goals of the correctional institution (*Wolff v. McDonnell* at 556). This balancing of interests implies that one side will win out depending upon the gravity of its claim. The primary objective of any correctional facility is security, and this objective is the greatest counterpoise to any claim that can be asserted by inmates. When evaluating an institution's security claim, courts must give "wide-ranging deference" to prison administrators "in the adoption and execution of policies and practices that in their judgment are needed to preserve internal order and discipline and to maintain institutional security" (*Bell* at 547–548; see also, *Jones v. North Carolina Prisoners' Labor Union* and *St. Claire v. Cyler*). This deference flows from a realization by the courts that corrections is a highly specialized area that demands great expertise: indeed, "courts are ill equipped to deal with the increasingly urgent problems of prison administration and reform (*Procunier* at 405).

Using this line of reasoning in the 1984 case of *Hudson v. Palmer*, the Supreme Court held that prisoners have no Fourth Amendment expectation of privacy in their prison cells. Chief Justice Burger, writing for the majority, concluded that "(w)e strike the balance in favor of institutional security, which we have noted is 'central to all other correctional goals' " (at 3201; citing *Pell* at 823).

While concepts such as "balancing," "mutual accommodation," and "wide-ranging deference" are all helpful in determining the validity of official policy vis-a-vis prisoners' rights, it was not until 1987, in *Turner v. Safley*, that the Court gave its most illuminating statement for evaluating inroads on retained rights. Strongly reiterating *Jones* and *Bell*, the Court gave a standard as well as criteria to assist in the evaluation process. Rejecting strict scrutiny, the test normally used in assessing alleged violations of fundamental rights, the Court held that "when a prison regulation impinges on inmates' constitutional rights, the regulation is valid if it is *reasonably related to legitimate penological interests*" (Id. at 2261, emphasis added). Reasonableness can be determined by asking certain questions. First, is there a nexus between the regulation in question and the "legitimate governmental interest" to which it is in response? There must be a "rational connection" between the policy and its "legitimate and neutral" objective (Id. at 2262). Second, does the policy leave alternative ways of exercising the residual right? Third, what effect will accommodation of the asserted constitutional right . . . have on guards and other inmates, and on the allocation of prison resources generally" (Id.)? And finally, is there an absence of "ready alternatives" to the policy at issue? The Court was quick to note that this *did not* mean that a least restrictive alternative test was mandated. As the Court concluded, "prison officials do not have to set up and then shoot down every conceivable alternative method of accommodating (a prisoner's) constitutional complaint" (Id., parenthesis added). Justice O'Connor, writing for the majority, reaffirmed the notion of judicial deference to corrections officials' decisions when applying these evaluative criteria based upon their expertise and location in the executive branch (i.e., separation of powers).

In *Turner*, the Court upheld policy related to a prohibition on inmate-to-inmate correspondence, but overturned a policy on marriage as overly restrictive. Two days later, the Court handed down its decision in *O'Lone v. Estate of Shabazz*. *O'Lone* involved a policy that had the effect of prohibiting Muslim inmates classified as "gang minimum" from attending Jumu'ah, a weekly service ordered by the Koran. Because of over-crowding, gang minimum inmates worked outside—away from the main building where Jumu'ah services were held each Friday. In upholding this incursion on the Free Exercise Clause of the First Amendment, the Court applied the *Turner* criteria of reasonableness. It was concluded that there was a nexus between the policy and the legitimate governmental interests of responding to overcrowding, easing tension, and curbing congestion at the gate through which the gang minimum inmates had to enter upon return from their work detail. Muslim inmates were given full opportunity to participate in *other aspects* of their faith; for example, congregation for prayer, pork-free meals, the provision of an imam, and special arrangements for fasting during Ramadan. Finally, the Court looked to the impact of accommodation concerning Jumu'ah on other inmates and staff. The development of "affinity groups" and perceived favoritism on the part of prison officials by non-Muslims, as well as the necessity of establishing extra supervisory personnel, made it clear to the Court that there were no "obvious, easy alternatives" to the policy in question.

The point to be made is that when correctional officials are considering a policy, notably in the AIDS area, that may limit some retained inmate right, they should methodically scrutinize it with the above considerations in mind. This reasonableness standard, along with great deference to prison officials' expert judgment, are hallmarks of the judiciary's approach to the following issue areas concerning the HIV dilemma.

MEDICAL ISSUES

Quality of Care

It is obvious that prisons are not designed to care for the terminally ill; punishment and intensive medical care are concepts that meld poorly (see *New York Times*, "Poor Care," 13 May 1988). For example, it was recently discovered that inmates with AIDS in the New York prison system survive only about one-third as long as others with the virus (*New York Times*, "Justice System," 7 February 1988). Shulman and Mantell (1988:983) note that "(t)he complexity and array of symptoms, mood disturbances, cognitive deficits, psychomotor retardation and personality changes associated with AIDS complicate and challenge staff's abilities to manage patient care." This recognition has led LaMarre (1988:127) to conclude that "(a)s the effects of AIDS continue to intensify, correctional agencies will find it more difficult to provide even the basics of adequate health care, opening the door for increased liability" (see also Vaid, 1987:246). To complicate matters, inmates themselves are often quite reticent about seeking timely medical treatment. They "invariably delay coming to sick call until the very last possible moment, going to great lengths to disguise their condition from other inmates and their families" (Coughlin, 1988:64). Fear of the disease itself and shunning or physical assault by other inmates are causes of such secretive, yet destructive, behavior. Not only does this prevent staff from responding properly to the inmate's needs, but also raises the worst case spectre of certain opportunistic diseases associated with HIV (tuberculosis, influenza, hepatitis, etc.) spreading to the general population. The only way to force medical care on such a recalcitrant inmate is by court order (Id.).

Once an inmate has been diagnosed as having AIDS, he or she can expect, as with any other medical condition of sufficient magnitude, a certain level of care that is guaranteed by the Constitution. This constitutionally mandated level of care is, however, quite low. One is entitled to reasonable or "essential" care, but not the best care available (see *Vinnedge v. Gibbs* and *Thomas v. Pate*). Inmates must show that prison officials have exhibited a "deliberate indifference to a . . . serious illness or injury" (*Estelle v. Gamble* at 104) when raising a medical claim under the Constitution. Note that this standard is bifurcated—a deliberate action or inaction concerning a serious medical problem. "Deliberate indifference" must be taken quite literally; that is, accident, unintended consequence, or negligence in diagnosis and/or treatment are not actionable as constitutional claims.[7] This type of indifference results "when prison officials have prevented an inmate from receiving recommended treatment or when an inmate is denied access to medical personnel capable of evaluating the need for treatment" (*Ramos v. Lamm* at 575). The fact that an inmate simply disagrees with a diagnosis or the treatment received does not meet the *Estelle* test and is not a basis for action. As the court stated in *Massey v. Hutto* (at 46), "claims of inadequate medical treatment which reflect a mere disagreement with prison authorities over proper medical treatment do not state a claim of constitutional magnitude" (see also, *Goff v. Bechtold*). To the extent that discomfort results from a constitutionally acceptable level of care, it is "the penalty that criminal offenders pay for their offenses against society" (*Rhodes v. Chapman* at 347). The bench has noted that "the Constitution does not mandate comfortable prisons" (Id. at 349).

As well, this indifference must be concerning a "serious" medical problem. A problem is deemed as being serious "if it is one that has been diagnosed by a physician as mandating treatment or one that is so obvious that even a lay person would easily recognize the necessity for a doctor's attention" (*Laaman v. Helgemoe* at 311). The denial of *non-emergency* care has been held to be nonactionable (*Feazell v. Augusta County Jail*; see also *Goff v. Bechtold* at 698). In contrast, the failure to provide post-operative treatment has been held to violate the *Estelle* standard (*West v. Keve*).

Implicit in *Estelle*, and explicit in actions under 42 U.S.C. 1983, is the notion that a prisoner must be harmed by the deliberate indifference. In *Thagard v. County of Cook*, a jail inmate requested an HIV test on four separate occasions. Although the staff agreed to provide the test, Thagard was transferred into state custody before it could be given. He contended that the failure to provide the requested test resulted in a lack of adequate medical treatment. The federal district court reasoned that Thagard had not met the requisite criteria—deliberate indifference to a serious medical need. He never alleged that he had AIDS, nor did he suffer any actual physical harm because he was not tested in the Cook County Jail. As the court concluded, while providing an HIV test to those requesting it may be good practice, federal courts are "not authorized . . . to enforce good medical practice" (*Thomas v. Pate* at 2).

Similarly, in *McDuffie v. Rikers Island Medical Department*, the plaintiff had spent five months in medical segregation because of a misdiagnosis of AIDS. Seeking redress, he tried to bring a claim of medical malpractice under 42 U.S.C. 1983. In holding that his claim did not reach the level of a constitutional violation, the court reiterated *Estelle* and noted that McDuffie had "not alleged that he suffered any physical harm due to the misdiagnosis nor that medical officials . . . deliberately ignored his serious medical needs" (at 330). Because of a lack of information, the court did not reach the question of "the degree of care that prison officials must exercise in confirming a medical diagnosis of AIDS before segregating an inmate" (Id.).

It is deliberate indifference to a serious medical problem that offends contemporary standards of decency and thus constitutes the "unnecessary and wanton infliction of pain" prohibited in *Gregg v. Georgia* (at 173). Only then does the violation rise to constitutional proportions.

There is no question that AIDS represents a "serious" medical problem for the afflicted inmate. This means that one-half of the *Estelle* standard has been met. A continual monitoring of policy and its impact should take place to ensure essential care. This monitoring should involve greater cooperation between corrections administrators and state health authorities. The judiciary defers to prison officials on correctional matters; so too should these officials give great weight to the opinions of the medical community as to what constitutes essential care in light of contemporary standards of decency and advances in medical knowledge. As such knowledge of the disease increases, what is adequate one year may be inadequate the next. An ongoing monitoring of conditions and quality of care would go far in demonstrating that incidents of alleged shortcoming are not the result of deliberate indifference. All of this will necessitate a greater financial outlay than has been historically allocated for inmate health care; this is the real dilemma for administrators. To better avoid liability, more attention must be paid to adequacy of care. Prison officials are now in the business of responding to the special needs of the terminally ill. Unless more emphasis is placed on responding to these needs, staff and facilities may be stretched to a point that constitutes a denial of essential care.

Confidentiality

In order to protect the inmate with AIDS from harassment and assault, as well as protect his or her interest in confidential medical treatment, actual diagnostic results should be made available only on a "need to know" basis. This, of course, is easier said than done. Guerrero and Koenigsfest (1986:130) found that any "inmate who merely develops suspect symptoms and receives a medical checkup is automatically labeled an AIDS carrier by other inmates and nonmedical staff." In addition, infected inmates often use the disease "for self-serving purposes such as acquiring medical clemency, special diet, various privileges, and more favorable housing" (Id. at 132), and in so doing destroy confidentiality.

In *Baez v. Rapping*, a federal district court speculated in *dicta* that "failure to issue a warning to prison officials to avoid contact with the body fluids of an AIDS carrier might itself be deemed a failure to perform official duties" (at 115) on the part of the physician involved. This does not mean that confidentiality must be breached. Inmates with the virus should be generically labeled, along with other appropriately ill inmates, as having an "infectious disease." This approach guards against a "private right of action" granted under Civil Procedure and Law Rules, Section 4, 504, for violations of medical confidentiality (Coughlin, 1988:64). Though a rather shallow euphemism, the "infectious disease" classification would trigger proper precautionary procedures developed by the Centers for Disease Control that are applicable to a wide variety of diseases (staph infection, hepatitis, etc.). Such a policy would show a good faith effort on the part of prison officials to avoid the blatant labeling of infected inmates while protecting staff.

SEGREGATION AND CONDITIONS OF CONFINEMENT

There is ample precedent to support the policy of segregating inmates with AIDS.[8] Quelling general contentions that diversity of treatment between inmate groups is *per se* a violation of equal protection, the Supreme Court stated in the 1977 case of *Jones v. North Carolina Prisoners' Labor Union* that "(t)here is nothing in the Constitution which requires prison officials to treat all inmate groups alike where differentiation is necessary to avoid an imminent threat of institutional disruption and violence" (at 136). The danger of the spread of the disease and the potential for assaultive behavior against HIV-positive inmates certainly poses an imminent threat of disruption.

In the groundbreaking case of *Cordero v. Coughlin*, a federal district court, speaking directly to a policy of segregation of inmates with AIDS, held that the equal protection clause "simply does not apply." Even if it did, such inmates are not a "suspect class," and "as long as there is a legitimate governmental end and the means used are rationally related to that end," there is no violation (at 10). Indeed, one district court, as *dicta*, suggested that "it may well be that prison officials might face a Section 1983 suit for failing to isolate a known AIDS patient or carrier, if the carrier infects another inmate who could show that such failure to isolate constituted grossly negligent or reckless conduct on the part of such officials" (*Judd v. Packard* at 743).

If, however, individuals *within* a class receive disparate treatment, then there is an equal protection claim. Corrections officials should see to it that "all members of the class (inmates who are known carriers . . .) are treated equally" and the "classification is non-arbitrary" (*Powell v. Department of Corrections* at 971).

Special care should also be taken to ensure that such segregation is nonpunitive in nature and remains as such over time. As Vaid (1987:243) warns, "(p)rison officials should remember that even when the decision to segregate is reasonable, conditions of confinement in segregation must be constitutionally adequate." Adequacy, in Eighth Amendment terms, refers to "adequate food, clothing, shelter, sanitation, medical care and personal safety" (*Wolf v. Levi* at 125). Such mandated treatment, however, does not mean treatment *identical* to other inmates'. The court, in *Cordero*, noted that "transfer of an inmate to less amenable and more restrictive quarters for nonpunitive reasons is well within the terms of confinement ordinarily contemplated by a prison sentence" (at 10).

In *Powell v. Department of Corrections*, an HIV-infected inmate alleged a number of constitutional violations resulting from his nonpunitive segregation from the general population. Among other things, he contended that he had been denied exercise, attendance at worship services, and family visit periods. The district court, citing *Hewitt v. Helms* (at 466–467), reasoned that the "due process clause does not implicitly create an interest in being confined in general population rather than administrative segregation." Courts are without power to intervene in prison affairs so "long as the conditions or degree of confinement are within the purview of the Constitution . . ." (*Powell* at 970). Rights may be limited in the interests of order and the accomplishment of legitimate policies and goals. Though limited in program participation, Powell still has access to work through his job in the infirmary and to worship through visits from the chaplain; that is, he had *alternative ways* of exercising his retained rights (see *Turner v. Safley, supra*).

Program participation may indeed be limited or curtailed if such action has a "rational basis" to legitimate correctional goals, and if participation in the program is not a right. In two separate cases, HIV-positive inmates challenged being removed from a conjugal visitation program and a community trustee work program, respectively (*Doe v. Coughlin* and *Williams v. Sumner*). The courts in each case noted that participation in such programs was a privilege (nonconstitutional) granted through the discretionary authority of prison officials. In *Williams*, had the Nevada legislature enacted "substantive regulatory limitations on the discretion" of such officials, then an employment interest would have been created; however, the law "stop(ped) far short of requiring that the director provide a job for each offender" (at 512).

Curtailment of participation in the conjugal visitation program in *Doe* was related to a substantial interest on the part of prison officials to prevent the spread of the disease. On review, the appellate court affirmed this holding by stating that "(g)iven the recognized danger of AIDS and the fact that (the prison officials) cannot guarantee the disease would not be spread to the nonprisoner if the petitioners are afforded conjugal visits, (the officials) had a rational basis for their determination . . ." (Ct. App. *Doe* at 788, parenthesis added).

Likewise, short of a state enacting "certain regulatory measures whereby a liberty interest is indeed created" (*Baez v. Rapping* at 115), transfer for medical reasons does not trigger any due process right to a hearing. In *Muhammad v. Carlson*, a federal inmate diagnosed as pre-ARC challenged his transfer without hearing to the U.S. Medical Center in Springfield, Missouri. In upholding the transfer process, the Eighth Circuit Court of Appeals ruled that the wording of the regulations in question gave no liberty interest, nor did they "specify any substantive limitations on prison officials' discretion" to transfer after medical recommendation (at 178). Transfer to segregation served the "legitimate purpose of isolating suspected AIDS carriers for diagnostic, treatment, and security purposes" (Id.).

Efforts by inmates to use the Rehabilitation Act of 1973 (29 U.S.C. 794) to challenge program limitations and segregation have been unsuccessful. The Act prohibits institutions or programs, as a *quid pro quo* of receiving federal assistance, from discriminating against otherwise qualified individuals because of their handicap. Inmates have thus claimed that official acts against them are discriminatively based on their alleged handicap—HIV infection. Since official discrimination is not of the invidious variety, strict scrutiny is unnecessary. The appropriate standard for review is "whether the challenged official action has a *legitimate purpose* and whether it was *rational* for the actors to believe that the treatment afforded the individual would promote that purpose" (*Judd v. Packard* at 743). Given the potential severity of the AIDS problem, particularly in the closed prison environment, the need for identification, diagnosis, and treatment are essential. Even if an inmate was considered "handicapped" by the disease,[9] the danger of transmission would lead one to "conclude that he was not 'otherwise qualified' to participate in the program due to the gravity of the disease and the potential of transmission" (*Doe* at 212).

FAILURE TO PROTECT AND LIABILITY FOR TRANSMISSION

A prison "is, at best, tense. It is sometimes explosive, and always potentially dangerous" (*Marchesani v. McCune* at 462). This danger includes sexual assault—an act particularly suited to the transmission of HIV. Inmates have a right to be protected from any harm or suffering that is not a concomitance of their incarceration. Should circumstances deteriorate beyond conditions deemed adequate by "evolving standards of decency," they would constitute the infliction of punishment beyond the boundaries of the Eighth Amendment. As the Tenth Circuit noted in *Woodhaus v. Virginia*, prisoners have "a right, secured by the Eighth and Fourteenth amendments, to be reasonably protected from constant threat of violence and sexual assault by (their) fellow inmates" (at 890, parenthesis added). The court did not have in mind isolated incidents of violence, but was speaking to "confinement in a prison where violence and terror reign . . ." (Id.). This does not mean a state of "anarchy" has to exist, but prisoners must at least have a "reasonable fear for their safety and to reasonably apprise prison officials of the existence of the problem and the need for protective measures" (*Withers v. Levine* at 161). Prison officials must exercise reasonable care to see that such conditions do not develop (see also, *Ramos v. Lamm*). Correctional administrators become open to liability when they are *"deliberately indifferent* to (a prisoner's) constitutional rights, either because they actually intended to deprive him of some right, or because they acted with *reckless disregard* of his right to be free from violent attacks by fellow inmates" (*Martin v. White* at 474, emphasis added). For an inmate to have an actionable claim, it must be shown that there exists "a pervasive risk of harm" and "a failure of prison officials to reasonably respond to that risk" (Id.).

Failure to protect is not simply limited to a concern for assaultive behavior, but also includes a certain protection from communicable disease. In *Lareau v. Manson*, the court held that a failure to screen for communicable diseases could be a "punishment" under *Bell v. Wolfish* since it "created an indiscriminate threat to all inmates" (at 109). AIDS is a communicable disease, though its legal recognition as such may be questionable,[10] and many prisons do screen all inmates for the presence of HIV. The ability of inmates to challenge the presence of seropositive inmates at their institutions has yet to meet with success. Many institutions keep asymptomatic HIV-infected inmates in general population, and some go so far as to house fit inmates with ARC in population as well (Coughlin, 1988:64–65). Some writers believe that seropositivity alone is not enough to mandate segregation. Only when an HIV-positive prisoner has a history of sexually violent behavior would they impose isolation (Vaid, 1987:246).

General population inmates, often operating under profound misconceptions and misinformation about the disease, have challenged the decision to keep seropositive inmates out of segregation. Their problem has been, however, that the courts require "(m)ore than the mere presence of 'possible' AIDS carriers in the prison" for an actionable constitutional claim (*Foy v. Owens* at 1–2; *Muhammad v. Frame* at 2). Prisoners must show, with some degree of specificity, how the conditions of confinement they are challenging put them "so at risk of contracting AIDS that constitutional rights are implicated" (*Muhammad v. Frame* at 2; see also, *Foy v. Owens* and *Jezick v. Frame*).

In *Glick v. Henderson,* an Arkansas prisoner alleged a failure and refusal of the prison system to protect inmates from exposure to the virus. He argued that since the Department of Corrections neither tested *all* inmates and personnel nor segregated those who did test positive, there was a danger flowing from the interaction of inmates and inmates and staff. As well, he alleged the presence of practicing homosexuals in the prison system. Glick sought an injunction to command that prison officials begin to:

1. test *all* inmates and staff for the virus;
2. hospitalize all those inmates that have AIDS;
3. segregate all inmates that are seropositive;
4. prohibit any contact between seropositive staff and inmates;
5. fire all staff with the disease; and
6. report all cases to various governmental agencies.

The court, in refusing to grant relief, went beyond the usual deference to corrections officials' judgments and declined "to involve itself in a medical controversy and to dictate medical guidelines in an area where the medical profession has not yet spoken" (at 2). Notwithstanding this refusal to make medical/correctional policy, the court stated that Glick's allegations were "based on unsubstantiated fears and ignorance," and that the chances of transmission by the means put forth were "simply too remote to provide the proper basis for (his) complaint as . . . framed" (Id. at 3, parenthesis added).

To allege an actual HIV infection in a failure to protect action, an inmate is required to "link transmission to a particular incident" and "establish that the correctional system was 'grossly negligent or reckless.' " (National Institute of Justice publication, 1988:105). The Supreme Court has ruled that mere negligence, some act or inaction that results in unintended loss or injury, does not warrant a constitutional claim (*Daniels v. Williams* at 663; see also *Davidson v. Cannon*). Gross negligence or recklessness involves a higher quantum of mental culpability than simply a "failure to measure up to the conduct of a reasonable person" (*Daniels* at 665). An inmate must show a deprivation of life, liberty, or property as the result of a *deliberate decision* of prison officials (Id.; see also, *Martin v. White, supra*). Even if a specific incident of transmission could be proven, showing that it was the result of a deliberate decision on the part of correctional officials would be a weighty burden with which to go forward.

CONCLUSION

Legal questions concerning AIDS in correctional institutions can, by and large, be answered by applying established (but evolving) case law to the new factual situations that are presented. This does not mean that dealing with the virus behind prison walls will become easy. It merely means that there are definite administrative guideposts put forth by the courts that will assist prison officials in "developing an integrated approach to administering equitable, judicially sanctioned AIDS policies and procedures" (Coughlin, 1988:63). Such an approach will go far in negating any allegation of deliberate indifference to the needs of inmates with AIDS or their noninfected counterparts. However, only so much can be accomplished by "reactive" policies. As Margolis (1988:61) notes, "(f)or more than 94 percent of those with AIDS, the disease is behaviorally transmitted, allowing for the possibility to alter the course of the epidemic through behavioral change." Proactive educational measures aimed at behavioral change "could work as the prison administration's best defense to liability suits" (Vaid, 1987:246). Through inmate and staff education about the disease, "prisons may well be able to meet their duty to warn and can thereby raise affirmative defenses such as assumption of risk" (Id.; see also, National Institute of Justice publication, 1988:105). This approach of combining sound reactive policy with a massive proactive effort is the only way to truly diminish liability; either approach standing alone is not enough.

NOTES

1 As is generally known, "the essential feature (of HIV) transmission involve(s) interchange of blood or body fluids containing the virus" (Bennett, 1987:531). Homosexual contact, IV needlesharing, and tattooing are common prison practices that carry the potential for exchange of such fluids.
    The total number of AIDS cases reported through February, 1989, was 86,656 (Centers for Disease Control, 1989:10). The CDC estimates that one to one and one-half million people are infected with the virus. The Hudson Institute, a private research group, contends that the range is actually two to three million (*New York Times*, "Research Group Says," 20 August 1988). AIDS cases are disproportionately male (91 percent of reported cases) and disproportionately black and Hispanic (41 percent of reported cases), according the CDC (at 10). For example, of all AIDS deaths in the New York prison system between 1984 and 1986, 43 percent were Hispanics and 43 percent were blacks (*New York Times*, "AIDS in Justice System," 7 February 1988).
2 HIV infection carries a complex symptomology. Those infected may not manifest any symptoms (asymptomatic). Early symptoms may include enlarged lymph nodes (PGL) and weight loss. ARC refers to "patients who develop prolonged symptoms of fatigue, fevers, night sweats, weight loss, and unexplained diarrhea. Almost all show evidence of T-cell disorders and chronic swollen glands" (Gong and Rudnick, 1987:13). The terminal phase is often referred to as "end stage" AIDS, where the patient falls victim to a variety of opportunistic diseases. A recent study suggests that one-half of those infected with the virus will develop AIDS within nine years. Another 25 percent will develop ARC during the same time period (*New York Times*, "AIDS Virus," 13 March 1989).
3 For examples of AIDS-specific statutes, see 1987 Ala. Acts 87–574, Section 21(c) and Fla. Stat. Ann. 384.24 and 384.34.
4 For example, in *U.S. v. Moore*, an HIV-infected inmate at the Federal Medical Center in Rochester, Minnesota, was charged with assault with a deadly weapon for biting two correctional officers. The indictment specifically stated that Moore was HIV-positive. The trial court judge declined to instruct the jury that the prosecution had to prove that HIV could be transmitted by a bite before it could

claim that the teeth were a deadly weapon. The Eighth Circuit, though allowing the charges to stand because of the danger posed by any human bite, refused to recognize that it was the HIV infection that made the teeth a deadly weapon. Mention of the disease in the indictment was held to be "surplusage." The court reasoned that "in a legal context the possibility of AIDS transmission by means of a bite is too remote to support a finding that the mouth and teeth may be considered a deadly and dangerous weapon . . ." (at 1168). See also, *U.S. v. Kazenbach.*

    A Georgia inmate received a fifteen-year sentence for biting a correctional officer who later tested negative for the disease. Prosecutors warned that they would "pursue attempted murder charges against any other inmate with the virus . . . who bites a guard" (*New York Times*, "15 Years," 9 October 1988).

    In related areas, an army private was acquitted of three counts of aggravated assault for having unprotected sexual relations after having tested positive for the virus. The court felt that there was a lack of intent to harm (*New York Times*, "Soldier," 29 July 1988). Joseph Markowski was acquitted on two counts of attempted poisoning for selling his infected blood to a plasma center. Here as well, the court felt that there was a lack of specific intent (*New York Times*, "Man with AIDS," 3 March 1988).

5 Vehicles for inmate civil actions, depending upon the inmate's location in the system, include:

  a. 42 U.S.C. 1983, which allows state inmates to seek redress in federal court for "deprivation of any rights, privileges, or immunities secured by the Constitution and laws." For discussions of related issues, see *Alabama v. Pugh* (11th Amendment sovereign immunity), *Davis v. Sherer* and *Storms v. Department of Corrections* (violation of a federally protected right necessary), *Baez v. Rapping* (qualified immunity), *Thomas v. Pate* and *Gibson v. McEvers* (actual harm requirement).

  b. 42 U.S.C. 1985, conspiracy to deprive one of a federally protected right.

  c. 42 U.S.C. 1981, deprivation of equal rights under the law.

  d. 28 U.S.C. 2680 (Federal Tort Claims Act). See *U.S. v. Shearer* for discussion.

  e. State tort law or state civil rights law.

  f. *Bivens v. Six Unknown Federal Narcotics Agents*, which gives victims of a constitutional violation by federal agents a right to seek damages in federal court even though no statute specifically confers the right.

6 See, for example, *Ruffin v. Commonwealth of Virginia.* A prisoner, "as a consequence of his crime, not only forfeit(s) his liberty, but all his personal rights except those which the law in its humanity accords him. He is for the time being the slave of the state" (at 796).

7 However, the prisoner may still pursue redress under state tort law.

8 Nor does an inmate have a liberty interest in the location of his segregation. See *Morris v. Meachum*, where a federal district court reasoned that an inmate "does not have a substantial personal right in the situs of his confinement . . ." Because of the nature of incarceration, such an "interest has been extinguished to the point that the state may confine him where it wishes" (at 1356).

9 See *School Board of Nassau County v. Arline*, where the Supreme Court refused to consider whether AIDS was a physical impairment, or whether contagiousness alone could be considered a handicap under the Act (at 1128, footnote 7). For discussions of the Act and *Arline*, see Kushen, 1988; Levy, 1988. However, a federal district court in Los Angeles expanded the definition of handicap to include HIV-positive individuals (*New York Times*, "AIDS Carriers," 9 July 1988).

10 See note 9, *supra.*

TABLE OF CASES

David v. Scherer. 104 S. Ct. 3012 (1984).

Doe v. Coughlin, 509 N.Y.S.2d 209 (A.D.3 Dept. 1986). Affirmed, Doe v. Coughlin. 523 N.Y.S.2d 782 (Ct. App. 1987).

Estelle v. Gamble. 429 U.S. 97 (1976).

Foy v. Owens, 1986 WL 5564 (not reported in F. Supp.).

Gibson v. McEvers. 631 F.2d 95 (7th Cir. 1980).

Glick v. Georgia. 428 U.S. 153 (1976).

Hewitt v. Helms. 459 U.S. 460 (1983).

Hudson v. Palmer. 104 S. Ct. 3194 (1984).

Jezick v. Frame. 1988 WL 2045 (not reported in F. Supp.).

Jones v. North Carolina Prisoners' Labor Union. 433 U.S. 119 (1977).

Judd v. Packard. 669 F. Supp. 741 (D. Md. 1987).

Kazenbach v. U.S. 824 F.2d 649 (8th Cir. 1987).

Laaman v. Helgemoe. 437 F. Supp. 269 (D.N.H. 1977).

Lareau v. Manson. 651 F.2d 96 (2d Cir. 1981).

McCray v. Maryland. 456 F.2d 1 (4th Cir. 1972).

McDuffie v. Rikers Island Medical Department. 668 F. Supp. 328 (S.D.N.Y. 1987).

Marchesani v. McCune. 531 F.2d 459 (10th Cir. 1976).

Martin v. White. 742 F.2d 469 (8th Cir. 1984).

Moore v. U.S. 846 F.2d 1163 (8th Cir. 1988).

Morris v. Meachum. 718 P.2d 1354 (1986).

Muhammad v. Carlson. 845 F.2d 175 (8th Cir. 1988).

Muhammad v. Frame. 1987 WL 16889 (not reported in F. Supp.).

O'Lone v. Estate of Shabazz. 107 S. Ct. 2400 (1987).

Powell v. Department of Corrections. 647 F. Supp. 968 (N.D. Okl. 1986).

Price v. Johnston. 334 U.S. 266 (1948).

Procunier v. Martinez. 416 U.S. 396 (1974).

Ramos v. Lamm. 639 F.2d 559 (10th Cir. 1980).

Rhodes v. Chapman. 452 U.S. 337 (1981).

Ruffin v. Commonwealth of Virginia. 62 Va. 790 (1871).

School Board of Nassau County v. Arline. 107 S. Ct. 1123 (1987).

Shearer v. U.S. 473 U.S. 57 (1985).

Smith v. Sullivan. 553 F.2d 373 (5th Cir. 1977).

St. Claire v. Cuyler. 634 F.2d 109 (3d Cir. 1980).

Storms v. Department of Corrections. 1986 WL 4704 (not reported in F. Supp.).

Thagard v. Cook. 1985 WL 1495 (not reported in F. Supp.).

Thomas v. Pate. 493 F.2d 151 (7th Cir. 1974).

Turner v. Safley. 107 S. Ct. 2254 (1987).

Vinnedge v. Gibbs. 550 F.2d 926 (4th Cir. 1977).

West v. Keve. 571 F.2d 158 (3rd Cir. 1978).

Williams v. Sumner. 648 F. Supp. 510 (D.Nev. 1986).

Withers v. Levine. 615 F.2d 158 (4th Cir. 1980).

Wolff v. McDonnell. 418 U.S. 539 (1974).

Wolf v. Levi. 573 F.2d. 118 (2nd Cir. 1978).

Woodhaus v. Virginia. 487 F.2d 889 (4th Cir. 1973).

REFERENCES

"AIDS Carriers Win a Court Ruling," *New York Times,* 9 July 1988, sec. 1, p. A6.

"AIDS Inmates Get Poor Care, Report Says," *New York Times,* 13 May 1988, sec. 2, p. B1.

"AIDS in Justice System, Searching for Fairness," *New York Times,* 7 February 1988, sec. 1, p. A56. "Correction," 28 February 1988, sec., 1, p. A3.

"AIDS Virus—Carriers Facing Dim Future," *New York Times,* 13 March 1988, sec. 1, p. A23.

Bennett, F. J. 1987. "AIDS as a Social Phenomenon." *Social Science Medicine* 25:529.

Centers for Disease Control, (1989). *HIV/AIDS Surveillance,* March.

Christel, Lois P. (1980). "An Ounce of Prevention. . ." *Corrections Today* 32 (February).

Coughlin, Thomas A. (1988). "AIDS in Prisons: One Correctional Administrator's Recommended Policies and Procedure." *Judicature* 72 (June–July):63.

Daniels, Victor G. (1987). *AIDS—The Acquired Immune Deficiency Syndrome.* Second edition. London: MTP Press, 1987.

Des Jarlais, Don C. and Dana E. Hunt. (1988). "AIDS and Intravenous Drug Use." National Institute of Justice *AIDS Bulletin* (February).

"15 Years for Biting Guard," *New York Times,* 9 October 1988, sec. 1, p.A28.

Guerrero, Isabel and Alan Koenigsfest. (1986). "AIDS in Prison." In Victor Gong and Norman Rudnick (eds.), *AIDS Facts and Issues.* New Brunswick: Rutgers University Press, p. 124.

Kushen, Robert A. (1988). "Asymptomatic Infection with the AIDS Virus as a Handicap Under the Rehabilitation Act of 1973." *Columbia Law Review* 88:563.

LaMarre, Madeline. (1988). "AIDS Inmates: A Management Dilemma." *Corrections Today* 98 (June).

Levy, Susan J. (1988). "The Constitutional Implications of Mandatory Testing for Acquired Immunodeficiency Syndrome—AIDS." *Emory Law Journal* 37 (1988):217.

"Man with AIDS Virus Cleared in Blood Sales," *New York Times,* 3 March 1988, sec. 1, p. A25.

Margolis, Steven. (1988). "The AIDS Epidemic: Reality versus Myth." *Judicature* 72 (June–July):58.

Messitte, Peter J. (1989). "AIDS, A Judicial Perspective." *Judicature* 72 (December–January):204.

National Institute of Justice. (1988). *AIDS in Correctional Facilities: Issues and Options,* Third edition. Washington, D.C.

"Research Group says AIDS Cases May Be Twice the U.S. Estimate," *New York Times,* 20 August 1988, sec. 1, p. A7.

Shulman, Lawrence C. and Joanne E. Mantell. (1988). "The AIDS Crisis: A United States Health Care Perspective." *Social Science Medicine* 26:979.

"Soldier with AIDS Acquitted of Assault on 3 Other Soldiers," *New York Times,* 29 July 1988, sec. 1, p. A6.

Sullivan, Kathleen M. and Martha A. Field. (1988). *Harvard Civil Rights—Civil Rights—Civil Liberties Law Review* 139.

Vaid, Urvashi. (1987). "Prisons." In Harlon L. Dalton, Scott Burris and the Yale AIDS Law Project, *AIDS and the Law.* New Haven: Yale University Press, p. 235.

19

Confidentiality, Legal, and Labor Relations Issues

Dana Eser Hunt, with assistance from Saira Moini and Susan McWhan

This chapter is divided into three sections. The first examines the issue of notification and disclosure, that is, who receives or should receive information on the HIV status of individuals under community corrections supervision. The second discusses the growing case law on AIDS as it applies to probation and parole departments. The concluding section provides summary guidelines for developing policies to protect confidentiality and minimize the liabilities of parole and probation services.

NOTIFICATION AND CONFIDENTIALITY

The need to form policies regarding disclosure of HIV antibody test results and notification of an AIDS or ARC diagnosis gives rise to some of the most pressing decisions that parole and probation services face. Community corrections staff often argue that they have both a need and a legal right to know test results, because of the perceived health risks associated with not knowing, the potential liabilities for failing to provide necessary services, and the failure to notify and thus prevent HIV infection of a third party. Seropositive individuals conversely assert their right to privacy. While there have been no cases brought specifically against community correction agencies or officers, it is reasonable to assume that indiscriminate circulation of a client's HIV status might entail a serious risk of liability.

Reprinted from *AIDS in Probation and Parole* (Chapter 5), Washington, D.C.: National Institute of Justice, June 1989.

Decisions regarding confidentiality and disclosure may be governed by state law or policy standards. California, for example, requires written authorization to release test results or other medical records. More often, however, there is room for discretion, and community corrections services face conflicting demands.

Community corrections administrators may feel a need to know test results in order to make informed classification and programming decisions. Probationers or parolees suffering from AIDS or ARC often do have special needs in obtaining medical attention, employment, housing, counseling or other support services. In these cases, officers may have a legitimate need to know in order to secure the necessary services. Notification to public health departments, other agencies within community corrections (such as residential facilities), or third parties, such as spouses, sexual partners, employers, or family are all considered important in releasing clients into the community responsibly. Disclosures may also reduce the system's legal liability should a probationer or parolee transmit HIV infection to others.

On the other hand, the most compelling reason for maintaining confidentiality is that persons known to have AIDS, ARC, or asymptomatic HIV infection may suffer discrimination in employment, housing, or insurance coverage, as well as possible ostracism by the community, family, or friends. Again, there is also the danger of complacency or a false sense of security if it is assumed that all those infected have been identified. By contrast, if "universal" blood and body fluid precautions are routinely followed, knowledge of antibody status will be unnecessary to protect staff from infection.

OVERVIEW OF NIJ SURVEY RESULTS

As preceding sections have reported, there are only a handful of community corrections systems that are currently testing or planning to test clients for HIV antibodies. Only three agencies currently do any systematic testing of parolees and two others are considering instituting testing. Five probation systems currently test some probationers and five plan to begin selective testing programs in the future. . . . (H)owever, most agencies do have access to test information from other sources. Thirty percent of the systems surveyed have access through prior incarceration records and 21 percent have access through medical reports.

Few community corrections systems have specific policies regarding the disclosure of HIV antibody test results. Only 21 percent of the probation agencies and 16 percent of the parole systems answered questions concerning disclosure of clients' HIV antibody test results. Again, it must be emphasized that the lack of a response to this question cannot be assumed to indicate a lack of a policy. Survey results indicate that when this information is available, some parole or probation officers, physicians, other medical staff, and departments of public health will be informed. Seven percent of the systems surveyed formally inform the officer and 5 percent formally notify the attending physician. Seven percent surveyed officially notify the department of public health, as is often required by law. Only one probation system and one parole system—both in Georgia—routinely disclose this information to an individual's spouse or family, and no systems report that they inform employers.

RANGE OF LEGAL OPTIONS REGARDING WHO RECEIVES INFORMATION

Sixteen states reported state laws governing notification. The laws vary widely in their restrictions on disclosure, from severely limited to more lenient.

Many states, including California, Florida, Illinois, Massachusetts, Oregon, and Wisconsin, have very restrictive laws regarding disclosure of HIV antibody test results. Under California law, only the subject is entitled to the results of the test unless he or she provides written authorization for their disclosure; written consent is also required for each subsequent disclosure. Without written consent, no one may identify the subject or divulge the results of any test. Test results are not subject to disclosure under California's employer "right-to-know" law and may not influence any decision regarding employment or insurability. In California, for example, blood banks and plasma centers submit monthly reports summarizing data concerning HIV antibody tests, but reference to the identity of individual donors is prohibited.

Under Wisconsin's law, only the subject, the subject's physician, laboratory personnel or other staff of health-care facilities, and the state epidemiologist can legally receive results of HIV antibody tests. A court order is required for all other disclosures. Therefore, in states such as California and Wisconsin, community corrections staff who are not health-care personnel have no right to obtain test results.

Medical staff, in particular an individual's attending physician, have an obvious need to know HIV antibody test results for diagnostic and treatment purposes. These individuals are in a crucial position for maintaining the confidentiality of this information within a correctional environment, as they may be the only persons legally authorized to obtain and disclose this information. If community corrections authorities are notified of a client's HIV seropositivity, the information often comes from correctional medical staff where the individual has been incarcerated.

Many community corrections services argue that both administrators and line officers need to know the results of HIV antibody tests in order to make classification and programming decisions and to protect themselves and the community from infection. The argument that an officer might need to know the HIV antibody test results of an individual under supervision rests on the need for that information in order to provide the necessary services: financial, housing, legal, medical, or counseling. It is essential, however, that policies define carefully who needs to know what and why. Universal precautions with all clients are adequate for the protection of staff in their day-to-day duties so that officers not associated with a client have no real need to know his or her HIV antibody status.

On the other hand, directly supervising officers concerned about provision of medical services or protection of third parties may feel strongly that they need to know. Because community corrections systems have few and usually broad policies regarding disclosure of information on HIV infection, every effort should be made to formalize procedures as precisely as possible. Vagueness inevitably causes problems, and while it may help protect the agency from liability, it serves only to increase the potential liability of an officer.

Moreover, policies should be both reasonable and enforceable, as an officer may be liable for not enforcing agency guidelines. For example, a condition of supervision prohibiting the transmission of bodily fluids (through unprotected sex, donation of blood, etc.) may place an impossible responsibility on officers to monitor the most intimate behaviors of clients.

Few community corrections services are aware of or could become aware of an individual's HIV antibody status, barring self-disclosure or evidence of either clinical indications or high-risk behaviors. However, most systems require that presentence reports include a description of the offender's mental, psychiatric, and physical condition. In New York State, the investigating probation officer looks for possible signs of AIDS or ARC when compiling such reports. If a defendant states that he or she has AIDS or ARC or if this information is passed on to the officer by a third party, the source and circumstances of the disclosure are recorded, along with an assessment of its reliability. If it is suspected that a defendant has AIDS or ARC, despite the absence of substantiation, guidelines suggest that the officer explain to the defendant why it is important that this information be communicated to the agency, although the officer must be careful not to deny the defendant his or her right to privacy.[1]

In the case of parole, if the offender has previously been incarcerated, the same prison systems notify the parole board of an individual's HIV antibody status. Although only a few prison systems conduct mass screening, many test on a limited basis—when clinically indicated, on request, or if inmates are believed to be at risk. A number of correctional systems, including Missouri, Maine, Iowa, and New York, routinely notify community corrections authorities of an individual's HIV antibody status. This information is often included in the medical report, as are diagnoses of AIDS or ARC, to ensure treatment or to secure other necessary services.

New York State provides for a formal exchange of medical information. The Department of Corrections provides institutional parole staff with medical discharge summaries. These reports include a diagnosis of the parolee's condition, a reference to living arrangements and employability where dictated by his or her current medical condition, an indication of whether the inmate has accepted his or her condition and is cooperating with treatment, and whether there is any need to develop or continue treatment. The Department of Corrections sends the Director of Parole a list of all inmates diagnosed with AIDS or ARC. In turn, senior parole officers receive a list of all those under parole supervision who have developed ARC or full-blown AIDS.[2]

The notification of the infected individual's supervising officer is based on the need to provide special services. It would be difficult to argue that *all* officers have a right to know when they are working with HIV-infected individuals based solely on a perceived health risk, since AIDS cannot be transmitted through normal officer-client interactions. As long as standard blood and body-fluid precautions are followed, the officer has little or no risk of infection. AIDS education and training and documented precautionary policies can successfully alleviate unfounded fears of HIV infection on the part of staff who are not directly involved in providing services.

Notification of Other Criminal Justice Agencies, Public Health Departments

Opinions vary on the need to notify other criminal justice agencies. The study highlighted two concerns in particular. One is whether it is necessary to inform residential facilities of a client's HIV antibody status. If these facilities segregate seropositives, disclosure could be required or strongly advised prior to placement. Alternatively, as is the case in Texas, parolees may be required to submit to an HIV antibody test prior to placement, and if they test positive, they may be refused placement. Jurisdictions with such policies defend them as efforts to protect a correctional institution from potential liability should staff or other individuals at the facility become infected. States that have special housing requirements include Wisconsin, Florida, Texas, Colorado, New Hampshire and Georgia. There is, of course, the potential liability from exclusion or special treatment of these clients inherent in this policy.

Another consideration is whether or not community corrections services should inform local police or other law enforcement officers of HIV-infected individuals under their jurisdiction. Some services, including New York, Massachusetts (to a limited degree) and Iowa have made specific provisions for disclosure to local jurisdictions in the event that an individual violates probation or parole and a warrant is filed for his or her arrest.[3] In some jurisdictions, the specific diagnosis may not be revealed, but officers may be warned to "take normal precautions," or they may be given vague disclosures regarding "infectious diseases" or "blood-borne diseases." While technically these warnings maintain confidentiality, since they can apply to diseases other than AIDS, they may in actuality be thinly-veiled codes. Because following "universal precautions" for blood-borne diseases should protect the arresting officer from infection, there may be no real argument in support of such policies.

Six percent of probation systems and 6 percent of responding parole systems routinely notify public health agencies when a client is known to be seropositive. Some states, including Colorado, Nevada, and Louisiana, have laws requiring notification of public health departments. Others, such as California, have laws requiring that summary, statistical information be reported without revealing a subject's identity.

Under the Colorado law, all positive HIV antibody tests must be reported to state and local public health agencies. The law is designed to alert public health authorities to the presence of potentially infectious individuals and to ensure counseling about test results and preventive measures. However, in Colorado, this information is to be held in the strictest confidence and is not disclosed to insurers or employers without permission of the subject.[4]

Notification of Sexual Partners, Spouses, Employers

Notification of sexual partners presents one of the most difficult problems for supervising officers. Many community corrections administrators feel that they may have a moral responsibility to notify the spouse or sexual partner(s) of probationers or parolees with HIV-related conditions, when there is evidence that the individual will not assume that responsibility. The real question is whether community corrections systems should take on a responsibility that is not required of institutions in the community at large, or whether they should rely on AIDS counseling and education to persuade clients to reveal their status to partners.

Some states require that an inmate give his or her written consent for disclosure to the spouse, in order to be eligible for parole. There are serious legal issues raised by such a policy, since mandated disclosure may contradict a constitutional right to privacy. Instead, in an effort to minimize the risk of liability, some agencies adopt written policies requiring the physician, health-care provider, or officer who may know of an individual's HIV seropositivity to counsel him or her. These providers or officials would advise the individual of the responsibility to inform all sexual partners of his or her medical condition, to use safer-sex techniques and if relevant, not to share needles and to disinfect them properly.

In cases in which subjects refuse to inform their spouse or sexual partners of their HIV status, the Federal Division of Probation and the American Parole and Probation Association recommend that community corrections officers refer the matter to the public health authorities. However, if after consultation with public health authorities an officer determines a specific, medical risk to a third party, and the public health department is unable or unwilling to make such a disclosure, *and state or local law does not prohibit such a disclosure,* the officer should provide a "discreet and confidential warning."[5]

Recent CDC guidelines similarly suggest that if an infected individual refuses to notify his or her sexual partners, the health-care professional should consider making a confidential disclosure. A recent law in California permits physicians to notify the spouses of HIV-infected persons. Community corrections systems should make sure that they are aware of state and local confidentiality laws before instituting policies governing third-party disclosures. Such guidelines must be precise, avoiding vague wording that leaves decisions to the "discretion of the officer" or to examination on a "case-by-case" basis.

Since AIDS cannot be transmitted casually, an employer cannot argue that a probationer or parolee poses a threat to the health and safety of others in the workplace. It is unlawful for an employer to discriminate against an employee who is HIV antibody-positive, unless that individual is incapable of performing the tasks required of the job. Therefore, there is no need for community corrections officers to disclose HIV status information to an employer. In fact, agencies may be held liable for defamation or invasion of privacy if the probationer or parolee is discriminated against in a work environment or refused employment as a result of the disclosure.

LEGAL AND LABOR RELATIONS ISSUES

Currently, legal issues pertaining to the treatment of AIDS cases in probation and parole systems are theoretical, as no cases have been filed. However, an examination of the rapidly growing case law on AIDS, in particular as it relates to AIDS in a correctional environment, may clarify the legal issues and liabilities facing community corrections services. This section summarizes case law and legal and labor relations issues raised by probationers and parolees, and by staff.

Issues Raised by Probationers and Parolees
- Challenges to parole eligibility
- Discrimination against those with HIV infection/AIDS
- Special conditions for those with HIV infection/AIDS
- Challenges to segregation in residential facilities
- Challenges to HIV antibody testing
- Confidentiality of medical information
Issues Raised by Staff
- Community corrections' liability for third-party HIV infection
- Testing in response to potential transmission incidents
- Labor relations issues
- Obligation to perform duties

CHALLENGES TO PAROLE ELIGIBILITY

It has been argued that inmates with AIDS should remain under the correctional system's medical care, without parole or pre-release placement in halfway houses or community-based programs, in order to ensure proper care, to minimize the risk of HIV transmission, and to reduce potential liabilities faced by the system. The question is whether or not a parolee's physical condition should alter sentences which were originally mandated by criminal acts and whether or not there are any legal implications associated with such a policy.

Persons who are mentally ill *and* who pose a threat to society or to themselves may be legally removed from society at large and may be committed for extended periods of time. The case of a person with AIDS, however, is very different as the danger of transmission rests largely on consensual acts rather than forcible victimizations. The violent sexual offender is, of course, the exception; he may require special efforts to ensure rehabilitation prior to release. When determining an inmate's eligibility for parole, it would seem reasonable to make an assessment of his or her medical condition as well as an assessment of the likelihood that he or she would engage in violent or other non-consensual acts by which the infection might be transmitted. However, it is unlikely that medical factors alone could legally warrant extending incarceration.

Early release and executive clemency are being considered by some states as the number of persons with AIDS in correctional facilities rises. No states currently report an early release policy for persons with AIDS, though all may use the discretionary early release provision for illness.

Although it may seem reasonable for an officer to recommend early discharge for a parolee dying of AIDS, such a recommendation, based solely on humanitarian reasons, may not be consistent with criteria established by law. Most states have laws dictating early discharge from community corrections services, depending on whether the individual has diligently complied with the conditions of the sentence, whether his or her release would jeopardize public safety (from criminal behavior, *not* from disease), and whether he or she is in need of continued guidance or other assistance as provided through community corrections services.[6]

While early release of individuals with AIDS or ARC is not necessarily recommended except in special circumstances, there may be legal grounds for establishing such special conditions for those with AIDS, ARC, or asymptomatic HIV infection. Community corrections services could be held liable if, as a result of supervision, a client is subject to conditions that adversely affect health. In this regard, an individual's medical condition might warrant changes or exceptions to supervision requirements. Persons with AIDS or ARC may experience periods of severe debility or illness, requiring hospitalization or periods of recuperation, during which time home visits may be the only reasonable method for making personal contacts. AIDS diagnosis alone is not necessary and sufficient to mandate reclassification, although a client's health may factor into such decisions.

DISCRIMINATION AGAINST PROBATIONERS OR PAROLEES WITH AIDS

In October, 1988, the U.S. Department of Justice was asked to issue an opinion on the scope of the existing antidiscrimination provisions of the federal Rehabilitation Act of 1973. This act prohibits federally funded employers from discriminating against employees with handicaps, provided they are otherwise qualified to work. It was unclear, however, whether both persons ill with AIDS and asymptomatic HIV carriers were protected.

The Justice Departments' opinion stated that the first group, those ill with the disease, were clearly protected according to the decision of the U.S. Supreme Court in *School Board of Nassau County v. Arline* (1987). The Court ruled that a contagious disease—in this case, tuberculosis—is a handicap protected by the Act. Notably, the court rejected arguments that fear of transmission was grounds for dismissal:

> It would be unfair to allow an employer to seize upon the distinction between the effects of a disease on others and the effects of a disease on a patient and use that distinction to justify discriminatory treatment. [The. . .] basic purpose [of the Act is] to ensure that handicapped individuals are not denied jobs or other benefits because of the prejudiced attitudes or the ignorance of others.[7]

The Justice Department opinion concurred with the Court and took the further position that even asymptomatic HIV-infected individuals should be protected.

The Office of Legal Counsel, which prepared the opinion, said it was guided by information from the Surgeon General. He contends that even asymptomatic HIV-infected individuals are "physically impaired," from a medical standpoint, and adds that the impairment of HIV infection cannot meaningfully be separated from clinical AIDS.[8]

Thus the Justice Department concludes that both those with full-blown AIDS and those asymptomatic but infected are included in the definition of handicapped for the purposes of the Act. The Department mentions further grounds for including the latter group: the Supreme Court concluded in *Arline* that "if a person is perceived by others as having a handicapping condition . . . that in itself could bring the person within the terms of the Act."[9]

In conclusion, the opinion reiterated earlier statements that HIV-infected employees should be treated on a case-by-case basis. So long as they pose no "threat to the health or safety of others [and are not] unable to perform the job," the Department feels employees should receive full federal antidiscrimination protection.[10]

In New York it is illegal to discriminate against a person with asymptomatic HIV infection, ARC, or AIDS. Last year in New York, the state Supreme Court ruled that AIDS is a disability and that individuals with AIDS, ARC, or asymptomatic HIV infection are protected by the New York State Human Rights Law

(Executive Law Art. 15) which prohibits discrimination against persons who are disabled or who are perceived to be disabled. AIDS has been characterized as a handicap in several other cases as well.[11]

As the trend is towards treating AIDS, ARC, and HIV antibody positivity as protected handicaps, it would seem that community corrections services must afford those with AIDS all the rights and opportunities available to others, and in particular, that discrimination in housing or employment would be unlawful.

Special Conditions of Supervision

In an effort to protect themselves from the threat of third-party liability, some agencies suggest imposing special conditions on HIV-infected individuals. Some advocate conditions which prohibit contact with bodily fluids of HIV-infected individuals. However, . . . the United States Parole Commission and the Federal Division of Probation maintain that to impose such a condition inappropriately extends the role of community corrections from the prevention of crime to the prevention of disease. Moreover, such a condition places the responsibility on officers to monitor the most intimate behaviors of their clients. As such it is perhaps an unenforceable condition, which serves only to further the liability of community corrections officers in the event of injured third parties. Only one state, Georgia, imposes such specific prohibitions as conditions of supervision.

Some agencies, including Georgia and Tennessee, require that infected clients disclose their status to spouses, prospective sex partners, or other persons in danger of being infected as a condition of parole or probation. A compelling argument against such a condition is that in many states, non-voluntary disclosure constitutes violation of state law. The Federal Division of Probation maintains that mandated disclosure as a condition of supervision by clients who have been exposed to HIV "is an unwarranted intrusion by criminal justice into the public health arena without any medical evidence that it would have any effect whatsoever on the AIDS epidemic."[12] However, the Federal Parole Commission suggests disclosure to third parties at risk in states where it is permissible.

Another condition of supervision used in some states is participation in AIDS education and training for probationers and parolees who are HIV-infected. As previously discussed, under most circumstances community corrections authorities are not permitted to disclose an individual's HIV antibody status to third parties. Thus, identifying persons for participation must be handled judiciously. It may be reasonable, for example, to establish a special condition requiring the successful participation of all clients in AIDS education, counseling, and treatment programs. Alternatively, such participation could be required of persons with a history of IV drug use, or sexual offenses. Unlike other conditions, this one is rehabilitative and supportive in nature, a role with which community corrections authorities may be more comfortable.

Challenges to Eligibility and/or Segregation in Residential Facilities

Residential facilities and prisons face similar programming decisions when attempting to ensure the health and safety of staff and individuals under their supervision. When dealing with HIV infection and AIDS in a secure environment, systems have a responsibility to protect staff and inmates from transmission. Those who are HIV seropositive must also be protected from threats and possible violence as a result of their antibody status. A brief examination of the existing case law for correctional facilities may clarify potential suits faced by residential facilities.

Many correctional facilities have chosen to segregate inmates with AIDS, ARC, or asymptomatic HIV in response to these concerns and, as a result, have faced suits filed by segregated inmates alleging that conditions of their confinement violate equal protection standards and/or constitute cruel and unusual punishment. Although several cases remain pending, the courts have upheld the discretion of correctional officials to segregate HIV-infected inmates and to deny them access to programs and privileges, such as rehabilitation or work-release programs, in an effort to advance medical, safety, and security objectives. In the context of community corrections, one could envision residential facilities faced with suits filed by parolees challenging their segregation at these facilities or their exclusion from these programs as a result of their HIV antibody status.

In *Cordero v. Coughlin*,[13] a group of segregated inmates with AIDS sued the New York State Department of Correctional Services alleging cruel and unusual punishment, deliberate indifference to their serious medical needs, and deprivation of equal protection of the laws, claiming that the conditions of their confinement produced depression and decline in their medical condition. The plaintiffs also argued that even though they had no absolute right to such things as rehabilitation programs, exercise or visitation, they were nonetheless entitled to equal access to those programs. The court held that inmates have no constitutional right to freedom from segregation enforced to further a legitimate institutional objective, in this case preventing HIV transmission. Any equal protection claims were denied because the court did not consider inmates with AIDS to be "similarly situated" as other inmates in the institution, as required by the Constitution.

A similar suit was filed in an Oklahoma case, *Powell v. Department of Corrections*.[14] In this case, an HIV antibody-positive but asymptomatic inmate alleged that he was segregated from the general prison population and denied access to worship services and exercise. Despite the different medical conditions of the plaintiffs, the court reached the same conclusion as in *Cordero* that the segregation policy sustained correctional objectives of protecting staff and inmates from HIV infection. In addition, the court asserted that inmates have no constitutional right to be in the general population and that the inmate was not denied equal protection, as he had not been treated differently from other seropositive inmates, even though he was the only identified seropositive inmate in the prison system.

In *Marsh v. Alabama Department of Corrections*,[15] an inmate alleged that he was unconstitutionally segregated and disqualified from work-release programs as a result of his HIV seropositivity. Citing *Cordero* and *Powell*, the court ruled in favor of the Alabama correctional system. Case law is quite extensive in this area and follows the patterns of the cases described here.[16]

In light of these decisions, it seems reasonable to expect that the courts would rule in favor of community corrections services, in the event that a parolee were to file suit alleging that he or she was unconstitutionally segregated or excluded from a residential facility as a result of his or her HIV antibody status. However, the expense of segregation and its ultimate utility in dealing with transmission may make such a policy untenable.

CHALLENGES TO HIV ANTIBODY TESTING

To date, there have been no suits challenging mandatory mass screening for antibodies to HIV, although such a suit might result if HIV status became a widespread criterion for determining eligibility for parole. There have been, however, several challenges to other antibody testing situations. In Connecticut an inmate tried to prevent blind epidemiological studies of the incidence of HIV in the correctional population in the case of *Durham v. Commissioner of Corrections*,[17] but the case was dropped by the plaintiff. In an Oklahoma case, an inmate claimed that he was tested against his will,[18] emphasizing the care which must be taken to define procedures carefully before conducting any kind of testing.

Numerous suits have been filed by inmates and staff of correctional facilities seeking mandatory testing and segregation of seropositives in order to ensure protection from HIV infection; these cases may have some relevance to the issue of screening for residential placement. The courts have upheld, thus far, correctional systems' policies not to institute mass screening, and are likely to be consistent in cases involving residential facilities.[19]

Confidentiality of Medical Information

As of yet, there have been no suits filed by clients or staff challenging the disclosure or the confidentiality of medical information regarding AIDS and HIV infection in a community corrections environment.

As has been the case with inmates in correctional facilities, probationers or parolees may challenge the disclosure of information about their HIV status. As the risks of transmission associated with confinement are not present for community corrections services, a client may well be able to invoke his or her right to privacy and build a potentially strong case against the agency and/or the officer responsible for making an unauthorized disclosure.

Additionally, a probationer or parolee could have grounds for claiming mistreatment, defamation or psychological hardship or damage as a result of the disclosure. Recent legislation suggests that an exception to such a ruling may be cases involving disclosure to spouses. For example, California has enacted laws permitting physicians to disclose a patient's HIV antibody status to his or her spouse. Should an individual refuse to inform a spouse of his or her medical condition, an agency may well have firm legal grounds for making a confidential disclosure.

On the other hand, there may be instances in which community corrections staff try to obtain lists of all seropositives within their system. Two such suits have been filed by staff of correctional facilities, one permitting and one limiting such disclosure. In Delaware, a group of inmates claiming to have had homosexual relations with an HIV-infected inmate volunteered to be tested with a guarantee of confidentiality. In response, officers filed a union grievance claiming that based on a provision of their contracts, they were entitled to know which inmates were "suspected of having any communicable disease." The court ruled that the correctional system, abiding by the terms of the contract, must disclose the names of the seropositives.[20] In Nevada, however, correctional officers have made several attempts to gain access to similar lists. The state's attorney general issued an opinion that disclosure was limited to those who "have a legitimate medical need to know in connection with the prevention and control of AIDS."[21]

Issues Raised by Staff: Community Corrections' Liability and Concerns

One of the most serious legal concerns for community correction services is the threat of liability should staff, probationers or parolees, or members of the community become infected with HIV as a result of contact with an infected individual. A federal district court judge noted that, in the case of prisons, "prison officials might face a §1983 suit for failing to isolate a known AIDS patient or carrier, if the carrier infects another inmate who could show that such failure to isolate constituted grossly negligent or reckless conduct on the part of such officials."[22]

Plaintiffs alleging HIV infection as a result of negligence face two serious problems. First, with the possible exception of blood transfusions and spouse infection, it is very difficult to link a particular incident to transmission. And secondly, as community corrections systems cannot be expected to monitor the most intimate acts of their clients or to enforce behavior changes, it would be difficult to establish that an agency or officer was negligent in allowing the incident to occur.

To avoid potential liability, community corrections services should attempt to prevent high-risk behavior among clients through AIDS education and training, particularly for those at risk of infection, including homosexuals, drug users, and sex offenders. All clients who are known to have AIDS, ARC, or asymptomatic HIV infection should be counseled regarding their responsibility to inform sexual partners of their medical condition. And, as previously discussed, in the event that a client refuses to make such a disclosure, the agency should consider making a confidential disclosure in keeping with laws and/or policies of the jurisdiction.

Residential facilities, like correctional facilities, may be held liable for damages resulting from homosexual rapes and other assaults.[23] However, correctional facilities have not been held liable for insuring the *absolute* safety of persons in their custody. In several cases, the courts have ruled that a facility can only be held liable for assaults it knew or should have known would occur.[24]

Although no cases of this kind have been filed, community corrections services may also be concerned with the liability involved should an employee be infected by a probationer or parolee under his or her supervision. Systems are not mandated by law to ensure the absolute safety of their employees, but are only held to a reasonable standard of care. An agency is not liable for injury incurred in the line of duty unless procedures are violated or the department is found to be otherwise negligent. While worker's compensation might well apply, negligence on the part of the agency would also have to be established in the case of HIV infection. Inadequate AIDS education and training or poor precautionary guidelines against HIV infection could be sufficient to establish such negligence. Training and procedures should be well documented as protection against future lawsuits.

The question of whether or not an individual may be compelled to be tested for HIV antibodies following an incident in which transmission may have occurred is complex. Some jurisdictions prohibit mandatory testing and it can be argued that forced testing violates a person's Fourth Amendment protection from search and seizure. Some recent state-level legislation suggests, however, that persons involved in aggressive or negligent acts can be required to undergo testing. For example, judges may issue a court order requiring testing and disclosure in special cases. In Houston, Texas, court orders requiring testing have been issued to sex offenders.[25] In Florida, search warrants are issued for "examinations" of persons with sexually transmitted diseases, including AIDS.[26]

Notably, at least two such cases have been decided in favor of the defendant. A Massachusetts trial judge ruled that an inmate who had allegedly scratched and spit on a guard could not be required to undergo HIV antibody testing based on a state law prohibiting forced testing and disclosure as well as on medical evidence against HIV transmission through saliva.[27] Similarly, a California court revoked a search warrant authorizing HIV antibody testing of a defendant charged with biting a police officer, based on a state law prohibiting the disclosure of test results without the subject's informed consent.[28]

Staff of community corrections services express two major concerns regarding AIDS. The first is the possibility of HIV transmission in the course of their jobs, and the second is the threat of personal liability as a result of actions taken or not taken regarding clients with AIDS, ARC, or asymptomatic HIV infection.

While survey results indicate that few community corrections staff have taken concerted action regarding HIV infection on the job, correctional facilities have had complaints, particularly by those working in special AIDS units, and have received demands for "hazardous duty" pay and/or reduced working hours. These fears—and demands—can only be addressed through AIDS education and training and through written policies which outline an agency's response to incidents in which transmission may have occurred. In one case reported in the NIJ survey, staff refused to participate in urinalysis testing procedures due to fear of HIV transmission from probationers and parolees. An education and training program took place and the issue was settled. In another instance, staff took concerted action to obtain training from the agency. In a third reported case, officers attempted to pressure the parole department to release HIV status of parolees under their supervision. No full legal action was pursued.

A frightening prospect for staff is the possibility of a lawsuit filed against a community corrections officer. Should such a case be filed, 75 percent of probation and 77 percent of parole agencies surveyed report that they would provide defense for the officer who acted within the line of duty; a few others would provide defense in all circumstances. Some systems (44 percent of probation and 35 percent of parole) have liability insurance to cover officers who are sued. Forms of coverage include state indemnification statutes, comprehensive general liability, or state insurance funds for risk management. In a limited number of jurisdictions, self-insurance is also available.

In most cases an officer's concerns can be alleviated through written policies which describe how agencies will respond to a lawsuit. Few agencies have state or local guidelines explaining potential criminal or civil liabilities. However, 44 percent of probation systems surveyed and 36 percent of the parole systems surveyed disseminate information to agency staff concerning general representation and damages.

OBLIGATION TO PERFORM DUTIES

Survey results indicate that only three probation systems and one parole system have faced potential work disruptions as a result of staff members who have refused to work with HIV-infected clients. In general, agencies have taken the position that fear of AIDS does not excuse employees from performing duties, as there is a very low risk of HIV infection associated with occupational activities. In response to the San Francisco Sheriff's Department request for a legal opinion as to whether officers were required to render CPR to inmates known or suspected to be HIV-infected, the city attorney's office asserted that deputies have an unequivocal responsibility to provide CPR whenever necessary, as failure to do so could make the city liable for any resulting injury and subject the employee to disciplinary action.[29]

Pregnant staffers, however, are an exception to this rule. In California, for instance, no pregnant women may be assigned duties involving the supervision or care of persons with AIDS. This is because of the risk of exposure to cytomegalovirus (CMV), commonly found in persons with AIDS, which can cause birth defects.

Precise and accurate AIDS education and training, coupled with policies calling for swift disciplinary action should an employee refuse to perform his or her duties out of fear of AIDS, can effectively allay most concerns and disruptions among community corrections staff. Legally, an employee cannot refuse work in other situations because of personal bias, such as work with a handicapped, female, or minority co-worker. Though not tested in the courts, the rulings may hold true for refusal to work with a co-worker or client with AIDS.

Policy Recommendations

In this chapter we have reviewed some of the legal issues involved in dealing with AIDS in community corrections. In the following sections, we summarize some of the key questions and answers.

- *What are the legal guidelines for disclosing the HIV status of someone under supervision to third parties such as spouses, other family members, potential residential placements or employers?*

   Each state has different laws regarding confidentiality of HIV status information. Many states require mandatory reporting to Public Health Departments by medical personnel identifying the condition; this does not include reporting by or to community corrections services. Community supervision staff should seek legal verification of the confidentiality and disclosure statutes in their state before any disclosure or special placement is made. For example, in most states staff may not disapprove of a client's residence plan if he or she refuses to disclose HIV status to the person with whom he or she will be living. Such a disapproval could be seen as a violation of the right to confidentiality.

- *Can staff refuse to supervise or work with HIV-infected persons?*

   No. Refusal to work with AIDS-infected persons could be interpreted as discrimination if the infected individual is otherwise carrying out his or her obligations, either job obligations or the requirement to report for supervision. Only in the case of a pregnant supervisory officer might this refusal be allowable.

- *What is the best protection against third-party suits in community corrections?*

   Suits can be mounted against corrections staff on grounds such as inappropriate disclosure of HIV status, failure to disclose with resultant third-party injury, or damages due to inadequate medical management resulting in injury. Detailed disclosure guidelines for protection of confidentiality and documented training in those guidelines provide the best protection in these instances. Similarly, the problems of inadequate medical management can be alleviated by training of staff in AIDS information and referral systems available. Failure to disclose, while troubling to many supervisory staff, is a problem generally dealt with by restrictions of state and federal law.

- *Can I require testing for an individual whom I suspect is HIV antibody-positive and who is involved in a transmission incident?*
  This depends on your state's laws. Some agencies currently can obtain a court order in cases of transmission incidents which can be used to force HIV antibody testing. Careful examination of the incident is urged prior to such action. For example, is it an incident in which a real risk exists, as in a rape, or a negligible or nonexistent risk, as in a biting or spitting incident? It may be more prudent to have the victim tested for a six-month period than to avoid possible legal action from the offender.
- *Can state residential placement facilities refuse to house HIV antibody-positive parolees?*
  Again, depending on state law, this may be legally possible. Case law nationally has upheld segregation of persons with AIDS in prisons and jails. A more cautious approach, however, argues that all individuals be treated as though seropositive since there is no way to determine the HIV status over time of the total population. Persons deemed acceptable at one point in time are possibly unacceptable (infected) at later points. These realities should be stressed to residential facilities, few of which have resources available for repeated testing of residents.

NOTES

1 *AIDS Policy Guidelines for Probation Departments and Alternatives Programs*, State of New York Division of Probation and Correctional Alternatives, Albany, New York, 1987, p. 3.
2 *AIDS Information Guide*, New York State Parole Operations, Albany, New York, April 1986, p. II–3.
3 *Ibid.*, p. III–11.
4 Colorado: H.B. 1177, Chapter 208, 1987 Laws.
5 D. Chamlee, Chief of the Federal Division of Probation, letter to Benjamin F. Baer, chief of the U.S. Parole Commission, September 29, 1987.
6 *AIDS Policy Guidelines*, Section 410.90 of the New York State Criminal Procedure Law; p. 16.
7 *School Board of Nassau County v. Arline*, 107 S. Ct. 1123 (1987).
8 D. W. Kmiec, Office of Legal Counsel, U.S. Department of Justice, Memorandum, October 6, 1988.
9 *School Board of Nassau County, op. cit.*
10 Kmiec, *op. cit.*
11 *Doe v. Charlotte Memorial Hospital*, Complaint No. 04-84-3096 (August 5, 1986); *Thomas v. Atascadero Unified School District*, Civil No. 86-6609, U.S. Dist. Ct. (C.D. California, November 7, 1986); *Shuttleworth v. Broward County*, 639 F. Supp. 654 (S.D. Florida, 1986); *American Federation of Government Employees Local 1812 v. U.S. Department of State*, 25 Govt. Empl. Rel. Reptr. (BNA) 612 (U.S.D.C. D.C. No. 87-0121, April 22, 1987).
12 Chamlee, *op. cit.*
13 607 F. Supp. 9 (S.D.N.Y., 1984).
14 U.S.D.C., N.D. Oklahoma, Nos. 85-C-820-C and 85-C-816-B, dismissed February 20, 1986.
15 U.S.D.C., N.D. Alabama, No. CV-86-HM-5592-NE. Decided April 20, 1987.

[16] *Farmer v. Levine* (U.S.D.C., Maryland, 1985), No. HM-85-4284, 19. Magistrates Report dated May 28, 1986; *Marioneaux v. Colorado State Penitentiary*, 465 F. Supp. 1245 (1979); *Johnson v. Fair* (U.S.D.C., D. Massachusetts, 1987). Civil Action NO. 87-0217 Mc; *Williams v. Sumner* 648 F. Supp. 510 (C.D. Nevada, 1986) *Doe v. Coughlin* 509 NYS 2d 209 (NY App. 1986). Buraff Publications, *AIDS Policy and Law*, December 2, 1987, 2:5.

[17] Hartford District Court, Civil No. H-87-623.

[18] *Dunn v. White* (U.S.D.C., N.D. Oklahoma) No. 87-C-753-C.

[19] For some examples see *Wiedmon v. Rogers* (U.S.D.C., E.D., North Carolina), No. C-85-116-G; *Maberry v. Martin* (U.S.D.C., E.D. North Carolina), No. 86-341CRT; *Potter v. Wainwright* (U.S.D.C., Middle Dist. Florida), No. 85-1616-CIV-T15; *Stalling v. Cave* (2d Circuit, De Leon County); *McCallum v. Staggers* (5th Circuit, Lake County), No. 85-1338-CAOI; *Bailey v. Wainwright* (8th Circuit, Baker County); *Lloyd v. Wainwright* (2d Circuit, De Leon County), No. 86-3144; *Jarrett v. Faulkner*, (U.S.D.C., S.D. Indiana), No. IP85-1569-C; *Herring v. Keeney* (U.S.D.C., Oregon), filed September 17, 1985, decided July 1987; *Piatt v. Ricketts* (U.S.D.C., Arizona), No. CIV-85-538-PHX); *Foy v. Owens* (U.S.D.C., E.D. Pennsylvania, 1986), Civil Action No. 85-6909; *Lareau v. Manson* 651 F. 2d 96 (2d Cir. 1981); *Bell v. Wolfish* 441 U.S. 520 (1979); *Estelle v. Gamble* 429 U.S. 97 (1976).

[20] *State Department of Correction v. Public Employees Council 82* (Del h. 1987), Civil Action No. 8462.

[21] *AIDS Policy and Law*, December 16, 1987; 2–5; *Carson City Nevada Appeal*, November 12, 1987, p. A–10.

[22] *Judd v. Packard*, (unreported opinion, U.S.C.D., Maryland), Civil Action No. S 87-1514, September 24, 1987. Cites *Withers v. Levine* 625 F.2d 158 (4th Cir.), cert denied, 449 U.S. 849 (1980).

[23] See *Redmond v. Baxley* 475 F. Supp. 1111 (U.S.D.C. E. Dist. Mich. 1979); *Garrett v. United States* 501 F. Supp. 337 (U.S.D.C. N. Dist. Georgia 1980); *Saunders v. Chatham County* 728 F.2d 1367 (11th Cir. 1982); *Kemp v. Waldron* 479 N.Y.S. 2d 440 (Sup. Ct. 1984); *Thomas v. Booker* 762 F. 2d 654 (8th Cir. 1985).

[24] See *Mosby v. Mabry* 699 F. 2d 213 (8th Cir. 1982); *O'Quinn v. Manuel* 767 F. 2d 174 (5th Cir. 1985).

[25] *Manual of Policies and Procedures for Health Services*, No. 3-39, October 1987, p. 6.

[26] §796.08 Florida Statutes (Supplement 1986). See Aylesworth, G. and Knabe, R., "Warrant for Examination for Sexually Transmitted Diseases," *Florida Police Chief*, December 1987, 13:63.

[27] *Dean v. Bowie*, Suffolk Sup. Ct. (Massachusetts), Civil Action #87-4745.

[28] *Barlow v. Superior Court* 236 Cal Rptr. 134 (Cal. App. 4th Dist. 1987).

[29] "Deputy Sheriff's Duty to Administer CPR," City Attorney George Agnost to Sheriff Michael Hennessey, July 1, 1985.

WE VALUE YOUR OPINION—PLEASE SHARE IT WITH US

Merrill Publishing and our authors are most interested in your reactions to this textbook. Did it serve you well in the course? If it did, what aspects of the text were most helpful? If not, what didn't you like about it? Your comments will help us to write and develop better textbooks. We value your opinions and thank you for your help.

Text Title _____ Edition _____

Author(s) _____

Your Name (optional) _____

Address _____

City _____ State _____ Zip _____

School _____

Course Title _____

Instructor's Name _____

Your Major _____

Your Class Rank _____ Freshman _____ Sophomore _____Junior _____ Senior

_____ Graduate Student

Were you required to take this course? _____ Required _____Elective

Length of Course? _____ Quarter _____ Semester

1. Overall, how does this text compare to other texts you've used?

_____ Superior _____Better Than Most _____ Average _____Poor

2. Please rate the text in the following areas:

	Superior	Better Than Most	Average	Poor
Author's Writing Style	_____	_____	_____	_____
Readability	_____	_____	_____	_____
Organization	_____	_____	_____	_____
Accuracy	_____	_____	_____	_____
Layout and Design	_____	_____	_____	_____
Illustrations/Photos/Tables	_____	_____	_____	_____
Examples	_____	_____	_____	_____
Problems/Exercises	_____	_____	_____	_____
Topic Selection	_____	_____	_____	_____
Currentness of Coverage	_____	_____	_____	_____
Explanation of Difficult Concepts	_____	_____	_____	_____
Match-up with Course Coverage	_____	_____	_____	_____
Applications to Real Life	_____	_____	_____	_____

3. Circle those chapters you especially liked:
   1 2 3 4 5 6 7 8 9 10 11 12 13 14 15 16 17 18 19
   What was your favorite chapter? _____
   Comments:

4. Circle those chapters you liked least:
   1 2 3 4 5 6 7 8 9 10 11 12 13 14 15 16 17 18 19
   What was your least favorite chapter? _____
   Comments:

5. List any chapters your instructor did not assign. _____

6. What topics did your instructor discuss that were not covered in the text?_____

   _____

7. Were you required to buy this book? _____ Yes _____ No

   Did you buy this book new or used? _____ New _____ Used

   If used, how much did you pay? _____

   Do you plan to keep or sell this book? _____ Keep _____ Sell

   If you plan to sell the book, how much do you expect to receive? _____

   Should the instructor continue to assign this book? _____ Yes _____ No

8. Please list any other learning materials you purchased to help you in this course (e.g., study guide, lab manual).

   _____

9. What did you like most about this text? _____

   _____

10. What did you like least about this text? _____

    _____

11. General comments:

    May we quote you in our advertising? _____ Yes _____ No

    Please mail to: Boyd Lane
                     College Division Research Department
                     P. O. Box 508
                     Columbus, Ohio 43216-0508

    Thank you!